EAT THIS NOT THAT! 2012

The No-Diet Weight Loss Solution
Completely Updated and Expanded

BY DAVID ZINCZENKO
WITH MATT GOULDING

RODALE

Eat This, Not That! is a registered trademark of Rodale Inc.

© 2011, 2010, 2009, 2008 by Rodale Inc.

Rodale books may be purchased for business or promotional use or for special sales. For information, please write to: Special Markets Department, Rodale Inc., 733 Third Avenue, New York, NY 10017

Printed in the United States of America

Rodale Inc. makes every effort to use acid-free ♾, recycled paper ♻

Book design by George Karabotsos

Cover photos by Jeff Harris / Cover food styling by Ed Gabriels for Halley Resources

Interior photo direction by Tara Long

All interior photos by Mitch Mandel and Thomas MacDonald/Rodale Images
Rodale Images food styling by Melissa Reiss with the exception of pages: 299, 301, 303, 305, 307, 309, 311, 313, 315, 317, 319, 321, food styling by Diane Simone Vezza

Illustrations by Jonathan Carlson

Library of Congress Cataloging-in-Publication Data is on file with the publisher

ISBN-13: 978-1-60961-065-4 paperback

Trade paperback and exclusive direct mail edition published simultaneously in August 2011.

Distributed to the trade by Macmillan

2 4 6 8 10 9 7 5 3 1 paperback

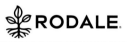

We inspire and enable people to improve their lives and the world around them.

www.rodalebooks.com

EAT THIS NOT THAT! 2012

DEDICATION

To the 8 million men and women who have made *EAT THIS, NOT THAT!*
a publishing phenomenon and who have spread the word to friends and
relatives about the importance of knowing what's really in our food.
Because of your passionate efforts, food manufacturers and restaurant
chains are waking up to the fact that more and more of us demand good,
solid information about our food, and healthy choices that will let us
drop pounds and stay lean for life.

And to the men and women working in America's fields, farms,
and supermarkets, waiting tables, and toiling in kitchens everywhere:
It is because of your hard work that Americans have so many options.
This book is designed to help us choose the best of what you've created.

—Dave and Matt

ACKNOWLEDGMENTS

This book is the product of thousands of meals, hundreds of conversations with nutritionists and industry experts, and the collective smarts, dedication, and raw talent of dozens of individuals. Our undying thanks to all of you who have inspired this project in any way. In particular:

To Maria Rodale and the Rodale family, whose dedication to improving the lives of their readers is apparent in every book and magazine they put their name on.

To George Karabotsos and his crew of immensely talented designers, including Courtney Eltringham, Laura White, Mark Michaelson, and Elizabeth Neal. You're the reason why each book looks better than the last.

To Clint Carter. Thanks for another huge effort. And to James Carlson, Andrew Del-Colle, Alex Howe, Hannah McWilliams, and Dana Ramirez. Your contributions are more valuable than you know.

To Tara Long, who spends more time in the drive-thru and the supermarket aisles than anyone on the planet, all in the name of making us look good.

To Debbie McHugh, whose ability to keep us sane and focused under the most impossible circumstances cannot be overstated.

To Agnes Hansdorfer. You make us all look good.

To the Rodale book team: Steve Perrine, Karen Rinaldi, Chris Krogermeier, Erin Williams, Sara Cox, Mitch Mandel, Tom MacDonald, Troy Schnyder, Melissa Reiss, Nikki Weber, Jennifer Giandomenico, Wendy Gable, Keith Biery, Liz Krenos, Brooke Myers, Nancy Elgin, Sonya Maynard, and Sean Sabo. You continue to do whatever it takes to get these books done. As always, we appreciate your heroic efforts.

—Dave and Matt

Check out the other bestselling books in the **EAT THIS, NOT THAT!**® and **COOK THIS, NOT THAT!**™ series:

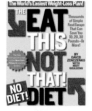

Eat This, Not That! for Kids! (2008)

Eat This, Not That! Restaurant Survival Guide (2009)

Cook This, Not That! Kitchen Survival Guide (2010)

Drink This, Not That! (2010)

Eat This, Not That! No Diet Diet (2011)

CONTENTS

INTRODUCTION

Welcome

BY PICKING UP YOUR COPY of *Eat This, Not That!*, you've just granted yourself membership in one of the most exclusive organizations in the country, a club that 65 percent of Americans simply can't get into.

Or, should I say, can't squeeze into.

I'm talking about the Sorority of the Slim, the Fraternity of the Fit, the League of Extraordinarily Toned Ladies and Gentlemen. I'm talking about men and women and even kids and teens who look and feel their very best and enjoy all the benefits—from more energy to bigger paychecks to more robust relationships—that come with being lean, fit, and healthy.

Just how exclusive is this club? More and more of us are locked out every year. Two out of every three American women—and three out of every four American men—are overweight or obese. Many have simply given up hope of ever looking and feeling the way they want.

But I'm here to tell you that you can do it—and the key to unlocking that elusive door is right here in your hands. Millions of Americans have experienced fast, effective, and permanent weight loss the *Eat This, Not That!* way (in fact, you'll meet many of them in the coming pages). I'm talking about folks just like you who have conquered weight gain, losing 10, 20, 30—some of them more than 100!—pounds using the No-Diet Weight Loss Solution.

And they did it not by dieting, not by sacrificing, but by eating all of their favorite foods, wherever and whenever they liked. All that these successfully slimmed-down folks needed was a few smart swaps that helped them strip away hundreds of calories a day, like magic.

Does the idea of losing weight and

to the club!

keeping it off seem impossible? It isn't, once you know a few secrets. But it does require having a bit of knowledge and making some smart decisions—and that's what this book is designed to help you do. Whether you're whipping up breakfast at home, popping into the drive-thru for lunch, ordering up delivery for dinner, or swinging by the ice cream shop for dessert, you'll know instantly how to indulge your cravings, satisfy your taste buds, and still strip away hundreds of calories a day—without ever feeling hungry, tired, or deprived.

Is it really that easy? Yes. But before you move on and discover the thousands of amazing, indulgent, and delicious foods, from fast-food burgers to supermarket desserts, that are going to help you strip away fat fast, I want to share some amazing—and, literally, life-altering—information with you.

As the editor-in-chief of *Men's Health*, I've spent the past 2 decades interviewing leading experts, poring over groundbreaking studies, and grilling top athletes, trainers, and celebrities for their health and fitness advice. And I've learned that what separates the fit from the fat, the slim from the sloppy, the toned from the torpid, is a set of rules: The 8 Immutable Laws of Leanness. And what's amazing is that none of them involves spending hours on a treadmill, eating nothing but grapefruit and tree bark, or having part of the small intestine replaced with fiberfill. Follow these rules, and the simple swaps in these pages, and weight loss will be automatic.

(Warning: These rules are so easy and so appealing that you'll invariably wind up smacking yourself on the forehead. If you are holding a sharp object, please put it down before reading on!)

Lean People Don't Diet.

→ What? Of course lean people diet! They're just magically better at denying themselves than the rest of us are, right?

No. In reality, studies show that the number-one predictor of future weight gain is being on a diet right now. Part of the reason is that restricting calories reduces strength, bone density, and muscle mass—and muscle is your body's number-one calorie burner. So by dieting, you're actually setting yourself up to gain more weight than ever. And a recent study in the journal *Psychosomatic Medicine* showed that tracking your diet in a food journal can actually boost your stress levels, which in turn increases your level of a hormone called cortisol, and it is linked to—you guessed it—weight gain.

Lean People Eat Breakfast.

→ A recent study of people who successfully lost weight and kept it off found that 78 percent of the weight-loss winners ate breakfast every single day.

Is there some kind of magic in waffles? No, but when you eat within 90 minutes of waking, you trigger your metabolism to start burning calories—and keep burning them all day long. When you skip your morning meal, on the other hand, you send the message to your body that food may be in short supply; as a result, you develop food cravings throughout the day. That's one reason why skipping breakfast has been shown to raise the risk of obesity by a whopping 450 percent!

Lean People Don't Go Fat Free.

→ A European study tracked nearly 90,000 people for several years and discovered that participants who tried to eat "low fat" had the same risk of being overweight as those who ate whatever they wanted.

Fat doesn't make you fat, period. Indeed, you need fat in your diet to help you process certain nutrients, such as vitamins A, D, and E. And many "fat free" foods are loaded with sugar, and therefore have even more calories than their full-fat cousins. Even the American Heart Association says that fat-free labels lead to higher consumption of unhealthy sweets. Fat keeps you full and satisfied. Fat free will send you running back to the fridge in an hour, hungry for more.

Lean People Sit Down and Eat.

→ In fact, the more you enjoy your food, the leaner you're going to be. Punishing yourself only makes you fat!

Greek researchers recently reported that eating more slowly and savoring your meal can boost levels of two hormones that make you feel fuller. And researchers

"I traded in my Plymouth van of a body and got a Ferrari."

For **Mike McGeever**, being overweight was normal—just the way of life in America. "You hear about people being depressed about being fat," he says. "I had more of a Santa Claus, jovial attitude about it." On a vacation to Disney World, Mike was forced to get off a ride when he failed to fit under the restraining belt, but even that didn't register as a problem. "I thought, 'How weird that they don't make them for normal-sized people.'" But when Mike returned home, he compared photographs from the trip with pictures from a Disney World vacation he'd taken in high school. Suddenly, he didn't feel so "normal." "I said, 'How did this happen? Who is this guy?'"

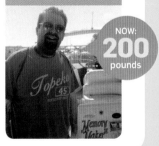

BEFORE:
290
pounds

VITALS:
Mike McGeever, 27
Location: Alexandria, VA

HEIGHT: 5'8"

TOTAL WEIGHT LOST: 90 lbs

TIME IT TOOK TO LOSE THE WEIGHT: 15 months

NOW:
200
pounds

THE TEST

At the time, Mike was working in an airport's publications department. *Eat This, Not That!* showed up in the bookstore, and he decided to see how well it worked with his daily lunch at the airport's restaurant chains. "I decided, maybe you can't just blame genes for everything. Maybe I hadn't even given myself a shot at being a different size." He was in his mid-twenties, overweight, and worried about his blood pressure. "Maybe life doesn't have to be this way," he thought. So Mike made a rule: He would no longer eat at any restaurant that *Eat This, Not That!* had graded a C+ or worse.

MAKING THE GRADE

Mike's *Eat This, Not That!* test was a success, and the weight began falling off with surprising ease. "*Eat This, Not That!* does the hard stuff for you," he says. "Now meals are like an open-book test. The test is, You've gotta eat. The book is—Hey, chief! Just don't eat that!" Now Mike's getting a big confidence boost from being slimmer. After he lost the weight, he returned to his hometown to celebrate homecoming. He likens the experience to the season finale of *The Biggest Loser*. "I walked into the bar and everyone was cheering," he says. "It's so weird—I'm 27 and I feel better than I did at 22. It's the healthiest I've ever been. I traded in my Plymouth van of a body and got a Ferrari."

at Cornell University found that when people sat down at the table with plates of food, they consumed up to 35 percent less than they did when eating family-style by passing around serving dishes. Imagine eating 35 percent less simply by being comfortable!

Lean People Know What They're Going to Eat Next.

→ Planning your responses to hunger may help you shed pounds faster, say Dutch researchers. They posed their subjects questions like "If you're hungry at 4 p.m., then...what?" Those who had an answer ("I'll snack on some almonds") were more successful at losing weight than those who didn't have an answer.

One of the best things about *Eat This, Not That!* is that you'll never be at a loss for what to eat. If you're in the mood for a munchie, we've got you covered, whether you're at the movie theater, pulling into the coffee shop, or running a gauntlet of vending machines. Know what you're going to eat before you go to eat, and you'll make the smart choice every time.

Lean People Eat Protein.

→ In a recent European study, people who ate moderately high levels of protein were twice as likely to lose weight and keep it off as those who didn't eat much protein.

A *New England Journal of Medicine* study looked at a variety of eating plans and discovered that eating a diet high in protein and low in refined starches (like white bread) was the most effective for weight loss. Protein works on two levels: First, you burn more calories to digest it. Second, because your body has to work harder to digest a steak than, say, a Ho Ho, you stay fuller longer.

Lean People Move Around.

→ I don't mean climbing Kilimanjaro, breaking the tape at the Boston Marathon, or joining 24 Hour Fitness and literally spending 24 hours there. I mean going for a short bike ride (20 minutes burns 200 calories), taking a leisurely walk (145 calories every 51 minutes), wrestling with your kids (another 100 calories smoked in 22 minutes), or fishing (there's 150 calories gone in an hour, even more if you actually catch something). Simply put, fit people stay fit by having fun. Scientists have a name for how you burn calories just enjoying yourself. It's called NEAT: non-exercise activity thermogenesis. Sounds complicated, like something only policy wonks at a global warming summit are qualified to discuss. But it's pretty simple: Pick a few activities that you enjoy, from tossing a stick for your dog to bowling with your best girlfriend

"People couldn't believe I wasn't taking weight-loss drugs."

As a manager for troubled-youth homes, **Jesse Leyva** didn't think much about the fact that many of the teenagers he worked with were overweight. He had been an overweight child himself, after all, and had never managed to slim down. Based on personal experience, he assumed weight loss was impossible for some people. "I had periods of going to the gym and trying to eat healthier," he says. "I'd lose 10 or 20 pounds, get complacent, and the cycle would start over." The extra weight dug a pretty big divot in his self-esteem, and he felt helpless to change.

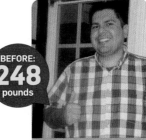

BEFORE: **248** pounds

THE GIFT OF MOTIVATION

For Christmas 2009, Jesse received clothes from his family, but they were all too small. Instead of hiding them in the back of a dresser, he made a pivotal decision. "I decided I was going make the clothes fit—that would be my goal," he says. He shared his objective with a friend, and the friend shared another gift: a copy of *Eat This, Not That!*. Jesse began making food swaps and jogging, and in time, his friends and colleagues took notice. "I started hearing, 'Hey, you've lost weight' more and more," he says. So he hopped on a scale and was shocked to discover that he weighed less than he had in high school. After that he sloughed off 10 more pounds—and sculpted his best body ever—just by sticking to *Eat This, Not That!* swaps. "People couldn't believe I wasn't taking weight-loss drugs."

SPREADING THE LOVE

As the weight came off, Jesse's self-esteem grew. Before, he had carried a fear of rejection that prevented him from becoming romantically involved, but today he's enjoying a happy and supportive relationship. What's more, Jesse is sharing his weight-loss secret with those who need it most. He took a copy of *Eat This, Not That!* to the staffer in charge of feeding the teens he works with. "I said, 'If it's not in this book, don't buy it,'" he says. "'I want everything in this book in the house.'" The effects were immediate: Three of the overweight teens have already lost more than 10 pounds.

VITALS:
Jesse Leyva, 28
Location: Costa Mesa, CA

HEIGHT: 5'9"

TOTAL WEIGHT LOST: 85 lbs

TIME IT TOOK TO LOSE THE WEIGHT: 1 Year

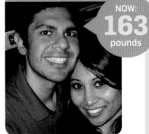

NOW: **163** pounds

to getting busy with the one you love, and just do it more often. The average person makes 200 decisions every day that affect his or her weight. If you choose the fun option more often than not, you'll see results.

Lean People Watch Less TV.

→ Instead of calling it the boob tube, maybe we should call it the man-boob tube. About 18 percent of people who watch less than 2 hours of TV a day have a body mass index (BMI) of 30 or more—the cutoff line for obesity, according to the Centers for Disease Control and Prevention. But of those who watch more than 4 hours of TV a day, nearly 30 percent have a BMI that high, according to a study in the *Journal of the American College of Cardiology*.

Look, I like TV. I watch *The Colbert Report* obsessively, I dedicate my Sunday nights to HBO, and I have a small voodoo altar in my den dedicated to getting Steve Carell to come back to *The Office*. But all things in moderation: In a study at the University of Vermont, overweight participants who cut their daily TV time in half (from an average of 5 hours to 2.5 hours) burned an extra 119 calories a day. Even reading this book right now is burning more calories than watching TV does. Amazing, right? And a recent study of people who successfully lost weight found that 63 percent of them watched less than 10 hours of TV a week. Want more? A study in the journal *Annals of Behavioral Medicine* reported that lean people have an average of 2.6 television sets in their homes. Overweight people have an average of 3.4.

Crazy, right?

So, bottom line: Don't diet. Enjoy your food more. Watch a little less TV. Take a kid fishing. And make the smart swaps you'll find populating the next 300 or so pages. That's all it takes to become part of the Society of the Slender, the Royal Order of the Ripped, the Knights of the Slightly Less Round Table.

It's an increasingly exclusive club. And you know what? We're really glad to have you.

Dig in!

"I really believe *Eat This, Not That!* saved my life."

Mike Kelley was a fit young man. In college, he maintained an impressive physique with rigorous tennis and weightlifting regimens, but upon leaving academia, fitness took a backseat to a new marriage and career. He began to accumulate flab in his 30s, but its growth was so slow that it seemed inconsequential. In his head, Mike was just a slightly heavier version of that fit college athlete. Then one day he looked down at the scale. The number looking up at him was 230, and he was suddenly struck by a disheartening realization. "When I was growing up, the scales only went to 230," he says. The fit young man inside him balked. Mike knew it was time for a change.

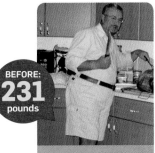

BEFORE:
231 pounds

VITALS:
Mike Kelley, 60
Location: Leesburg, FL

HEIGHT: 5'9"

TOTAL WEIGHT LOST: 72 lbs

TIME IT TOOK TO LOSE THE WEIGHT: 10 months

THE POWER OF A NO-DIET DIET

Mike resolved to lose weight, but he was skeptical of diets. What's more, his physician warned him that at his age, a slowed metabolism would make weight loss difficult. Then Mike stumbled upon *Drink This, Not That!* in the supermarket. He was intrigued by the idea that losing weight could be as simple as making smarter beverage choices, so he purchased the book, changed his drinking habits, and lost 25 pounds in just 3 months.

Encouraged, he bought the rest of the *Eat This, Not That!* series and started dropping a solid 6 to 8 pounds every month. "I went from a size 46 pant to a 32 in 10 months," he says. "I'd walk into JCPenney and the gal would go, 'No, not you again!'"

A MEDICAL MIRACLE

By warning that it would be difficult for Mike to lose weight at his age, Mike's doctor had presented him with a challenge, and he overcame it. "I'm not genetically gifted; I just followed everything in the books."

Mike's weight-loss success was so robust that his tennis partner didn't recognize him on the court. "I've gotten 'Are you Mike Kelley?!' from several people now," he says, laughing. Plus he's sleeping better, breathing easier, and feeling healthier. And the doc? "He finds it incredible that I could do this without some sort of 'secret.'" Mike's cholesterol dropped from the high 200s to the low 100s. "I really believe *Eat This, Not That!* saved my life," he says.

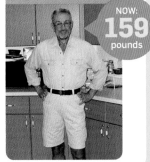

NOW:
159 pounds

Who Moved My Cheeseburger?

A beef patty, a bun, and an epic journey from mere value meal to becoming part of YOU

IF YOUR BODY were a Fortune 500 company, it would be the envy of CEOs everywhere. Not that it's perfect, mind you, but it is astoundingly efficient. No matter what happens outside your epidermis, your body charges full steam ahead 24 hours a day, 7 days a week, 52 weeks a year. It doesn't take time off during the holidays or get tangled up with lawmakers over corporate regulations. When the stock market crashes, it pushes ahead without wavering. Neither snow nor rain nor gloom of night prevent it from achieving its mission, and so long as you continue to feed it raw materials, it will continue to produce its product.

So what is this elusive product? Energy. You can't see or touch it, but your muscles, cells, and brain consume it the way preteen girls consume Robert Pattinson movies. To meet its own ongoing demand, your body must produce a constant supply. The raw material it uses to do this is food. Your body transforms the proteins, fats, and carbohydrates contained within each bite of food into the energy you need to crawl out of bed in the morning, daydream about the beaches in St. Barts, and uncork a bottle of wine after you trudge home from work. Understanding how this process works, knowing how your body produces energy from food, can illuminate many of the secrets behind why you gain weight. To that end, let's walk through the production cycle for one meal—a nice, juicy cheeseburger. Turns out the process begins before you even take a bite.

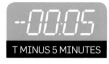

T MINUS 5 MINUTES

As you open the door to your local burger joint, the scintillating scent of sizzling beef meets your nostrils and sends a relay message to your brain. This triggers glands in your mouth to begin pumping out the enzyme amylase, which stands ready to deconstruct the bun's carbohydrates. Your body is now ready for the first step in energy production.

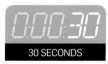

30 SECONDS

The cheeseburger passes your lips and your teeth begin pulverizing it into smaller pieces, which allows saliva's enzymes to work more efficiently. After a few seconds of chewing, you swallow, and the cheeseburger shrapnel glides down the conveyor belt of your esophagus and then lands with a plop in your stomach.

1 MINUTE

Although no longer resembling a cheeseburger, the raw materials that arrive in your stomach are still relatively intact. But they won't be for long. With rhythmic ripples of the stomach's wall, your body churns and mixes the cheeseburger into a uniform soup in a process that takes about 3 hours. At the same time, hydrochloric acid unwinds the beef's coiled proteins and begins ripping away the bonds of the complex carbohydrates in the lettuce and tomato. For now, fat is left untouched.

20 MINUTES

Despite having churned the cheeseburger chowder for nearly as long as it takes to play the extended version of "Shine On You Crazy Diamond," your stomach only now gets around to sending the fullness signal to your brain. Too bad you already ordered that ice cream dessert, right? This delay is an obvious glitch in the production cycle, because it causes you to consume more calories than your body truly needs. (In other words, if you can wait for 20 minutes after finishing your meal to think about dessert, you'll often find that you're not in the mood.)

The stomach can empty the bulk of the pasty mixture of food and stomach juices—what dietitians unappealingly call "chyme"—

within an hour or two, but the more protein, fiber, and yes, even fat you consume, the longer this process takes. That's good, because it means you stay full longer and burn more calories digesting the food. If your meal consisted entirely of sugar, on the other hand, your blood sugar would spike dramatically and induce what you might recognize as a sugar rush. That's why soda makes you feel good, even though the effect is short-lived. The solution is simple: It's okay to have some sugar, but you've also got to have some fat and protein mixed in. Ice cream, anyone?

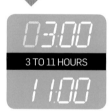

The cheeseburger milk shake slowly exits the stomach and eventually gets to the small intestine. This is where energy extraction takes place. The small intestine mixes in pancreatic enzymes to further undress the structures of the complex carbohydrates and proteins you ate. Carbohydrates that began as long strings of chemically fused sugars are now broken down into smaller units and proteins are unraveled into individual amino acids.

In the small intestine's processing plant, bile is among the key instruments. While you're most likely snacking on your next meal, this bitter fluid flows over from the liver and attacks all the fatty triglycerides you consumed hours ago. Once broken down into individual fatty acids, these tiny particles pass through the intestinal wall along with the rest of your meal. If the cheeseburger was consumed at dinnertime, you are likely now asleep. But your body's assembly line is in full production mode.

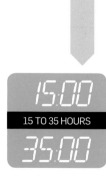

Fiber, the only macronutrient that never passes through the intestinal wall, continues on to the large intestine along with other undigestible particles and any other nutrients that happened to slip through. Some 5 to 10 percent of the calories you consume aren't absorbed, and the more fiber you take in, the higher this number climbs. That means that if your burger contained 400 calories, 20 to 40 of them likely slipped through undigested.

"People ask me what surgery I had. I tell them I learned how to eat!"

It wasn't a lack of motivation that kept **Nichole Storms** overweight. She regularly ran for exercise, and she followed whatever food and nutrition tips she could pick up from friends and family. The problem was, some of those tips followed unhealthy conventions. "I had never even heard of high-fructose corn syrup," she says. "I would eat the yogurt with fruit because, hey, it's got fruit. Everything that everyone told me was completely wrong."

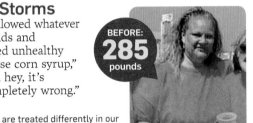

BEFORE: **285** pounds

THE KEY MOMENT

Nichole's big moment came when she and her friends booked plane tickets for a vacation to Mexico: She realized she'd become so large that she might not fit into a single airplane seat. "I was absolutely mortified," she says, and she asked herself, "Am I going to be embarrassed in front of my friends?" Nichole resolved to simply exercise more, but one day in the bookstore, she serendipitously dropped her keys near a copy of *Eat This, Not That!* She noticed the book as she went for the keys, and she decided on a whim to give it a shot.

Nichole quickly learned to distrust food marketing. She was shocked to learn that low-fat peanut butter is made by removing the heart-healthy fat from peanuts and replacing it with sugar. As the weight came off, Nichole set her sights on a particular pair of jeans. "Every month I visited the store to see if they fit yet. Finally, when I put them on, I sat in the store with my girlfriend and just cried."

THE ADVANTAGES OF BEING THIN

Now almost unrecognizably thinner, Nichole is experiencing the upside of a sad reality: Overweight people are treated differently in our society. "Before, people shunned me and assumed I had no feelings," she says. "Now strangers are much more respectful and engaged. It's an amazing difference; guys hold doors open for me now. That never happened before." What's more, Nichole's success has been motivating the neighbors on her block. "When I jog, people will literally run out of their houses to ask me what surgery I had or what pills I'm taking," she says. "I tell them I learned how to eat!"

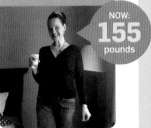

VITALS:
Nichole Storms, 39
Location: Glencoe, MN

HEIGHT: 5'8"

TOTAL WEIGHT LOST: 130 lbs

TIME IT TOOK TO LOSE THE WEIGHT: 1 year

NOW: **155** pounds

Meanwhile, as fiber sinks deeper into the holding tank of the large intestine, the nutrients that passed through the walls of the small intestine are sent out into the bloodstream, the body's comprehensive distribution center.

The simple sugars ride the bloodstream to the liver, where they're converted into glucose. If you've recently worked out and your muscles are depleted of glucose, it travels to the muscle cells to prepare you for the next bout of exercise. If not, it hangs out in the liver. Total, your body stores about 2,000 calories' worth of carbohydrates at any given time. If you have more than that entering your bloodstream and your body can't immediately use it as energy, then you have a problem of oversupply. Your body responds the way any decent company would: It boxes it up (in the form of fatty acids) and sticks it in storage (in the form of body fat). There is essentially no limit to the amount of fat your body can hold in long-term storage, which is why many of us walk around with belly flab that seems to grow outward each year.

The amino acids, the pieces pulled from protein, are still floating around in the bloodstream. These are the body's maintenance crew; they can fix almost anything. In response to various hormone triggers, they hightail it to areas in need of repair, be it minor shaving wounds that need closing; faulty heart cells that need replacing; or, if you've been in the weight room, shredded muscles that need mending.

Finally, anywhere from 24 to 72 hours after that big, juicy cheeseburger passed your lips, your body has fully deconstructed and converted it into energy or waste. Like Marvel Comics' Tony Stark and Iron Man: You are the cheeseburger, the cheeseburger is you. But the work isn't finished. It's never finished. There's always another meal coming down the production line.

"I don't feel like I'm on a diet; this is just the way I live now."

Donna Smith comes from an overweight family, so she resorted to dieting to combat her genetic fate. The challenge was her job. As a Lutheran minister, she was expected to partake in frequent communal meals. The result was an ongoing yo-yo diet—the weight dropped off, and then it came right back on. She says, "I always joked that I was so much a yo-yo that you could nickname me Duncan."

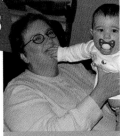

**BEFORE:
213
pounds**

DIABETES STRIKES

Two years ago Donna was diagnosed with diabetes. "There's no diabetes in my family," she says. "I was disgusted with myself—I thought, 'I did this. I got fat.' I hated to look at myself." Donna decided it was time to take a different approach. She picked up *Eat This, Not That!* and found a refreshing alternative to the diet advice she was used to. "I've always hated nutritionists—they're the model of conditional love," says Donna. "I'd tell them, 'I had wheat toast this morning!' They'd say, 'But what did you put on it?' Nothing was ever good enough."

Donna's intention was simply to get healthy and combat diabetes: She was pleasantly surprised when her weight began dropping. "Never in my life did I imagine I would lose weight after 50," she says. When she was on a 2-week cruise, *Eat This, Not That!* helped her overcome the formidable challenge of limitless access to buffets and fancy meals. She spent 14 days on a luxury ship, and in that time gained a paltry 2 pounds. "Now I know the food industry layers everything in salt, fat, and sugar," she says. "You don't realize you're basically addicting yourself to this stuff. It's an innocent green bean—why fry it? What'd it ever do to me?"

THE TURNAROUND

Donna's doctors are thrilled with her progress. She's managed to drop one diabetes medication entirely and reduce her dosage of another. Nothing, though, was as satisfying as taking six trash bags full of obsolete clothes to Goodwill. "I was so tired of plus-size clothing," she says. "Not having to shop in the fat-girl section of the department store was a champagne moment. I don't feel like I'm on a diet; this is just the way I live now."

VITALS:
Donna Smith, 57
Location: Champaign, IL
HEIGHT: 5'4"
TOTAL WEIGHT LOST: 40 lbs
TIME IT TOOK TO LOSE THE WEIGHT: 1 year

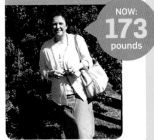

**NOW:
173
pounds**

Everything Is Bigger!

WANT MORE EVIDENCE that our obesity crisis is getting entirely out of hand? Everything around us seems to be getting bigger, except our bank accounts. And there's a direct relationship: Nearly 10 percent of all American medical dollars are now spent on obesity. In fact, people who are obese spend almost $1,500 more each year on health care—about 41 percent more than average-weight people. Everything from our insurance costs to the price of airline tickets is increasing, in part because of obesity. So you can either laugh or get ticked off when you realize…

➤ Buses are getting bigger!

The Federal Transit Administration wants to raise the assumed average weight of bus passengers from 150 to 175 pounds, claiming that previous assumptions were built on people looking as they did during the Mad Men era. In addition, the FTA also suggests increasing the space allotment for standing bus passengers to 1.75 square feet of floor space, up from the current 1.5 square feet, "to acknowledge the expanding girth of the average passenger," according to the *New York Times.*

➤ Boats are getting bigger!

The Coast Guard now says that fewer of us can fit on standard-size boats, so it's increasing the assumed average weight per person (the aptly abbreviated "AAWPP"!) to 185 pounds. This Halloween, try the Coast Guard's new game: bobbing for apple-shaped people.

➤ Bosoms are getting bigger!

The bra size needed by the average American woman has gone up 2 cup sizes since the mid-1980s. Fifty years ago, DD was the largest size you could find, but today lingerie shops stock bras with K, L, and even O cups, according to the Intimate Apparel Council. Last year, according to the

"*Eat This, Not That!* is the single best weight-loss tool I've found."

David Pool is a marketing man, and when the economy soured in the recent recession, he found himself turning to comfort foods to cope with worries about the future. "The problem was, I saw all food as comfort food," he says. "I guess I figured that if I could buckle my pants, I was okay—conveniently ignoring the gut that was hanging over the belt." It wasn't until he saw himself in a photo that he realized the impact of his recession-era diet. In the photo, David was riding a horse. "I was practically as big as the horse!" he says. He resolved to find his way back to pre-recession numbers. He set a 2010 New Year's resolution to get back to his college weight by 2011.

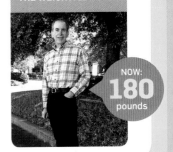

BEFORE:
258 pounds

VITALS:
David Pool, 57
Location: Albuquerque, NM

HEIGHT: 6'2"

TOTAL WEIGHT LOST: 78 lbs

TIME IT TOOK TO LOSE THE WEIGHT: 11 months

NOW:
180 pounds

BROTHERHOOD OF THE LOOSENING PANTS

With weight loss in his cross-hairs, David bought a copy of *Eat This, Not That!* He went through the book and picked foods he liked that added up to a maximum of 1,800 calories a day. As he started executing his plan, it dawned on him that the more healthy foods he ate, the easier it was to stay the course. "I'm crazy about nectarines," he says, "but if I have one, I don't want another. If I have three Oreo cookies, I want more! Feeling full is so much easier with real food." David weighed himself from time to time, but decided to gauge his progress more by the fit of his clothes than the sweep of the needle. "The scale can be a tyrant if you weigh yourself too frequently. The daily ups and downs are enough to make you crazy." Week by week, his pants became easier to slide into, and within a couple of months they started feeling downright baggy.

NEW YEAR, NEW BODY

David reached his weight-loss goal a week before Thanksgiving, and with the *Eat This, Not That!* no-diet approach as his guide, he managed to keep it off through the holidays. "The moment you use the word 'diet,' you're doomed; it automatically suggests a temporary program," he says. "I can easily say that *Eat This, Not That!* is the single best tool that I've found."

founder of the Intimacy retail chain, almost a quarter of all bras it sold were sizes G and up. And, in apparently related news...

➤ Babies are getting bigger!

One-third of infants in the United States are obese or at risk for obesity, according to a Wayne State University study. But don't let your baby get hung up on his or her weight. We've got the perfect solution.

➤ Cats and dogs are getting bigger!

More than half of all domestic pets are now overweight or obese. "Roll over. Stay. Good dog."

➤ Military recruits are getting bigger!

Which at first sounds like a good thing—who wouldn't want to send a battalion of supersized soldiers off to face the commies, or the fascists, or the terrorists, or whomever we're fighting next? But our soldiers aren't supersized in quite the right way. "Overall only 1 in 4 of our young adults between the ages of 17 and 24 is eligible for military service," says retired Rear Admiral James Barnett. Obesity is one of the main reasons, he says.

➤ Movie theaters are getting bigger!

Theaters now spend nearly a third more on their building space than they did just 20 years ago, the result of having to accommodate larger moviegoers. The average seat has increased from 20 inches to as wide as 26 inches. Perhaps smaller tubs of popcorn would help?

➤ Ambulances are getting bigger!

Boston's emergency services department put in a request for a new ambulance capable of ferrying people of up to 850 pounds. Geez, that's seven 1950s—era humans! But of course, getting an 850-pound patient safely to the hospital is just half the battle...

➤ Gurneys are getting bigger!

New "bariatric cots" made to carry patients weighing up to 1,000 pounds are being introduced around the country, although they cost four times as much as simple cots. Talk about your tax dollars being eaten up!

➤ Coffins are getting bigger!

Just in case your community hasn't invested in one of those bariatric cots, there's a backup plan: Goliath Casket makes models of up to 52 inches wide, capable of holding the 1,000-pound body those cots would have been transporting. "In the last year, business has gone up at least 30 percent," says the company's president. Of course, we're going to need some bigger graves...

"Now I can go out and play with my daughters without sucking wind."

David Terrall worked in manufacturing, and the physical labor kept him fit. But when he decided to go back to school, his new routine had some unintended consequences. "When I left my physical job to go back to finish my degree, I did a lot of sitting and studying," he says. "I was getting older but eating the same, and the pounds started creeping on." David had never found it necessary to think about his diet before, but that changed when he returned from a vacation. As he flipped through pictures from the trip, David paused at a photograph of himself and his girlfriend under a waterfall—a vision of paradise, marred by his unexpected girth. "I said, 'Wow, that is just not right. I've got to do something.'"

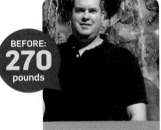

BEFORE:
270
pounds

VITALS:
David Terrall, 38
Location: Stoughton, WI
HEIGHT: 6'2"
TOTAL WEIGHT LOST: 70 lbs
TIME IT TOOK TO LOSE THE WEIGHT: 1 year

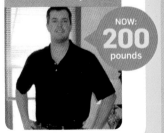

NOW:
200
pounds

OUT WITH THE "THAT'S"

David had seen *Eat This, Not That!* on the *Today* show. He was drawn to it because it offered realistic alternatives instead of drastic lifestyle changes. When he purchased the book, he suddenly realized how poorly he was eating. "All the things I used to order in restaurants were on the wrong side of the page!" Once David lost 5 pounds—and kept it off through the holidays—he seized his new power to make better choices. "I started paying attention to not only the number of calories, but the quality as well. I was learning that not every calorie is created equal."

HIGH AND DRY

Before losing weight, David was in dire sartorial territory—he'd taken to not fully drying his pants just so he could more easily squeeze into them. After losing weight with *Eat This, Not That!*, David needed a new belt and smaller pants—and he's free to dry them as much as he likes. "I feel so much better now," he says. "Now I have more energy, and I can actually go out and play with my daughters without sucking wind."

How to lose weight with this book

If you want to shed belly fat, there's only one formula you need to know, and luckily for you, it's easier than anything you encountered in ninth-grade algebra.

The magic formula is this: Calories in − calories out = total weight loss or gain. This is the equation that determines whether your body will shape up to look more like a slender 1 or a paunchy 0, a flat-bellied yardstick or a pot-bellied protractor. That's why it's absolutely critical that you have some understanding of what sort of numbers you're plugging into this formula.

On the "calories out" side, we have your daily activities: cleaning house, standing in line at the post office, hauling in groceries, and so on. Often when people discover extra flab hanging around their midsections, they assume there's something wrong with this side of the equation. Maybe so, but more likely it's the front end of the equation —the "calories in" side—that's tipping the scale. That side keeps track of all the cookies, fried chicken, and piles of pasta that you eat every day.

In order to maintain a healthy body weight, a moderately active female between the ages of 20 and 50 needs only 2,000 to 2,200 calories per day. A male fitting the same profile needs 2,400 to 2,600. Those numbers can fluctuate depending on whether you're taller or shorter than average or whether you spend more or less time exercising, but they represent reasonable estimations for most people. (For a more accurate assessment, use the calorie calculator at mayoclinic.com.)

Let's take a closer look at the numbers: It takes 3,500 calories to create a pound of body fat. So if you eat an extra 500 per day—the amount in one Dunkin' Donuts' multigrain bagel with reduced-fat cream cheese—then you'll earn 1 new pound of body fat each week. Make that a habit—like so many of us do unwittingly—and you'll gain 52 pounds of flab per year!

That's where this book comes in. Within these pages are literally hundreds of simple food swaps that will save you from 10 to 1,000 calories or more apiece. The more often you choose "Eat This" foods over "Not That!" options, the quicker you'll notice layers of fat melting away from your body. Check this out:

• A single cup of APPLE CINNAMON CHEERIOS cereal has 160 calories. Switch to KELLOGG'S APPLE JACKS five times per week and you'll drop 4½ pounds this year.

• A GRANDE JAVA CHIP FRAPPUC-CINO from Starbucks has 440 calories. Switch to an ESPRESSO FRAPPUCCINO three times per week and you'll shed 5½ pounds in 6 months.

• STOUFFER'S ROASTED CHICKEN FROZEN DINNER has 460 calories. Switch to Banquet's version of the same meal four times per week and you'll drop more than 2 pounds every 4 months.

• An ORIENTAL CHICKEN SALAD from Applebee's packs an astounding 1,340 calories. Instead, order the PARADISE CHICKEN SALAD three times per week—or make a comparable swap at some other restaurant—and you'll blast away nearly 7 pounds of body fat in just 2 months.

And here's the best news of all: These swaps aren't isolated calorie savers. If you commit yourself to just the four on this list, the cumulative calorie-saving effect will stamp out 1 pound of body fat every week this year. Take that, multigrain bagel! Check out more of our favorite calorie-squashing, fat-melting Top Swaps on the following pages.

TOP SWAPS

Burger

Not That!
Ruby Tuesday
Avocado
Turkey Burger
886 calories
54 g fat
2,712 mg sodium

Eat This!
Carl's Jr. Guacamole
Turkey Burger
490 calories
21 g fat
(6 g saturated)
1,120 mg sodium

Save!
396 calories
and
33 g fat!

The potential for excess is every bit as high with turkey as it is for any other burger. If the patty is riddled with fat and buried under calorie-dense accoutrements, it's going to cause damage, and that's true whether the meat comes from turkey, ostrich, or organic parakeet. Thanks to an oversized patty and an excessively buttered bun, Ruby's take on turkey has just 173 fewer calories than its hulking Bacon Cheeseburger. In your own kitchen you can construct a turkey burger with a quarter-pound patty, a slice of cheese, and a big scoop of guacamole for 400 to 500 calories, so that's exactly what you should expect when you eat out. Thankfully, that's what Carl's Jr. delivers.

Caesar Salad

Save!
310 calories
and 1,280 mg
sodium!

Protected by the public's perception of salad as a "healthy" entrée, Wendy's has pumped the fat and sodium levels up to heights unimaginable in such an unassuming dish. Compared with the Grilled Chicken Caesar Signature Salad on Panera's menu, the Spicy Chicken on Wendy's has 5.5 times the fat and nearly a third less protein, and thanks in large part to the massive chunks of Asiago cheese, Wendy's doles out more than 75 percent of your day's saturated fat with every Caesar sold. Not even the Baconator is that dangerous.

Pasta

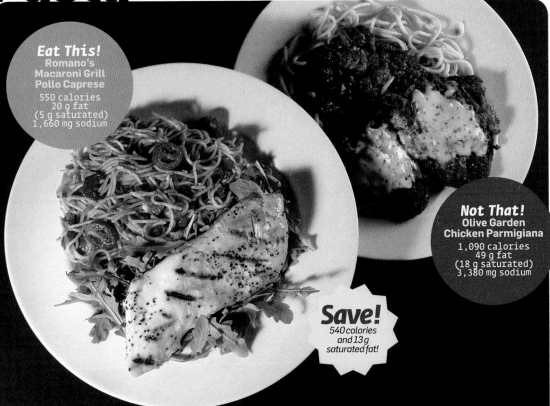

Eat This!
Romano's
Macaroni Grill
Pollo Caprese

550 calories
20 g fat
(5 g saturated)
1,660 mg sodium

Not That!
Olive Garden
Chicken Parmigiana

1,090 calories
49 g fat
(18 g saturated)
3,380 mg sodium

Save!
540 calories
and 13 g
saturated fat!

Here are two chicken dishes with roots in Southern Italy, but by the time they leave their respective kitchens, one has nearly twice as many calories as the other. "Caprese" denotes the deep-flavor trio of tomato, basil, and mozzarella, and Macaroni Grill serves it alongside a juicy piece of grilled chicken. "Parmigiana," on the other hand, is a dish that appears to have drawn more culinary inspiration from the southern states of America than from the southern tip of Italy. Notice how it has nearly four times as much saturated fat as the Caprese? That's because it's been dunked in a deep fryer, just like the french fries, onion rings, and chicken-fried steaks that help make one in three Americans obese.

Pizza

Save!
320 calories
and
24 g fat!

Pizza, more so than any other food, suffers unjustly from a bad reputation, and much of that owes to the harm inflicted by thick-crusted pies. Pizza Hut's Supreme Pan Pizza is a prime example; each slice has 80 more calories than a 6-inch BLT from Subway. When it comes to pizza, a thin crust begets a thin belly. That's why we love Domino's Brooklyn Style crust. It's stretched thin, yet it's as soft and pliable as the thick crusts we're accustomed to. Rather than opting for one of Domino's specialty pies, though, construct your own supreme pizza by pairing one meat option (we love chorizo, since it has less than a third of the calories of normal sausage) with a battery of fresh vegetables. Make this swap and you'll eliminate 160 calories from every slice of pizza you pick up.

Wings

Eat This!
Applebee's
Buffalo Chicken Wings,
Southern BBQ

710 calories
49 fat
(14 g saturated)
2,000 mg sodium

Save!
640 calories
and
59 g fat!

Not That!
Uno Chicago Grill
3 Way Buffalo Wings

1,350 calories
108 g fat
(24 g saturated)
3,540 mg sodium

For all the chatter about them being junk food, wings can actually be a sensible start to a meal. With 61 grams of protein, these Southern-style wings from Applebee's may help you cut calories from your overall meal by frontloading your dinner with belly-filling protein. But choose the wrong chicken and you'll pay the price. Uno's version packs roughly twice the calories and fat, yet for all the excess only brings 5 extra grams of protein to the table. As a rule of thumb, if you order an appetizer, make sure your portion doesn't exceed 250 calories.

Steak Sandwich

Eat This!
Subway
Steak & Cheese Sub
(6")

380 calories
10 g fat
(4.5 g saturated)
1,060 mg sodium

Not That!
Quiznos Prime Rib
and Peppercorn Sub
(small)

620 calories
36 g fat (11 g saturated,
1 g trans)
1,240 mg sodium

Save!
240 calories
and
26 g fat!

Judging by the rapidly expanding line of prime rib subs at Quiznos, we're guessing that the second-largest sandwich chain in America has hit it big with beef. Too bad, since these are consistently the worst sandwiches on the entire menu. Both of these subs are stuffed with steak and cheese, yet Subway's delivers less than a third of the fat. The difference is due primarily to an oil-heavy condiment Quiznos calls "mild peppercorn sauce." In fact, whether you ask for it or not, Quiznos slathers all of its subs with some sort of sauce, and in some cases that can add more than 350 calories to your lunch. At Subway, this sandwich starts out as nothing but steak and cheese, onto which you're free to pile as many vegetables (we like onions, tomatoes, and sweet and spicy peppers) as you can fit. Feeling especially hungry? Double up on the steak and you'll still save 130 calories.

Fish Tacos

Eat This!
Baja Fresh
Baja Fish Tacos
(2)

500 calories
26 g fat
(4 g saturated)
840 mg sodium

Not That!
Long John Silver's
Baja Fish Tacos
(2)

720 calories
46 g fat
(9 g saturated,
7 g trans)
1,620 mg sodium

Save!
220 calories
and
7 g trans fats!

The nutritional deficiencies of Long John's tacos trace back to the hot oil burbling in the kitchen. See, LJS is one of the few fast-food chains still filling its fryers with trans fats. That's especially worrisome considering that the chain tops each Baja Fish Taco with a big scoop of "Crumblies," the deep-fried shards of trans fatty batter that might qualify as the least heart-friendly food on the planet. Baja Fresh, on the other hand, manages to both fry its fish and embellish it with tangy sauce without inflicting a gram of trans fatty damage. And instead of Crumblies, Baja tops its tacos with pico de gallo, a nutritionally rich flavor enhancer with just a handful of calories.

Classic Kids' Food

Save!
870 calories and 50.5g saturated fat!

Not That!
The Cheesecake Factory Kid's Menu Macaroni & Cheese

1,210 calories
N/A g fat
(53 g saturated)
687 mg sodium

Eat This!
Olive Garden Children's Menu Macaroni & Cheese

340 calories
6 g fat
(2.5 g saturated)
1,000 mg sodium

The childhood obesity rate has more than tripled over the past 3 decades, and much of that owes to the obscenely caloric entrées being served by unscrupulous chain restaurants. Unless you were nutritionally clairvoyant, you'd never guess that one of these bowls contains 165 percent more saturated fat than a full-grown adult should consume in an entire day. Kids' menus should be bastions of safe eating, but not one of Cheesecake Factory kids' meals has fewer than 500 calories, and at least five exceed 900. Order from Olive Garden's menu instead and you'll cut the caloric tariff by two-thirds. Top it with a few spears of broccoli—kids will eat veggies as long as cheese is invovled.

Smoothie

Eat This!
Jamba Juice
**Light Strawberry
Nirvana**
(Power size, 30 fl oz)
300 calories
0.5 g fat
58 g sugars

Portion distortion! These two cups differ by only 2 fluid ounces, yet Jamba's is a large and Smoothie King's is a medium. Order a "large" at Smoothie King and you'll receive a 40-ounce bathtub of a smoothie. That would have qualified as slapstick comedy 50 years ago, but today it's become standard fare. What is shocking is the part you can't see: Roughly a quarter of the sugar in the Lemon Twist Strawberry comes from added sweeteners. That's 150 unnecessary calories. In contrast, Jamba's smoothie earns the majority of its 58 grams of sugar from real fruit or fruit juice. And the 30-ounce cup you see here? It's the biggest you can order. That's good, because if you need more than 30 ounces of smoothie, you should probably consider sitting down to a real meal.

Save!
357 calories
and
98 g sugar!

Not That!
Smoothie King
**Lemon Twist
Strawberry**
(32 fl oz)
657 calories
0 g fat
156 g sugars

Ice Cream Bar

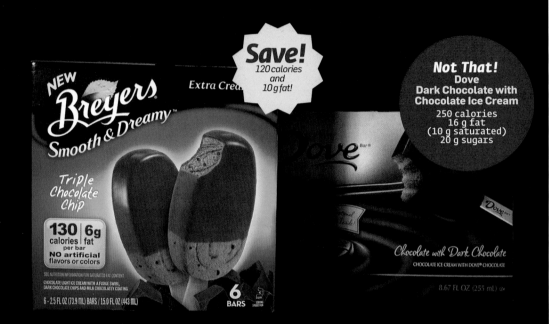

NEW
Breyers®
Smooth & Dreamy™

Triple Chocolate Chip

130 calories | **6g** fat
per bar
NO artificial
flavors or colors

SEE NUTRITION INFORMATION FOR SATURATED FAT CONTENT

CHOCOLATE LIGHT ICE CREAM WITH A FUDGE SWIRL,
DARK CHOCOLATE CHIPS AND MILK CHOCOLATELY COATING

6 - 2.5 FL OZ (73.9 mL) BARS / 15.0 FL OZ (443 mL)

6 BARS

Extra Crea...

Save!
120 calories
and
10 g fat!

Not That!
Dove
Dark Chocolate with
Chocolate Ice Cream
250 calories
16 g fat
(10 g saturated)
20 g sugars

Chocolate with Dark Chocolate
CHOCOLATE ICE CREAM WITH DOVE® CHOCOLATE

8.67 FL OZ (255 mL)

Eat This!
Breyers
Smooth & Dreamy
Triple Chocolate Chip
130 calories
6 g fat (4 g saturated)
13 g sugars

You know what sets "premium" ice cream products apart from standard supermarket varieties? Simple answer: fat and sugar. High-end purveyors like Dove, Ben & Jerry's, and Häagen-Dazs aren't shy either, consistently putting out bars with twice as many calories as you should settle for when searching for dessert. Fortunately, reasonable treats are there for the taking, and Breyers' products are consistently the safest way to soothe an aching sweet tooth thanks to the skim milk that forms the base of its Smooth & Dreamy line of ice creams and bars. As a result, this Triple Chocolate Chip bar delivers a heavy helping of indulgence for fewer calories than you'd find in three Oreo cookies.

Cheesecake

Eat This!
Romano's
Macaroni Grill
Ricotta Cheesecake

370 calories
23 g fat
(13 g saturated)
34 g carbohydrates

Not That!
PF Chang's
New York–Style
Cheesecake

920 calories
58 g fat
(36 g saturated)
94 g carbohydrates

Save!
550 calories
and 23 g
saturated fat!

Cheesecake is a dessert rarely executed with anything less than a stratospheric load of fat, and Chang's is no exception. The offending ingredient here is cream cheese, which is the base of any "New York"–style cheesecake. Eat one slice from Chang's and you'll take in more saturated fat than you'd find in two Bacon Deluxe Singles from Wendy's. So if you're a fan of cheesecake (c'mon—who isn't?), then get your fix at Macaroni Grill. The Italian eatery makes its cheesecake like every Italian eatery should—with ricotta, an Italian cheese that's naturally low in fat and high in protein. It's still hugely indulgent, but it's far less damaging than what you'll find on any other chain restaurant menu in the country.

What If Food Ads Told the TRUTH?

The food industry spends $40 billion a year on advertising, much of it to peddle junk disguised as health food. But what if food execs took a dose of truth serum before releasing their next ad campaigns? Here are five examples of what a bit of honesty might look like.

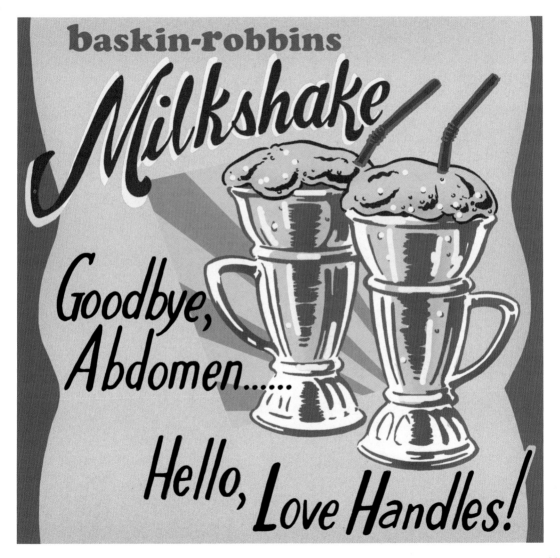

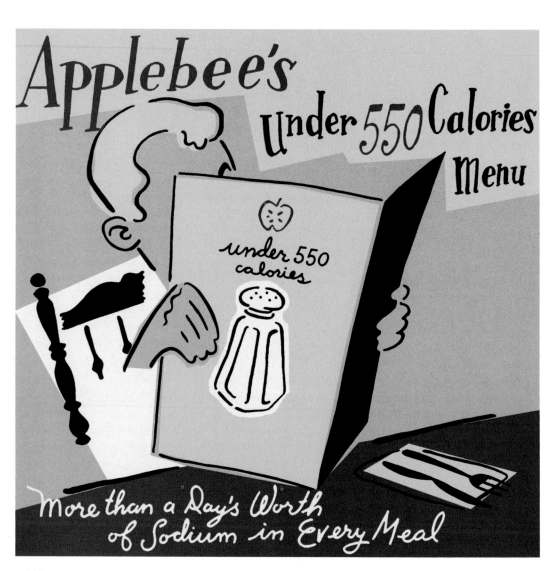

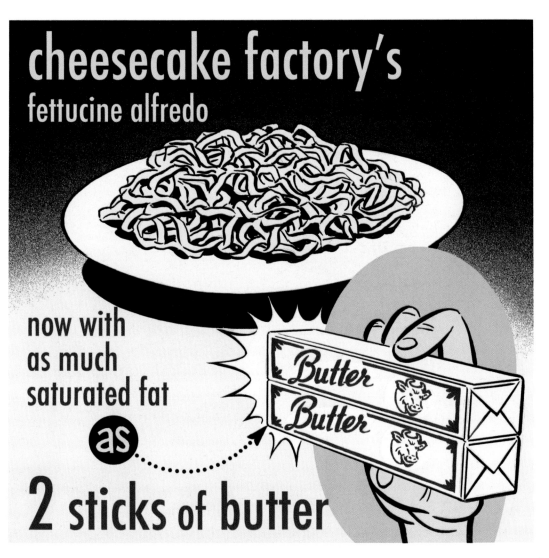

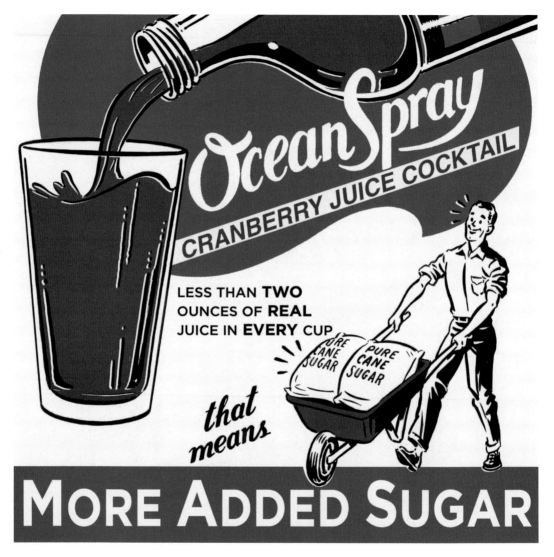

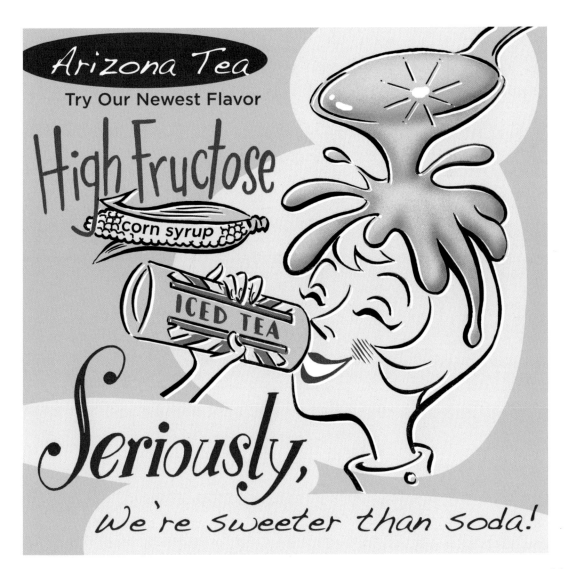

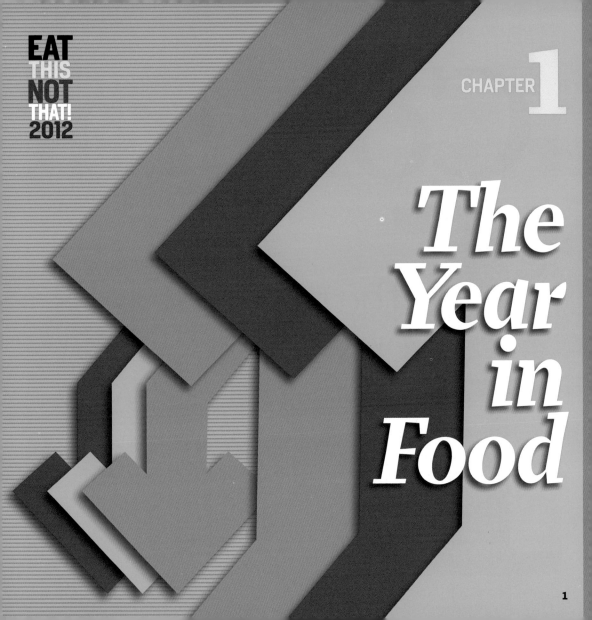

CHAPTER 1

EAT
THIS
NOT
THAT!
2012

The Year in Food

Congrat

I

n the past 12 months, you've helped make the world a healthier place, and you deserve a round of applause.

ulations!

What's that? You weren't aware that you'd changed the world for the better? Well, you did. Simply by being part of the *Eat This, Not That!* family, you've made a major impact on the future of nutrition. By making our little handbook a bestseller year in and year out, you've proven that eating healthy is at the tops of the minds of millions of Americans. By making smart food choices in restaurants, you've inspired giant multinational corporations to alter their foods and make healthier options more readily available. And by being better informed about what goes into the foods available at supermarkets and other places, you've helped to inspire federal, state, and local governments to keep an eye on marketers who are trying to damage our country's health.

But there's still a lot of work to be done. What follows is a brief look at what happened in the food industry in the past year, including plenty of high points—and more than a few lows.

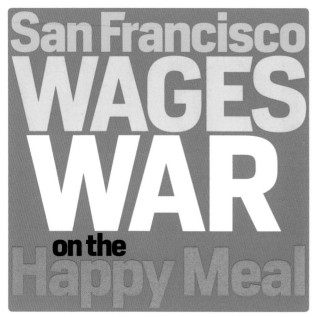

San Francisco WAGES WAR on the Happy Meal

IN A BOLD EFFORT TO STRIKE AGAINST childhood obesity, San Francisco's Board of Supervisors voted to prohibit toys in fast-food meals that don't meet certain nutritional criteria. Now, if you use a drive-thru at a McDonald's in San Fran, you'll have to decide between a Happy Meal with no toy and a Happy Meal with a toy and fewer than 600 calories, 640 milligrams of sodium, and 0.5 milligrams of trans fats. Oh, and it must also contain ½ cup of a fruit and ¾ cup of a vegetable, and not more than 35 percent of its total calories can come from fat.

Hmm, sounds complicated. And it leads some folks to ask the obvious question: Should the government be interfering with our food choices? Well, first of all, by subsidizing particular crops (corn, for example), the government already interferes with our food choices by making certain foods, like those you get at a drive-thru, cheaper, and other foods, like fruits and vegetables, comparatively more expensive. As a result, we've turned fast food from an occasional indulgence into a part of our daily lives. During the last 30 years of the 20th century, fast-food consumption among children increased by 400 percent. What's more, a Yale study found that preschoolers see 21 percent more fast-food ads on television today than they did in 2003, and that the overwhelming majority of those kids' meals fail to meet age-appropriate nutritional requirements. By allowing toys in only the healthier kids' meals, San Francisco hopes to encourage fast-food purveyors to make healthy foods more prevalent.

☑ ETNT APPROVED

ZOMBIE FOODS
Invade Suburbia

REAL FOODS COME FROM NATURE— things that grow, things that breathe. Zombie foods come from crazy food scientists. And this year, the trend in restaurants was straight out of *Dawn of the Dead*.

You might think nothing could top KFC's Double Down as the most absurd and grotesque food item in America. (If you need a refresher, the Double Down is the sandwich that uses two slabs of fried chicken as the bun and mashes between them bacon, cheese, and a fatty, mayo-based sauce. If you've ever eaten one, then you know what a heart attack tastes like. Salty, right?) But this year, things got even creepier. Here are the latest nutritional weapons now being served in America's restaurants:

➤ **Denny's Fried Cheese Melt,** a grilled American cheese sandwich stuffed with deep-fried mozzarella cheese sticks. The price is cheap, $4, but the nutritional toll is anything but. When the accompanying fries are taken into account, this dish has 1,260 calories and more than a full day's worth of saturated fat.

➤ **Friendly's Ultimate Grilled Cheese BurgerMelt,** a hamburger that replaces each half of the bun with a full grilled cheese sandwich. Yes, that's correct: It's two grilled cheese sandwiches encasing one big hunk of beef, which is why it weighs in at a flab-inducing 1,500 calories and 97 grams of fat.

➤ **Burger King's New York Pizza Burger,** which consists of four $1/4$-pound patties layered with pepperoni and mozzarella, smeared with marinara and pesto, and wrapped in a behemoth sesame seed bun that stretches nearly 10 inches in diameter. Thankfully, the Pizza Burger is available only in New York City, because each one contains 2,530 calories and 144 grams of fat.

➤ **Applebee's Provolone-Stuffed Meatballs with Fettuccine,** a dish of fat-heavy meatballs piped with molten cheese and plopped onto a bed of butter- and cream-loaded noodles. Net impact: 1,530 calories, 3,820 milligrams of sodium, and more than 2 days' worth of saturated fat.

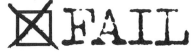

☒ FAIL

Nutella's
HAZELNUT SPREAD
Gets a Hazing

YOU'D BETTER SIT DOWN FOR THIS ONE. This year we learned that Nutella, the beloved chocolate-hazelnut spread, might not be the health food we all thought it was.

Wait...since when did we think Nutella was a health food?

The truth is, we didn't, but we write nutrition books for a living. It's our job to know these things. But one woman (not a nutrition author) wasn't so lucky. She had been regularly feeding Nutella to her child for breakfast when some friends clued her in to the fact that the brown paste is little more than spreadable sugar and fat. So in early 2011, she filed a lawsuit against Nutella's parent company, Ferrero. Her outrage was fueled by Ferrero's claim that Nutella is part of a "balanced breakfast" and by the company's advertisements that depicted healthy families eating the spread alongside whole-wheat toast and fruit. The woman claimed the ads are misleading, and she's asking the company to pay back all the profits it earned by using misleading marketing.

Okay, so it's easy to smirk at knee-jerk lawsuits like this, but take a look at Nutella's Web site. It's rosily marketed as "the original hazelnut spread," and touted as part of a balanced breakfast. But the first two ingredients are sugar and palm oil. By that standard, an ice cream cone could be considered part of a balanced breakfast, as long as you eat enough healthy food to "balance" the junk you are consuming.

Will the angry mom win? Probably not. But will she cause Nutella enough headaches that its manufacturer, and other food marketers, will think twice about selling us garbage and calling it gold? Maybe, and for that reason, this lawsuit is...

☑ ETNT APPROVED

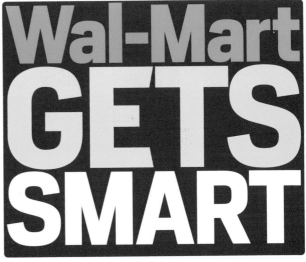

Wal-Mart GETS SMART

FIVE YEARS AFTER VOWING TO EXPAND its organic-food offerings, Wal-Mart has outlined an ambitious plan to improve the nutritional value of the processed foods on its shelves. The plan was inspired by Michelle Obama's Let's Move! campaign, and it commits Wal-Mart to reducing sodium levels by 25 percent, cutting added sugars by 10 percent, and eliminating trans fats in thousands of its suppliers' and its own brand's packaged foods by 2015. The company will also reduce the prices of healthier items like whole-wheat pasta so they match those of the traditional versions. This pledge has major ramifications for the future of your pantry. Wal-Mart is the biggest grocery retailer in America, and as manufacturers bend their products to meet Wal-Mart's specifications, the healthier fare will likely spread to other grocery stores.

Critics of the big-box behemoth bemoan these initiatives as money driven, and following the organics expansion announcement in 2006, a Wal-Mart official seemed to confirm their suspicion. In an interview with the *New York Times,* Wal-Mart's head of perishable food, Bruce Peterson, said, "This is like any other merchandising scheme we have, which is providing customers what they want." Our take? Of course it's money driven! That's the point! The more that consumers like you demand healthier foods, the more big companies will start catering to your needs— and the healthier we'll all get. Consider this major change a feather in your own cap!

☑ ETNT APPROVED

IF THE FEDERAL TRADE COMMISSION
gets its way, Count Chocula, Cap'n Crunch, and Tony the Tiger will soon be standing in the unemployment line.

As part of the government's effort to curb childhood obesity, the FTC has proposed asking food companies to rethink the products they advertise to children. Gone will be the sugar-loaded cereals and fruit snacks, and in their place will be a healthier new crop of products made with produce, low-fat dairy, and whole grains. What's more, these foods will have to fall below set thresholds for unhealthy nutrients like sugar, saturated fat, and sodium. (A *Los Angeles Times* editorial appropriately suggested the guidelines be referred to as "Advertise This, Not That!")

The implications here are potentially vast. According to a 2009 study from the *Journal of Nutrition Education and Behavior*, about 20 percent of television commercials targeting kids are for food, and of those, 70 percent are for foods high in fat and sugar. Another study, conducted by researchers at the Kaiser Family Foundation, found that children who are between the ages of 8 and 12 see an average of 21 food-related television commercials *every single day*. No wonder one-third of children are now overweight or obese.

The guidelines' only drawback is that they would be voluntary, but industry pressure would likely spur most companies to comply. Once they decide to do so, they will have 5 to 10 years to either ditch the cartoon mascots or reformulate their products to meet the new, healthier standards.

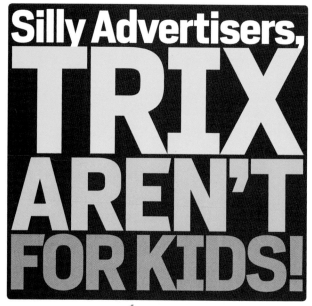

Silly Advertisers, TRIX AREN'T FOR KIDS!

ETNT APPROVED

America's Healthiest
FAST-FOOD CHAIN
Becomes
EVEN HEALTHIER

YOU KNOW THAT KID IN GRADE SCHOOL who sat in the front row and always raised her hand before the teacher even finished the question? Annoying kid, right? Well, now that student is the head of some major corporation and pulling in a six-figure income. While the rest of the class was doing just enough to get by, she was building herself up to be a leader. In the classroom of fast-food restaurants, that kid is Subway.

Since the first edition of *Eat This, Not That!* hit shelves in 2007, Subway has been an industry leader in healthy eating, and over the past 2 years it has grown even healthier. In 2010 the chain launched a breakfast menu that we lauded as the "nation's leanest line of fast-food breakfast sandwiches," and in 2011, it announced that it will make avocado available in all of its stores and decrease sodium counts across the entire menu. For the regular menu, Subway cut 15 percent of the sodium, and for the Fresh Fit items, it slashed a massive 28 percent.

Why would Subway, already America's most reliable source of a quick and healthy lunch, do such a thing? Apparently it realizes what few other chains have: that we consumers will go out of our way for a healthy meal. Along with the push for an even healthier healthy menu, in 2011 Subway also became the world's biggest fast-food restaurant, surpassing even McDonald's in total number of stores. Let this be a lesson to you other fast-food chains: It pays to be healthy.

☑ ETNT APPROVED

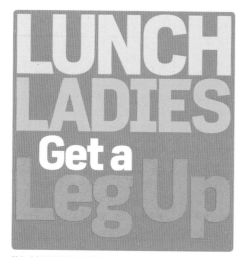

LUNCH LADIES Get a Leg Up

IN JANUARY 2011, hoping to implement the advice of the Dietary Guidelines for Americans, the USDA proposed the first major nutrition upgrade to the school lunch program in 15 years. Here are the big proposals:

→ The amounts of fruits and vegetables served to each child will be doubled.

→ Each week, each child from kindergarten through the eighth grade will receive a $\frac{1}{2}$ cup each of dark greens, orange vegetables, and legumes; older students will get a cup of each a week.

→ Starchy vegetables will be limited to 1 cup per week per child.

→ At least half of all grains served will be whole grains.

→ No milk served will contain more than 1 percent fat.

→ No ingredient will contain more than 0.5 gram of trans fats.

→ Sodium levels will be decreased by more than 50 percent in the next decade.

Ultimately, this leaves less room for grease-spotted pizzas, oil-drenched french fries, and butter-soiled biscuits. The only tragedy is that these regulations have been so long in the making. Since the last changes to school lunches, the Centers for Disease Control and Prevention says, the rate of childhood obesity has risen by 70 percent, and today's children consume as many as half of their daily calories at school. If the new rules are approved, they'll take effect at the start of the 2012–2013 school year. Angry parents, rejoice!

☑ ETNT APPROVED

TACO BELL
Proudly Pronounces
Its Meat
88% MEAT!

CALIFORNIA GURLS are really angry! (One too many annoying Katy Perry songs will do that to you.) While one West Coast mom was suing Nutella, another was suing Taco Bell for allegedly watering down its taco meat with junk-food fillers. According to the woman's claim, private testing of Taco Bell's "seasoned beef" found it to contain only 35 percent actual beef. The other 65 percent was "binders and extenders." If true, this meant Taco Bell's meat didn't meet the federal requirements to be labeled beef—not to mention that it's just gross.

Taco Bell was quick to counter the accusation by claiming that its taco meat is actually 88 percent beef, more than enough to meet the federal requirements. The other 12 percent breaks down like this: 3 percent water, 4 percent spices, and 5 percent processing ingredients like "isolated oat product" and "autolyzed yeast extract." When *Good Morning America*'s George Stephanopoulos asked how the processing ingredients improve the quality of the beef, Taco Bell president (now CEO) Greg Creed explained, "I'm not a food scientist, but what I can assure everybody is that every ingredient is in there for a purpose."

The lawsuit was withdrawn before it went to trial, but regardless, we're just plain creeped out that 12 percent of the "meat" we're eating isn't actually meat—and that Taco Bell thinks that's just dandy.

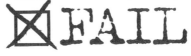

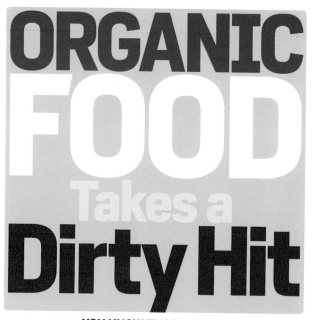

ORGANIC FOOD Takes a Dirty Hit

YOU KNOW THOSE ORGANIC STRAW-BERRIES you've been paying top dollar for? Turns out they might not be quite as "organic" as you thought. In March 2010, the USDA released a report showing that organic regulations are being poorly enforced.

Between 2006 and 2008, for instance, the National Organic Program failed to act for up to 2½ years on the results of investigations that found five operators were marketing products as organic that failed to meet the standard. During the interim, the products continued to be improperly marketed.

The report also noted that California, which tills the most organic acreage in the country, doesn't have the required compliance and enforcement mechanisms in place to ensure that organic food is actually, you know, organic. What's more, none of the certifying agents—the people who make sure producers are meeting organic standards—that the USDA looked at were conducting residue testing for pesticides and other nonorganic toxic chemicals, so the produce might have contained substances prohibited for use in organic products by federal law. According to the report, there's no reason to believe that residue testing is taking place at any of the approximately 28,000 certified organic farms worldwide.

Does that mean your organics are laced with pesticides? Probably not, but the dire picture painted by the USDA's report means we need to get serious about organics.

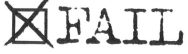

YOUR TYPICAL 12-OUNCE BEER

can have fewer than 80 calories or more than 220, but you'd never know which one it's closer to by looking at the bottle. The reason: Alcoholic beverages are exempt from nutrition labeling laws. That might change if the federal Alcohol and Tobacco Tax and Trade Bureau (TTB) goes through with a proposal to require labels on booze.

It's an idea that enjoys almost universal support. A 2003 poll of 600 American adults showed 89 percent supported including calorie content on alcohol labels. Exactly how the proposed labels might look and what information would be included is up for debate. The TTB is still seeking public comments. Not everyone in the industry is enthused, but the idea does have the backing of the biggest spirits company in the world—Diageo, maker of the Smirnoff, José Cuervo, and Johnnie Walker brands. "It's sort of bizarre," Diageo's executive vice president, Guy L. Smith, recently told the Associated Press, "that alcohol's the only consumable product sold in the United States that you can't tell what's inside the bottle."

We agree. (A toast to you, Mr. Smith!) For those of us who enjoy an evening drink but still want to keep our bellies flat, this kind of info can help us make better choices. And the unintended effect might be that it pushes manufacturers to consider creating lower-calorie drinks.

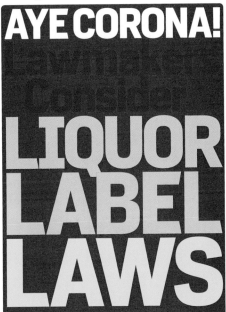

AYE CORONA! Lawmakers Consider LIQUOR LABEL LAWS

☑ ETNT APPROVED

McDONALD'S
Takes a Mushy Step into Health Food

DESPITE THE BEVY OF EGREGIOUS foods to sprout from America's menus this year, the biggest stir arose over a humble bowl of fast-food oatmeal. In early 2011, McDonald's added Fruit & Maple Oatmeal to its menu. Problem was, the oats didn't contain real maple, and a product sold in the state of Vermont can't have "maple" in the name if it doesn't have the real stuff. McDonald's, which used an imitation flavor, was violating Vermont law.

To make matters worse, Mark Bittman from the *New York Times* chastised the company for selling oatmeal containing unnecessary ingredients and more sugar than a Snickers bar, igniting a battle that brought other prominent writers to McDonald's defense. Despite—or maybe because of—the controversy, the Fruit & Maple oatmeal sold well in its early months, and McDonald's eventually did right by Vermonters by allowing them to ask for real maple syrup or sugar in addition to the artificial stuff already mixed in. Only in Vermont, though —we still get only "natural flavoring" outside the Green Mountain State.

Bottom line: If you want really healthy oatmeal, make it at home. (Spend 30 minutes cooking up a pot of steel-cut oats, put the mush in a container in the fridge, and each morning, nuke some for 60 seconds with a splash of milk. For about 85 cents, you've got a whole week's worth of the main ingredient for the ultimate super-cheap, super-healthy breakfast.) But if you're on the road, you could do worse than McDonald's version. For just 290 calories, McDonald's oatmeal serves up 5 grams of heart-healthy fiber. Order it without brown sugar and you eliminate 30 calories and 14 grams of sugar. Eat this bowl every day in place of your usual Sausage Biscuit and you'll cut about 5,100 calories (i.e., a pound and a half of fat) from your monthly intake.

☑ ETNT APPROVED

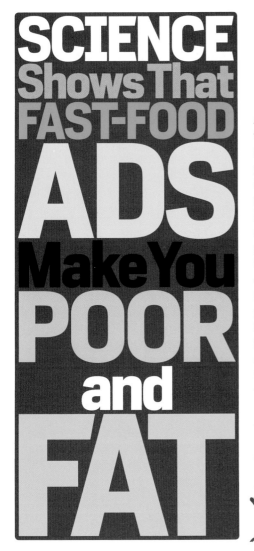

SCIENCE Shows That FAST-FOOD ADS Make You POOR and FAT

AN INTERESTING 2010 STUDY showed that fast-food signs and logos can trigger unconscious responses in the brain. A study published in the journal *Psychological Science* broke a group of students into two groups. One group studied McDonald's and KFC logos and the other reviewed the signs of similarly low-cost local diners. The two groups were then offered a series of gambits that involved receiving immediate but small cash payouts or waiting a week to receive larger amounts of money. The students primed with the fast-food signs were more likely to accept the smaller payments—which is clearly the worse option. The study's authors concluded, "Fast food seemed to have made people impatient in a manner that could put their economic interest at risk."

The way we see it, people already pay a steep price when they walk into a fast-food restaurant and sacrifice the chance to eat a truly healthy meal, but now you might actually stand to lose money by eating cheap food. So much for the "value menu."

☒ FAIL

Cheeseburger Bill Aims to PROTECT JUNK-FOOD PURVEYORS

MINNESOTAN HOUSE MEMBERS recently passed legislation that would make it impossible for citizens to sue fast-food chains for contributing to their obesity. (It's still awaiting a vote in the Senate before it becomes law, but 23 other states have enacted similar measures.) The legislation raises two interesting questions: How much responsibility should fast-food chains shoulder for their menu items' effects on our bodies? And, considering everything else that's going on in the world, why are lawmakers so concerned about protecting Colonel Sanders from a handful of fat kids?

Fast-food obesity lawsuits have been around since 2002, when the parents of two girls sued McDonald's (which often shoulders the brunt of our fast-food aggression) for making their two daughters portly. They didn't win, but such lawsuits run up high legal bills and damage a chain's reputation. What's interesting about this is that fast-food joints—while by no means innocent—aren't the sole causes of America's obesity. What about sit-down and fast-casual restaurants? Just about every family restaurant chain sells appetizers with more than 1,000 calories apiece, and at The Cheesecake Factory, you're more likely to find an entrée with more than 2,000 calories than you are to find one with fewer than 1,000. And then there's the junk food sold in supermarkets—cereals ruined with sugars, juices laced with high-fructose corn syrup, and whole foods that have had their natural nutrients replaced with cheap filler calories.

It's difficult to pin down one cause in the obesity crisis, but the legal system is where we debate and decide how we, as a society, should address our various ills. If lawsuits lead to healthier restaurant fare, more attention paid to obesity issues, and a general awareness of the pitfalls of fast food, then so be it. We think lawmakers should focus on protecting citizens from corporations—not the other way around.

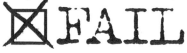 FAIL

Is Michelle Obama Stalking Us?

NEW EVIDENCE SUGGESTS THE FIRST LADY may be wiretapping the ETNT offices. *You* decide!

It's preposterous.

It's ludicrous.

It's outrageous.

Yet the evidence is overwhelming. Michelle Obama is stalking us!

It's true! Thanks to many hours of performing exhaustive research, playing golf with Donald Trump, and/or paging through back issues of the *National Enquirer*, we've accumulated conclusive evidence that behind Michelle Obama's elegant and glamorous demeanor lies a dark genius of covert nutrition ops! She's the Manchurian Candidate of calories, the Don Draper of diet, the Keyser Söze of... well, you get the point. And who knows what else she's up to?

Shhh! There could be a listening device hidden in this very book. Don't believe me? Consider the evidence:

EAT THIS, NOT THAT!: Publishes a book declaring war on childhood obesity

MICHELLE OBAMA: Declares war on childhood obesity

IN 2008, WE PUBLISHED *EAT THIS, NOT THAT! FOR KIDS* in response to our concerns about the number of overweight teenagers having nearly quadrupled since the late '70s. We also uncovered data showing that only a third of students were meeting their recommended activity requirements and that adolescent participation in physical education had dropped by 21 percent over a 14-year span.

Entirely by "coincidence," in February 2010, Michelle initiated the Let's Move! campaign, which aims to reduce the prevalence of childhood obesity to 5 percent by 2030, the rate it was at...in the late '70s! She also began encouraging the advertising arm of the food industry to direct ads for healthy foods at kids instead of the usual sugar-loaded garbage. Hmm...funny.

ETNT:
Pressures restaurants to disclose calories

MO:
Forces restaurants to disclose calories

When we published the first *Eat This, Not That!*, we ran into a problem: Not all restaurants were willing to cough up the nutritional numbers behind their foods. So we urged readers to help us protest, and we posted a blog on the home page of Yahoo! listing the e-mail addresses and phone numbers of all the chain restaurants that had dodged our requests for nutrition transparency. Since then, we've published a restaurant report card every year, and all restaurants that refuse to reveal their calorie information earn nonnegotiable Fs.

In March 2010, President Barack Obama signed into law a massive health care reform act. Buried deep inside it was a small mandate forcing any restaurant with 20 or more locations to print each item's number of calories conspicuously on menus and menu boards and to provide numbers like fat and sodium content on request. Granted it was the president who actually signed the bill, but we can't be sure that Mrs. Obama wasn't the little bird on his shoulder. You know the subject came up at some point, probably while the Obamas were eating homegrown Swiss chard at the First Dinner Table.

ETNT:
Works with the food industry to develop healthier foods in restaurants

MO:
Works with the food industry to develop healthier foods in supermarkets

When Jamba Juice began rolling out new food items in 2008, company spokesman Tom Suiter wrote a letter to *Eat This, Not That!* announcing that the company was determined to become "the healthiest restaurant chain in America." And last year, when Hardee's and Carl's Jr. decided they wanted to add healthier burgers to their menus, they asked *Eat This, Not That!* to help them design a line of big-flavor turkey burgers with fewer than 500 calories apiece.

So how does Obama react? In early 2011, Wal-Mart announced a 5-year plan to reduce levels of salt, sugar, and unhealthy fats in all of the foods on its shelves. But get this: The company's announcement came only after Michelle marched in to spearhead the discussion, also helping to push the retailer into a strategic effort to lower the costs of the fruits and vegetables it sells.

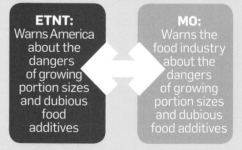

ETNT:
Warns America about the dangers of growing portion sizes and dubious food additives

MO:
Warns the food industry about the dangers of growing portion sizes and dubious food additives

In February 2011, the *New York Times* revealed that Michelle was holding private talks with the National Restaurant Association, and in March 2010, she gave the keynote speech at the Grocery Manufacturers Association's biggest annual event. She urged the association's members to develop healthier products and shift advertising dollars away from sodium- and sugar-filled junk foods. It was a wonderful speech. So good, in fact, that we might have written it ourselves. See what you think:

MO:
"Our kids today lead a very different kind of life. Those walks to and from school have been replaced by car and bus rides. Gym class and school sports have been cut, replaced by afternoons with the TV, and video games, and the Internet."

ETNT:
"When we were kids, we cared more about fishing nets than the Internet, played our tennis games on actual courts instead of virtual ones, and even walked to our friends' homes on the other side of the neighborhood."
Eat This, Not That! for Kids!, August 2008

ETNT:
"[When Keebler] took out 1 gram of fat, they replaced it with 3 grams of refined flour and sugar."
Eat This, Not That! Supermarket Survival Guide, December 2008

ETNT:
"The average American consumes 82 grams of added sugars every day, which contribute 317 empty calories to our daily diet."
Eat This, Not That! 2010, October 2009

MO:
"While decreasing fat is certainly a good thing, replacing it with sugar and salt isn't."

MO:
"Today, the average American is actually eating 15 more pounds of sugar [a year] than they were back in 1970."

Coincidence? Perhaps. And perhaps it's also coincidence that Abraham Lincoln and John F. Kennedy both had VPs named "Johnson." But we're not totally convinced. All we know is that, conspiracy or not, we admire the First Lady's dedication to cutting childhood obesity, and we're pretty sure the feeling is mutual. Once we get done proving the Moon landing was a fake, we're going to send her a note.

But meanwhile, Michelle, if you're reading this, you don't have to hide in that tinted SUV parked out on the street. Feel free to come in and say hello. And bring some of that organic chard with you, okay?

5 Dumbest Things Said About Food (Recently)

WHAT THEY SAID:

"Fat makes you fat."
—University of Iowa Hospitals and Clinics

"If we're supposed to go out and eat nothing, if we're supposed to eat roots and berries and tree bark and so forth, show us how."
—Radio talk show host Rush Limbaugh

FOOT-IN-MOUTH ALERT!

Fat contains more calories by weight than carbohydrates, true. But fat is also filling, and certain fats—like those found in nuts, olives, and fish—are really good for you. When will so-called experts learn: Eating fat won't make you fat any more than eating money will make you rich.

In our ridiculously partisan world, Michelle Obama could save Washington by catching a nuclear bomb in her teeth and Limbaugh would somehow find fault with her dental work. But in criticizing Obama's crusade against childhood obesity, the rotund radio ranter just looks silly. Nobody's recommending a menu of tree bark, least of all the burger-loving Obamas.

WHAT THEY SHOULD HAVE SAID:

"Eating too much—of any kind of food—makes you fat."

"As someone who's struggled with my own weight-related health issues—from a heart scare to painkiller addiction caused by back pain—I know firsthand that overweight children carry a heavy health burden into adulthood. Trying to change all that sounds like a good idea."

> "High-fructose corn syrup...provides many consumer benefits."
> —SweetSurprise.com, a publicity front for—you guessed it—the Corn Refiners Association

> "No consumer could reasonably be misled into thinking Vitaminwater was a healthy beverage."
> —Attorney representing the beverage's maker, Coca-Cola

> "I am eating a healthy diet."
> —Ninety percent of the 1,234 American adults surveyed by *Consumer Reports*

Besides changing the group's name from "Sweet Surprise" to "Nasty Surprise," this corn syrup flack attack would be much more honest if they admitted that HFCS has allowed the food industry to cheaply oversweeten legions of our snacks and staples, accelerating our junk-food-fueled descent into obesity.

"High-fructose corn syrup is not that different from sugar. And neither one is good for you."

Really? "Vitaminwater" doesn't sound like "a healthy beverage"? What's their next marketing strategy, renaming Fanta "Nice Shiny Teeth Drink"? In reality, Vitaminwater is nothing more than the latest slick sugar-delivery vehicle. The minor benefits of the vitamins mixed in are vastly outweighed by the damage these sweetened drinks can cause. We were relieved when a federal judge ruled the packaging misleading.

"Vitaminwater? Oh, we meant to call it 'Sugarwater.' Our bad!"

Two out of three women and three out of four men in America are overweight or obese. We have become so fat that even contestants on *The Biggest Loser* look somewhat normal. In reality, only about 33 percent of Americans eat enough fruits and 27 percent eat enough vegetables every day, according to the Centers for Disease Control and Prevention.

"Eating a healthy diet is very difficult in America today. But having Eat This, Not That! *sure helps!"*

The Truth About Your Food

What's in Your

LIFE USED TO BE SO SIMPLE. Home ownership was the best way to invest a paycheck; *Leave It to Beaver* represented the classic American family; and "eating out" meant gathering the family into the old Buick, cruising down to the local diner, and sipping a small soda while a clean-cut fella in a paper hat hand-pressed raw chuck into hamburger patties.

Somewhere between then and now, life took a sharp left turn toward chaos. Home ownership became more volatile than Texas hold'em, the Cleavers were replaced by the Kardashians, and that local burger was ousted by a frozen hockey puck shaped halfway across the country.

More than credit default swaps and Kim and Khloe chicanery, it's the changes in our food that have had the most impact on our happiness and well-being. Compared with their normal-weight peers, overweight people are 30 percent more likely to have asthma, 44 percent more likely to have high blood pressure, and 64 percent more likely to be hospitalized for diabetes. The fact is, we're heavier than we've been at any other time in history.

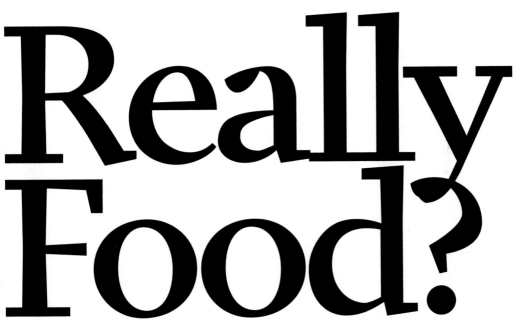

Really Food?

Sure, Americans have changed, but not nearly as much as American food has. Consider this: A 1950s ice cream sundae contained about 8 or 9 different ingredients. Today you can walk into any Baskin-Robbins in the country and order a sundae with 50 or more additives, most of them junk-food fillers that you would never stock in your pantry at home (unless of course you cook with polysorbate 80 and hydrogenated coconut oil).

The point is, food today is nothing like it was 60 years ago. The portions are bigger, the nutrients are fewer, and it requires a PhD in food chemistry to understand the intricacies of half the ingredients. More and more our favorite foods are being tweaked and manipulated in laboratories rather than roasted and sautéed in kitchens. And that has serious implications for all of us.

So before you mindlessly chew your way through another value meal, turn the page to unravel the mystery behind these freakish foods. Sometimes the truth is tough to swallow.

Kentucky Fried Chicken's Chunky Chicken Pot Pie?

CHICKEN POT PIE FLAVOR

Food processors know that if the flavor isn't correct, sales will suffer, and that presents a formidable challenge. See, after making room for emulsifiers, stabilizers, thickeners, and preservatives, the natural flavors in this pie are muted. To battle the blandness, KFC turned to chemists who specialize in what food should taste like. That means that when you take a bite, you're tasting the result of meetings and e-mails exchanged between KFC execs and guys in lab coats. Your taste buds register something like chicken and vegetables, but the driving force is an onslaught of chemicals derived from cheap commodity crops—corn, soy, and wheat—that have been laced with a proprietary "flavor," steeped in stock, and thickened with carbohydrates. It underscores the vicious cycle of our industrial food system: When artificial additives create problems, the solution is to invent more artificial additives.

GELATIN

Hard to believe, but the stuff that gives Jell-O its jiggle comes from the collagen found inside animals' skin and bones. Here, it's used as a gelling agent to give the sauce a more viscous consistency.

Chicken Stock

Potatoes (with sodium acid pyrophosphate to protect color)

Carrots

Peas

Heavy Cream

Modified Food Starch

Contains 2% Or Less Of Wheat Flour, Salt, Chicken Fat, Dried Dairy Blend (whey, calcium caseinate)

Butter (cream, salt)

Natural Chicken Flavor With Other Natural Flavors (salt, natural flavoring, maltodextrin, whey powder, non-fat dry milk, chicken fat, ascorbic acid [to help protect flavor], sesame oil, chicken broth powder)

Monosodium Glutamate

Liquid Margarine (vegetable oil blend [liquid soybean, hydrogenated cottonseed, hydrogenated soybean], water, vegetable mono and diglycerides, beta carotene [color])

Roasted Garlic Juice Flavor (garlic juice, salt, natural flavors)

Gelatin

Roasted Onion Juice Flavor (onion juice, salt, natural flavors)

Chicken Pot Pie Flavor (hydrolyzed corn, soy and wheat gluten protein, salt, vegetable stock [carrot, onion, celery], maltodextrin, flavors, dextrose, chicken broth)

Sugar

Mono and Diglycerides

Spice

Seasoning (soybean oil, oleoresin turmeric, spice extractives)

Parsley

Citric Acid

Caramel Color

Yellow 5

Enriched Flour Bleached (wheat flour, niacin, ferrous sulfate, thiamin mononitrate, riboflavin, folic acid)

Hydrogenated Palm Kernel Oil

Water

Nonfat Milk

Maltodextrin

Salt

Dextrose

Sugar

Whey

Natural Flavor

Butter

Citric Acid

Dough Conditioner

L-Cysteine Hydrochloride

Potassium Sorbate and Sodium Benzoate (preservatives)

Colored With Yellow 5 & Red 40.

Fresh Chicken
Marinated With:
Salt
Sodium Phosphate and
Monosodium Glutamate
Breaded With:
Wheat Flour
Salt
Spices
Monosodium Glutamate
Leavening
(sodium bicarbonate)
Garlic Powder
Natural Flavorings
Citric Acid
Maltodextrin
Sugar
Corn Syrup Solids
With Not More Than
2% Calcium Silicate Added
as an Anti Caking Agent

OR

Fresh Chicken Marinated
With:
Salt,
Sodium Phosphate and
Monosodium Glutamate
Breaded With:
Wheat Flour
Salt, Spices
Monosodium Glutamate
Corn Starch
Leavening (sodium
bicarbonate)
Garlic Powder
Modified Corn Starch
Spice Extractives,
Citric Acid
2% Calcium Silicate added
as Anticaking Agent

OR

Fresh Chicken Marinated
With:
Salt
Sodium Phosphate and
Monosodium Glutamate
Breaded With:
Wheat Flour
Sodium Chloride and
Anti-caking Agent
(tricalcium phosphate)
Nonfat Milk
Egg Whites
Colonel's Secret Original
Recipe Seasoning

OR

Potato Starch
Sodium Phosphate
Salt
Breaded With:
Wheat Flour
Sodium Chloride and
Anti-caking agent
(tricalcium phosphate)
Nonfat Milk
Egg Whites
Colonel's Secret Original
Recipe Seasoning

OR

Potato Starch
Sodium Phosphate
Salt
Breaded With:
Wheat Flour
Salt
Spices
Monosodium Glutamate

Leavening
(sodium bicarbonate)
Garlic Powder
Natural Flavorings
Citric Acid
Maltodextrin
Sugar
Corn Syrup Solids
With Not More Than
2% Calcium Silicate Added
as an Anti Caking Agent

OR

Potato Starch
Sodium Phosphate
Salt
Breaded With:
Wheat Flour
Salt
Spices
Monosodium Glutamate
Corn Starch
Leavening
(sodium bicarbonate)
Garlic Powder
Modified Corn Starch
Spice Extractives
Citric Acid
and 2% Calcium Silicate
Added As Anticaking Agent

OR

Seasoning (salt, monosodium glutamate, garlic
powder, spice extractives, onion powder)
Soy Protein Concentrate
Rice Starch and Sodium
Phosphates.
Battered With:
Water
Wheat Flour
Leavening (sodium acid
pyrophosphate,
sodium bicarbonate,
monocalcium phosphate)
Salt
Dextrose
Monosodium Glutamate
Spice and Onion Powder
Predusted With:
Wheat Flour
Wheat Gluten
Salt
Dried Egg Whites
Leavening (sodium acid
pyrophosphate, sodium
bicarbonate)
Monosodium Glutamate
Spice and Onion Powder.
Breaded With:
Wheat Flour
Salt
Soy Flour
Leavening (sodium acid
pyrophosphate, sodium
bicarbonate)
Monosodium Glutamate
Spice
Nonfat Dry Milk
Onion Powder
Dextrose
Extractives of
Turmeric and Extractives
of Annatto.
Breading Set in
Vegetable oil.

chicken
celery
carrot
onion
potato
chicken broth
butter
flour
milk
salt
black pepper

L-CYSTEINE HYDROCHLORIDE

Used as a dough conditioner in industrial food production, this nonessential amino acid is most commonly derived from one of three equally surprising sources: human hair, duck feathers, or a fermented mutation of E. coli. Yum.

RED 40 (NATURAL RED #40)

Red 40 is a crimson pigment extracted from the dried eggs and bodies of the female Dactylopius cocus, a beetlelike insect that preys on cactus plants. It's FDA-approved and widely used as a dye in various red foods, especially yogurts and juices. Still, it's hard to get excited about a beetle pot pie.

27

What's really in...

Dunkin' Donuts Boston Kreme Donut?

Donut:

enriched unbleached wheat flour (wheat flour, malted barley flour, niacin, iron as ferrous sulfate, thiamin mononitrate, enzyme, riboflavin, folic acid)

palm oil

water

dextrose

soybean oil

whey (a milk derivative)

skim milk

yeast

contains less than 2% of the following: salt

leavening (sodium acid pyrophosphate, baking soda)

defatted soy flour

wheat starch

mono and diglycerides

sodium stearoyl lactylate

cellulose gum

soy lecithin

guar gum

xanthan gum

artificial flavor

sodium caseinate (a milk derivative)

enzyme

colored with (turmeric and annatto extracts, beta carotene)

eggs

XANTHAN GUM It's not dangerous, but it is funky. Xanthan gum is a thickener and emulsifier derived from sugar through a reaction with Xanthomonas campestris, a slimy bacterial strain that often appears as black rot on broccoli and cabbage. Worldwide production of xanthan gum is about 20,000 tons a year, so there's a decent chance you'll find some in whatever you eat next today.

ARTIFICIAL FLAVOR Denotes any of hundreds of allowable chemicals such as butyl alcohol, isobutyric acid, and phenylacetaldehyde dimethyl acetal. The exact chemicals in flavorings are the propriety information of food processors, and they use them to imitate specific fruits, spices, fats, and so on. Ostensibly every ingredient hiding under the blanket of "artificial flavor" must be approved by the FDA, but because you have no way of knowing what those ingredients are, you can't simply avoid something you'd rather not eat.

Boston Kreme Filling:

water

sugar syrup

modified food starch

corn syrup

palm oil

contains 2% or less of the following: natural and artificial flavors

glucono delta lactone

salt

potassium sorbate and sodium benzoate (preservatives)

yellow 5

yellow 6

titanium dioxide (color)

agar

Chocolate Icing:

sugar

water

cocoa

high-fructose corn syrup

soybean oil

corn syrup

contains 2% or less of: maltodextrin

dextrose

corn starch

partially hydrogenated soybean and/or cotton-seed oil

salt

potassium sorbate and sodium propionate (preservatives)

soy lecithin (emulsifier)

artificial flavor

agar

flour

milk

sugar

yeast

eggs

butter

cream

whipped cream

BOSTON KREME FILLING

Note the "K" in "Kreme." That's a not-so-subtle acknowledgement that there's no actual dairy in this filling. Bavarian cream, the real stuff, is made with milk, eggs, cream, and whipped cream. But those are high-dollar ingredients that require special storage accommodations, so Dunkin' Donuts stocks its doughnut case with a loose interpretation. Gone are the famous ingredients that make Bavarian cream a deeply satisfying and memorable indulgence, and in their place is a crude sludge made mostly from palm oil, modified food starch, and two types of syrup. If it weren't for the "natural and artificial flavorings" injected alongside it, your tongue wouldn't pick up much besides fat and sugar.

McDonald's Big Mac?

100% PURE USDA INSPECTED BEEF The fact that McDonald's beef is "USDA inspected" isn't surprising; it would be illegal to sell it otherwise. By dropping this trivial detail onto the official ingredient statement, McDonald's seems to be trying to distance itself from the criticisms facing industrially processed beef. For starters, the cows killed for industrial beef are routinely treated with antibiotics, a practice that cuts costs for farmers but leads to resistant strains of bacteria that doctors can't effectively treat. But what's equally odious— and less acknowledged—is what happens to this antibiotic-fueled beef after slaughter. Before making its way onto the value menu, fast-food beef passes through the hands of a company called Beef Products, which specializes in cleaning slaughterhouse trimmings traditionally reserved for pet food and cooking oil. The fatty deposits in these trimmings are more likely to harbor E. coli and salmonella, so Beef Products cleans the meat with the same stuff the cleaning crew at Yankee Stadium might use to scrub the toilets— ammonia. Every week, Beef Products pumps some 7 million pounds of ground beef through pipes that expose it to ammonia gas that could potentially blind a human being. The tradeoff is that we don't have to worry about pathogens, right? Wrong. According to documents uncovered by the New York Times, since 2005 Beef Products' beef has tested positive for E. coli at least three times and salmonella at least 48 times.

Beef patty:
100% pure USDA inspected beef
seasoning (salt, black pepper)

Bun:
enriched flour (bleached wheat flour, malted barley flour, niacin, reduced iron, thiamin mononitrate, riboflavin, folic acid, enzymes)
water
high-fructose corn syrup
sugar
soybean oil and/or partially hydrogenated soybean oil
contains 2% or less of the following:
salt
calcium sulfate
calcium carbonate
wheat gluten
ammonium sulfate
ammonium chloride
dough conditioners (sodium stearoyl lactylate, datem, ascorbic acid, azodicarbonamide, mono- and diglycerides, ethoxylated monoglycerides, monocalcium phosphate, enzymes, guar gum, calcium peroxide, soy flour)
calcium propionate and sodium propionate (preservatives)
soy lecithin
sesame seed

Pasteurized Process American Cheese:
milk
water
milkfat
cheese culture
sodium citrate
salt
citric acid
sorbic acid (preservative)
sodium phosphate
artificial color
lactic acid
acetic acid
enzymes
soy lecithin (added for slice separation)

Our ingredient list...

ground beef

salt

pepper

Thousand Island dressing

shredded lettuce

American cheese

pickles

onion

hamburger buns (one top and two bottoms)

Big Mac Sauce:

soybean oil

pickle relish [diced pickles, high fructose corn syrup, sugar, vinegar, corn syrup, salt, calcium chloride, xanthan gum, potassium sorbate (preservative), spice extractives, polysorbate 80]

distilled vinegar

water

egg yolks

high-fructose corn syrup

onion powder

mustard seed

salt

spices

propylene glycol alginate

sodium benzoate (preservative)

mustard bran

sugar

garlic powder

vegetable protein (hydrolyzed corn, soy and wheat)

caramel color

extractives of paprika

soy lecithin

turmeric (color)

calcium disodium EDTA (protect flavor)

Lettuce

Pickle Slices:

cucumbers

water

distilled vinegar

salt

calcium chloride

alum

potassium sorbate (preservative)

natural flavors (plant source)

polysorbate 80

extractives of turmeric (color)

chopped onions

BIG MAC SAUCE

Mickey D's so-called "secret sauce" turns out to be more prosaic than years' worth of myth and mystery suggest. Soybean oil combines with egg yolk to make mayonnaise, which is in turn spiked with mustard, high-fructose corn syrup, and pickle relish. Surprisingly enough, the pink hue appears to come from two relatively nutritious spices, paprika and turmeric, not ketchup as most people assume. While a few of the industrial additives (like propylene glycol alginate, a thickener derived from kelp) creep us out, it's a relatively innocuous concoction that contains fewer calories than straight mayonnaise.

CALCIUM DISODIUM EDTA

This compound is complex, but here's all you need to know: It's really good at gathering metal ions in liquid. This gives it many functions, but in food, the trait allows it to prevent microscopic pieces of metals from discoloring or spoiling the liquid.

What's really in...

Chick-fil-A's Chicken Sandwich?

SODIUM/ SALT More than three-quarters of the sodium in the American diet comes from processed, packaged, and prepared foods, and here's a perfect example of why. Salt is undoubtedly the predominant source of dietary sodium, but by no means does it act alone. The chicken by itself, before you add bun and pickles, delivers three other sources of sodium: baking soda (aka "sodium bicarbonate,"), monosodium glutamate (aka "MSG"), and sodium stearoyl lactylate. Some sodium compounds are added for reasons other than flavor, but by and large, your taste buds are the target. That's why fast-food chains regularly brine their patties, and in many instances they rely on mechanically operated syringes to drive sodium deep into the muscle tissue. Ideally, most people in America wouldn't consume more than 1,500 milligrams of sodium in any given day, but with 10 sources of sodium in this sandwich, it packs in 1,410 milligrams on its own.

DIMETHYLPOLYSILOXANE

Go ahead, try to pronounce it. We'll wait... Ready? Okay, dimethylpolysiloxane is a silicone-based antifoaming agent added to fried foods to keep the oil from turning frothy. You'll also find it in a range of products from shampoos to Silly Putty. While no adverse health effects have been identified, there's something unsettling about the thought of Silly Putty in our chicken.

Their ingredient list...

Chicken:
100% natural whole breast filet
seasoning (salt, monosodium glutamate, sugar, spices, paprika)
seasoned coater (enriched bleached flour {bleached wheat flour, malted barley flour, niacin, iron, thiamine mononitrate, riboflavin, folic acid}, sugar, salt, monosodium glutamate, nonfat milk, leavening {baking soda, sodium aluminum phosphate, monocalcium phosphate}, spice, soybean oil, color {paprika})
milk wash (water, whole powdered egg and nonfat milk solids)
peanut oil (fully refined peanut oil with TBHQ and citric acid added to preserve freshness and methyl-polysiloxane an anti-foaming agent added)

Bun:
enriched flour (wheat flour, malted barley flour, niacin, reduced iron, thiamin mononitrate {Vitamin B1}, riboflavin {Vitamin B2}, folic acid)
water
high fructose corn syrup
yeast
contains 2% or less of each of the following: liquid yeast
soybean oil
nonfat milk
salt

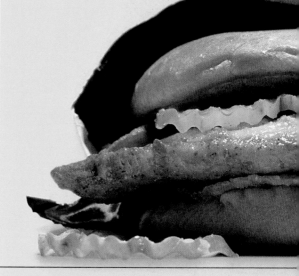

wheat gluten

soy flour

dough conditioners (may contain one or more of the following: mono- and diglycerides, calcium and sodium stea-royl lactylates, calcium peroxide)

soy flour

amylase

yeast nutrients (mono-calcium phosphate, cal-cium sulfate, ammonium sulfate)

calcium propionate added to retard spoilage

soy lecithin

cornstarch

butter oil (soybean oil, palm kernel oil, soy lecithin, natural and artificial flavor, TBHQ and citric acid added as preservatives, and artificial color)

Pickle:

cucumbers

water

vinegar

salt

lactic acid

calcium chloride

alum

sodium benzoate and potassium sorbate (preservatives)

natural flavors

polysorbate 80

yellow 5

blue 1

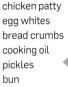

chicken patty

egg whites

bread crumbs

cooking oil

pickles

bun

TBHQ (TERT-BUTYLHYDROQUINONE)

An organic preservative that also can be found in dog food, perfumes, varnishes, and resins. Due to potential links with cancer and DNA damage, the FDA limits the use to 0.02 percent of the oil or fat in any single food item. Studies on its long-term safety have been contradictory, but as with all dubious additives, it's best to limit your exposure whenever possible.

BLUE #1 (BRILLIANT BLUE)

In an effort to make listless food look more appealing, processors regularly add artificial coloring to everything from breads and crackers to fruits and vegetables. The reason is simple: They know that we taste first with our eyes. If food looks boring, it's liable to taste boring, too. The problem is that many artificial colors have been linked to health problems. The Center for Science in the Public Interest recommends caution in consuming brilliant blue and avoidance of its cousin indigotin (blue #2) because they've been loosely linked to cancer in animal studies. And two British studies implicated the dye along with yellow #5 (also in Chick-fil-A's pickles) as possible causes of hyperactivity in children. But as long as it's legal and it makes food look pretty (though it's still unclear exactly why Chick-fil-A would choose blue to gussy up its iconic sandwich), don't expect fast-food companies to stop coloring anytime soon.

What's really in...

Baskin-Robbins Oreo Layered Sundae?

Oreo Cookies 'n Cream Ice Cream :
cream
nonfat milk
oreo chocolate cookies pieces
(sugar, enriched flour [wheat
flour, niacin, reduced iron, thiamine mononitrate, riboflavin,
folic acid]
vegetable shortening [partially
hydrogenated soybean oil],
cocoa [processed with alkali],
high fructose corn syrup,
corn flour, whey,
[from milk] corn starch,
baking soda, salt,
soy lecithin [emulsifier],
vanillin—an artificial flavor,
chocolate)
sugar
corn syrup
whey
n&a vanilla flavor
cellulose gum
mono and diglycerides
guar gum
carrageenan
polysorbate 80
annatto color
Oreo Cookies:
sugar
enriched flour
(wheat flour, niacin,
reduced iron, thiamine mononitrate (vitamin b1)riboflavin
(vitamin b2),
folic acid)
palm and/or high oleic
canola and/or soybean oil,
cocoa processed with alkali
high-fructose corn syrup
baking soda
cornstarch
salt
soy lecithin (emulsifier)
vanillin—an
artificial flavor
chocolate

VEGETABLE SHORTENING

Shortening is simply a code name for partially hydrogenated oil, which shows up three times on this ingredients list. The reason that's bad: Partially hydrogenated oils are the predominant source of trans fats in our diet, and research has shown a strong link between trans fat consumption and heart disease. A few years back the Institute of Medicine issued a report that stated that the only sensible trans fat recommendation the organization could make was zero grams. This sundae may only have 1 gram, but in our book, that's 1 gram too many.

CELLULOSE GUM

This additive is made from cotton or wood pulp, and in Baskin's sundae, it helps prevent the formation of ice crystals. Cellulose gum isn't dangerous, but its versatility as an additive makes for some strange applications. Toothpaste, shampoo, detergent, laxatives, and lubricant are but a few of the products in which it's used. When lumped in with that disparate group, this sundae begins to look less like food and more like any other commodity.

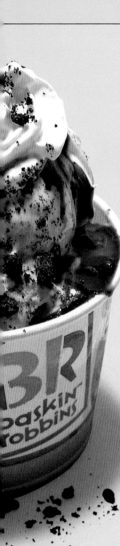

Hot Fudge Sauce:
sugar
corn syrup
water
partially hydrogenated coconut oil
partially hydrogenated soybean oil
cocoa (treated with alkali)
nonfat milk solids
modified food starch
salt
sodium bicarbonate
potassium sorbate (as preservative)
natural and artificial flavors
lecithin
propyl paraben–as a preservative)

Marshmallow Sauce:
corn syrup
sugar
egg whites
modified food starch
artificial flavor
sodium sulfite & sodium bisulfite (preservatives)

Whipped Cream:
cream
milk
sugar
dextrose
nonfat dry milk
artificial flavor
mono and diglycerides
carrageenan
mixed tocopherols [vitamin e] to protect flavor
propellant: nitrous oxide

milk
vanilla
sugar
chocolate
Oreos
whipped cream

SUGAR Sugar, in its various forms, appears 12 times in this sundae. That's 146 grams in total, which is more than you'd consume if you sat down to two full pints of Häagen-Dazs Butter Pecan ice cream. The impact of that sugar can't be overstated; if you stripped this cup of every ingredient except sugar, you'd still be left with nearly 675 calories. (As it's served, this sundae packs a staggering 1,330.) So why does Baskin-Robbins go to such destructively sweet lengths? Think about it: The store attracts customers on the promise of sugar, but outside of a few whole foods, almost everything we eat is loaded with the stuff. Bagels, deli meats, canned fruits, condiments, peanut butter—they're all laced with sugar. In order to create novelty, ice cream shops have to push the sugar to increasingly dangerous heights. The more sugar you eliminate from your diet, the less you'll need to satisfy your sweet tooth.

PROPYL PARABEN Parabens are a class of compounds used to preserve food, cosmetics, and pharmaceuticals. It's been well documented that parabens act as mild estrogens, and according to the Environmental Working Group, they can disrupt the natural balance of hormones in your body. In a Japanese study, male rats fed propyl paraben daily for 4 weeks suffered lower sperm and testosterone production, and other studies have found that the compounds concentrate in breast cancer tissues.

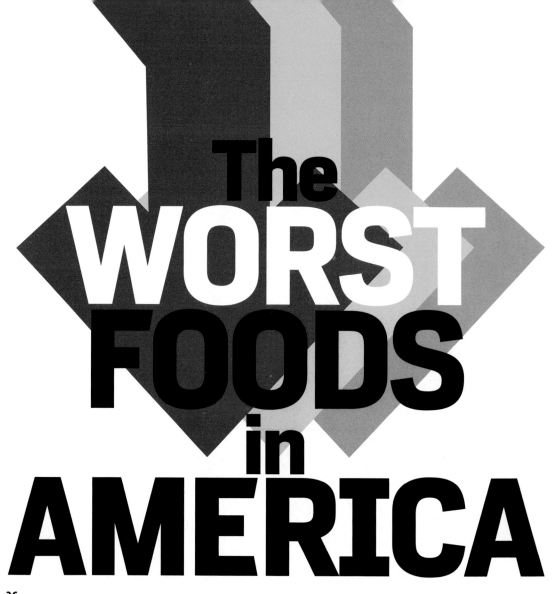

The WORST FOODS in AMERICA

We, the American eaters, are the perky blondes in horror movies who are always running up the stairs when we should run down. We never fail to unlock the dietary door when a knock comes in the middle of the night. And we continue to peek at the darkest corners of the appetizer menu even though we are suspicious of what's lurking behind those sordid descriptions. Because we, like the slasher-film scream queens, are notorious for ignoring imminent danger. We need help.

Research says we are woefully ill-equipped to calculate what we're putting in our bodies. A 2006 study in the *American Journal of Public Health* showed that unhealthy restaurant foods contained an average of 642 calories more than people estimated. If you're like the average American who eats out five times a week, that's 47 pounds a year you didn't know you were consuming.

Now look at what our ignorance has wrought: The top three killers of Americans are heart disease, cancer, and stroke—all three of which are strongly rooted in lifestyle. Translation: Our diets stink. It's time for us to put an end to the horror show. The list on the following pages presents the 20 most cunning villains in a world filled with shadowy characters. So be wise. Next time one of these nutrition nightmares comes knocking on your door, double-bolt it and turn off the lights.

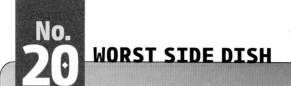

No. 20
WORST SIDE DISH

What appears to be two potatoes' worth of mash is corrupted with fat, fat, and more fat. First, they're whipped with butter and cream and then they're blanketed with Cheddar cheese and finally pelted with bacon pieces. This would be a poor entrée order. As a side, it's just gross. Because Friday's won't supply any nutritional information other than calories, we can't tell you how much of a fat toll this feast will take on your gut. It can't be light. We do know it will chew up half your calories for the day.

TGI Friday's Loaded Mashed Potatoes
930 calories

CALORIE EQUIVALENT:
6 Taco Bell Fresco Crunchy Beef Tacos

Eat This Instead! > Basket of Sweet Potato Fries
400 calories

WORST SUPERMARKET FOOD

Mammoth pieces of fried chicken, sweet corn, mashed potatoes, and a chocolate brownie add up to what the box proudly proclaims is "1 lb" of food. Every bit of it—minus the corn—is loaded with trans fat–heavy partially hydrogenated oils. How much of the sludgy stuff? You don't know because despite a 2006 FDA requirement, Hungry-Man doesn't list the trans fat content on its box-length list of ingredients.

Hungry-Man Pub Favorites Classic Fried Chicken
1,030 calories
62 g fat
(14 g saturated)
1,610 mg sodium

CALORIE EQUIVALENT:
Half a tray of homemade meatloaf

Eat This Instead! **> Marie Callender's Honey Roasted Turkey**
320 calories, 11 g fat (3.5 g saturated), 920 mg sodium

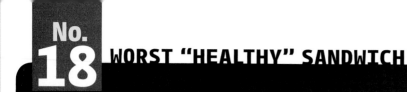

Quiznos Veggie
(large)

1,090 calories
61 g fat
(19 g saturated)
2,540 mg sodium

FAT EQUIVALENT:
4 Snickers bars

In most people's minds, "veggie" is synonymous with "healthy," which is what makes this sandwich such a sly beast. You might think it's a welterweight, but topped as it is with the trio of mozzarella cheese, Cheddar cheese, and guacamole —which together provide a full day's worth of fat—this sub fights its way into the big boys' division. If it's vegetables you seek at Quizno's, it's either the Pan Asian Chopped Salad or a fistful of fat.

Eat This Instead! > Pan Asian Chopped Salad (regular)

430 calories, 17.5 g fat (4 g saturated), 1,915 mg sodium

WORST FAST-FOOD BREAKFAST

Platters are meant to feed groups, not individuals. But serving size isn't the King's only flagrant foul. He hacks away at your arteries with buttered eggs, fried potatoes, gristly sausage, and a trans fat–filled biscuit. (And we're not even talking about the diabetic debacle that is the pile of pancakes and syrup.) You'd better have run 12 miles before queuing up for this breakfast at BK. That's what it would take for the average person to burn through this platter's 1,300 calories.

**Burger King
BK Ultimate
Breakfast Platter**

1,310 calories
72 g fat
(26 g saturated,
1 g trans)
2,490 mg sodium

**SODIUM
EQUIVALENT:**
Nearly 2 pounds of
oil-roasted peanuts

Eat This Instead! > Ham, Egg & Cheese Croissan'wich

350 calories, 17 g fat (7 g saturated), 1,100 mg sodium

WORST FRANKENFOOD

Used to be that only carnivals served ill-advised food mash-ups. No longer. KFC's 2010 release of the Double Down, a sandwich of bacon and cheese nestled between two fried chicken strips, opened food innovation doors that should have remained closed. Friendly's has taken up the audacious challenge with its new riff on the basic patty melt. A galling use of grilled cheese sandwiches as buns forms what appears to be three full meals stacked together. Not surprisingly, then, this burger is also loaded with more fat than three people should eat in one sitting.

**Friendly's
Grilled Cheese Burger**
1,540 calories
92 g fat
(35 g saturated)
2,490 mg sodium

**FAT
EQUIVALENT:**
10 McDonald's
Hamburgers

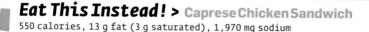

Eat This Instead! > Caprese Chicken Sandwich
550 calories, 13 g fat (3 g saturated), 1,970 mg sodium

WORST SALAD

California Pizza Kitchen Waldorf Chicken Salad
with Blue Cheese Dressing

1,561 calories
N/A g fat
(31 g saturated)
1,821 mg sodium

SATURATED FAT EQUIVALENT:
2 whole California Pizza Kitchen Traditional Cheese pizzas

After we castigated its Santa Fe Chopped Salad for years, TGI Friday's finally removed them from its menu. Unfortunately, there are plenty of unsettling salads to take its place. None are worse than this tangled heap of trouble from CPK. And the potential it had! The first half of this menu description reads like nutritional poetry—field greens, fresh grapes, sliced apples—but it stops there. Sugar-coated walnuts, Gorgonzola, and a flood of blue cheese dressing all conspire to saddle this salad with more calories than any of CPK's whole pizzas.

Eat This Instead! > Classic Caesar Salad with Grilled Shrimp
649 calories, N/A g fat (15 g saturated), 1,338 mg sodium

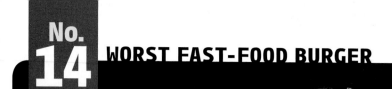

WORST FAST-FOOD BURGER

The recent unveiling of this menacing burger marks a new low for a chain already firmly entrenched among America's worst eateries. Before you even nosh a fry or sip a soda, you've packed in three-fourths of your day's calories. The bacon strips and onion rings will corral much of the criticism, but it's the less-flashy components that hold the hidden danger. Next to the half pound of beef, the two slices of Cheddar cheese and the double slather of mayo account for a third of the fat. (That's not to mention the "bun oil" squeezed on.) There are less perilous ways to get your burger fix.

Sonic Ring Leader Loaded Burger Double Patty

1,660 calories
120 g fat
(44 g saturated,
4 g trans)
1,450 mg sodium

SATURATED FAT EQUIVALENT:
29 slices of
Oscar Mayer Center
Cut Bacon

Eat This Instead! > Jr. Deluxe Burger with Bacon and Green Chilies

425 calories, 25 g fat (8 g saturated, 0.5 g trans), 705 mg sodium

WORST CHINESE ENTRÉE

Consider this: Experts recommend that endurance athletes consume no more than 300 mg of sodium per hour of exercise. At that rate, you would need to exercise for 25 hours to utilize the salt found in this one dish. While by no means low calorie, it's the noodles' status as the Saltiest Dish in America that truly terrifies us. Eat this and you don't need another milligram of sodium for 5 days.

SODIUM EQUIVALENT:
202 Premium Saltine crackers

PF Chang's Double Pan-Fried Noodles Combo
1,820 calories
84 g fat
(8 g saturated)
7,692 mg sodium

Eat This Instead! > Shanghai Shrimp with Garlic Sauce
390 calories, 40 g fat (4 g saturated), 2,100 mg sodium

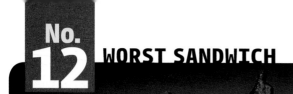

The Cheesecake Factory Grilled Shrimp & Bacon Club
1,890 calories
N/A g fat
(24 g saturated)
2,964 mg sodium

CALORIE EQUIVALENT:
315 medium shrimp

It's hard to blame a diner for thinking he or she might be taking a safe route by opting for this sandwich based on its menu description: "Charbroiled Shrimp, Bacon, Lettuce, and Tomato with Our Special Dressing." Only through a feat of dark nutrition arts did the Cheesecake Factory cram more calories than the worst fast-food burger has into such an innocuous-sounding sandwich. (In fact, you can have the hearty Factory Burger and save nearly 1,200 calories.) Why would a restaurant knowingly subject its loyal customers to such punishment?

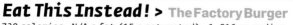

Eat This Instead! > The Factory Burger
730 calories, N/A g fat (15 g saturated), 1,016 mg sodium

WORST DESSERT

When Baskin-Robbins began to phase out its catastrophic line of Premium Shakes (the worst of which contained an eye-popping 2,600 calories), we cheered what we thought was the beginning of a more health-conscious corporate strategy. But this thick gulp of caloric excess is a reminder of just how deep their arsenal of belt-buckling treats runs. We might even go as far as to call this 24-ounce orgy of soft-serve, brownie, and hot fudge the most nutritionally imbalanced food in America, punishing ice cream hounds with not just an excess of calories and saturated fat, but also a concerning dose of trans fats, a dizzying amount of sugar, and, most disturbingly, more than half a day's worth of sodium.

SUGAR EQUIVALENT:
9 Hershey's Milk Chocolate bars

Baskin-Robbins Fudge Brownie 31° Below
(large)

1,900 calories
80 g fat
(39 g saturated,
1.5 g trans)
1,350 mg sodium
225 g sugars

Eat This Instead! > Premium Churned Light Aloha Brownie Ice Cream (4 oz)
250 calories, 8 g fat (4.5 g saturated), 33 g sugars

How do you make deep-fried potatoes even more detrimental to your health? Easy. Glob on a ladleful of gooey cheese and a pile of chili and dip the whole mess in ranch dressing. We know Americans love their fries (we eat more potatoes in this form than any other single vegetable), but this version veers into the farcical. With multiple food threats in one dish, it's best to choose the tamer side of original fries.

**Chili's
Texas Cheese Fries
with Chili and Ranch**

2,120 calories
144 g fat
(69 g saturated)
5,920 mg sodium

**CALORIE
EQUIVALENT:**
53 Pizza Hut
All American
Traditional Wings

Eat This Instead! > Homestyle Fries

380 calories, 13 g fat (3 g saturated), 1,210 mg sodium

WORST MEXICAN MEAL

Mexican food at its best can be a well-balanced cuisine built around fresh vegetables, grilled meats and fish, and healthy condiments like fresh salsa and guacamole. Unfortunately, the faux-Mexican food dished out by monster chains like Chili's, Chevys, and On the Border bears little resemblance to the real stuff, reliant as it is on deep-frying, cream-based sauces, and the ubiquitous blankets of melted cheese. These tacos represent what happens when an irresponsible corporate kitchen hijacks an entire culinary culture.

On the Border Dos XX Fish Tacos

2,150 calories
144 g fat
(31 g saturated)
3,740 mg sodium

FAT EQUIVALENT:
5 pints of Breyers All Natural Chocolate Ice Cream

Eat This Instead! > 3 Chicken Tostadas

390 calories, 15 g fat (6 g saturated), 1,050 mg sodium

No. 8

WORST FISH MEAL

Frying anything is a bad idea, but frying fish is a debasement of one of nature's purest foods. Why ruin what could be a protein-packed, muscle-building meal by sticking it in a vat of bubbling oil? But Culver's doesn't stop with its battered and oiled cod filets; it ups the risk to your waistline and overall well-being by adding heaping helpings of the default sides of cole slaw, fries, tartar sauce, and a dinner roll. We challenge more restaurants to do what's right with fish: buy it fresh, cook it with minimal flourishes, and let diners enjoy the simple beauty of a lean, well-cooked meal. Until Culver's takes up the challenge, make it the roasted chicken sandwich and tomato soup and move on.

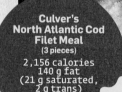

Culver's North Atlantic Cod Filet Meal
(3 pieces)

2,156 calories
140 g fat
(21 g saturated,
2 g trans)
2,378 mg sodium

FAT EQUIVALENT:
3 orders of
Applebee's
Mozzarella Sticks

Eat This Instead! > Flame Roasted Chicken Sandwich with Mashed Potatoes and Gravy
449 calories, 10 g fat (2 g saturated), 1,374 mg sodium

Chili's Jalapeño Smokehouse Bacon Burger with Ranch

2,210 calories
144 g fat
(46 g saturated)
6,600 mg sodium

SODIUM EQUIVALENT:
18 large orders of McDonald's french fries

The average burger-and-fry combo at Chili's packs 1,786 calories—about 85 percent of your daily allotment if you're an active female and more than two-thirds of an active male's caloric allowance. That's a heavy price to pay for a staple the average American consumes up to 150 times a year. Of course, this tricked-out number takes the havoc to a new high. Laced with more bells and whistles than a Michael Bay blockbuster (tortilla strips, bacon, Cheddar, mayo, and jalapeño-ranch dressing), this burger punishes partakers with more than 2 days' worth of saturated fat and as much sodium as you'd find in 6 pounds of McDonald's french fries.

Eat This Instead! > Margarita Grilled Chicken
550 calories, 14 g fat (4 g saturated), 1,870 mg sodium

WORST PIZZA

Chicagoans beam with pride when claiming rights to the deep dish pizza, as if the invention of one of the world's most dangerous foodstuffs is somehow a source of civic satisfaction. The problem starts, of course, with the crust, which is bathed in oil, rich in refined carbohydrates, and about three times thicker than normal pizza in order to support the onslaught of toppings it invariably houses. Tack on oozing layers of mozzarella, Romano, and sausage (the "classic" topping of choice), and you have an individual pizza with more calories than you'd consume if you took down an entire extra-large Domino's Thin Crust chorizo pie. If it's pizza you seek at Uno's, turn to the admirable new thin five-grain crust to avoid total catastrophe.

CALORIE EQUIVALENT:
11 slices of a medium Domino's Hand Tossed Crust ham and pineapple pizza

Uno Chicago Grill Chicago Classic Deep Dish Pizza
(individual)

2,310 calories
165 g fat
(54 g saturated)
4,650 mg sodium

Eat This Instead! > Thin Five-Grain Crust Roasted Eggplant, Spinach & Feta Pizza (½ pie)
435 calories, 17 g fat (5 g saturated), 600 mg sodium

No. 5

WORST APPETIZER

Applebee's Appetizer Sampler
2,430 calories
166 g fat
(48 g saturated)
6,070 mg sodium

SODIUM EQUIVALENT:
225 Nabisco Ritz Crackers

Sample platters are the lairs wherein all menu miscreants hang out, and nearly every chain offers a criminal version. Applebee's is the undisputed kingpin. Its repository of cheap, fried, monochromatic foods is a lesson in the perils of restaurant eating. It begins with chips and spinach-artichoke dip, a euphemism for a crock of cream and cheese with a few token shards of vegetable matter. From there, it gets worse: fried chicken wings, fried mozzarella sticks, and greasy cheese quesadillas. You could eat the celery on the plate to make yourself feel better, but by that point, the damage is done.

Eat This Instead! > Chicken Wonton Tacos

590 calories, 24 g fat (4.5 g saturated), 2,150 mg sodium

WORST BREAKFAST

IHOP
Big Country Breakfast
with Country Fried Steak
& Country Gravy

2,440 calories
145 g fat
(56 g saturated)
5,520 mg sodium

SATURATED FAT EQUIVALENT:
37 KFC
Original Recipe
Drumsticks

This smorgasbord is an unabashed siren call to gluttons everywhere. It's a 12-ounce steak breaded, fried, and dripping with gravy; three eggs; hash browns; and three pancakes crowned with an ice cream scoop of butter and a sugary tide of syrup. Heck, this meal wears its pride in its name. You could feed a small nation with the Big Country, though doing so would be grounds for UN intervention.

Eat This Instead! > Simple & Fit Spinach, Mushroom & Tomato Omelette
330 calories, 12 g fat (5 g saturated), 690 mg sodium

WORST RIBS

TGI Friday's Caribbean Rockin' Reggae Ribs

2,450 calories
N/A g fat
(52 g saturated)
3,810 mg sodium

SATURATED FAT EQUIVALENT:
Three 11.5-ounce bags of Doritos Nacho Cheese chips

Of all the foods on this list—burgers, fries, pasta, ice cream—no food is more consistently catastrophic than a rack of restaurant ribs. Part of that is due to the fact that ribs comprise a nutritionally flawed cut of meat, redolent as they are with both external and intramuscular fat. But restaurant cooking methods, which invariably involve layer after layer of oily, sugar-dense barbecue sauce, only compound the problem. Want ribs? Fire up the grill in the backyard and use our recipe for Dr Pepper Ribs in *Cook This, Not That!* It will save you 2,050 calories. In the meantime, cut your losses and order the sirloin.

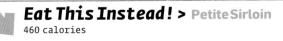

Eat This Instead! > Petite Sirloin
460 calories

No. 2

WORST CHICKEN ENTRÉE

Weighed down with more 2,000-plus-calorie meals than any other chain in America (26 at last count), the Cheesecake Factory offers diners a Russian roulette of choices, only with worse odds. Every time you pick up your fork, you risk absorbing days' worth of unsavory macronutrients. Take the Chicken and Biscuits for example. It's a classic like Grandma used to make—that is, if your grandma used every form of fat in the pantry and doled it out by the bathtubful. Even worse, the Factory seems to patronize those seeking to go lighter by putting its lower-calorie choices on the Weight Management menu. Anyone order a side of condescension?

CALORIE EQUIVALENT:
7 Wendy's
Jr. Bacon
Cheeseburgers

The Cheesecake Factory Chicken and Biscuits

2,580 calories
N/A g fat
(68 g saturated)
2,621 mg sodium

Eat This Instead! > Weight Management Spicy Chicken Salad

440 calories, N/A g fat (1 g saturated), 771 mg sodium

56

WORST FOOD IN AMERICA

The Cheesecake Factory Bistro Shrimp Pasta

2,730 calories
N/A g fat
(78 g saturated)
919 mg sodium

CALORIE EQUIVALENT:
14 Krispy Kreme Original Glazed Doughnuts

The Cheesecake Factory has earned the title of America's Worst Restaurant for the 4th year running. No establishment better represents the confluence of factors that have saddled America with an ever-worsening obesity crisis. First, portion sizes are large enough to feed an NFL offensive line. Second, the use of cheap sources of flavor—oils, butter, cream, salt, and sugar—knows no limit. Finally, the percentage of dishes fit for consumption is absurdly small (we count 8 on a menu of more than 200 dishes). Amidst the carnage, one dish sinks below all the rest: the Bistro Shrimp Pasta. Tangled up in these noodles are more calories than you'd consume if you ate three sticks of butter for dinner.

Eat This Instead! > Fresh Grilled Salmon
490 calories, N/A g fat (6 g saturated), 290 mg sodium

CHAPTER 3

At Your Favorite Restaurants

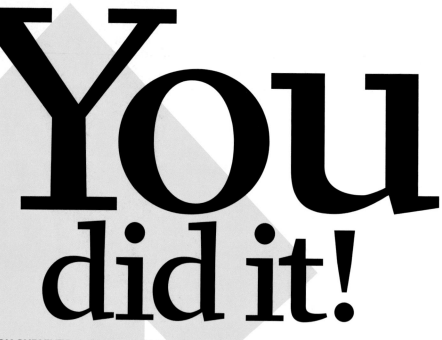

You
did it!

YOU SURVIVED A TOUGH DAY AT WORK/ a challenging commute/another family drama/a 6-hour marathon of *Keeping Up with the Kardashians*!

You deserve to celebrate/cut loose/ drown your sorrows/indulge while you dissect Khloé's relationship!

You should order the appetizer/ all-you-can-eat platter/dessert special/ enormous pitcher of fizzy stuff!

It's a special occasion!

Okay, really, it's not. It's just dinner. Or lunch. Or even breakfast. But if you've gone out to a restaurant for this meal, chances are you're going to feel like celebrating—even if there isn't anything to really celebrate. Experts call it the "special occasion mentality," and it sets in almost every time we set foot in a restaurant.

Of course, all restaurant meals feel special—the clinking of the glasses, the wafting scent of a sizzling supper, the overtired waitstaff marching down the aisle singing that happy-birthday song, over and over. Restaurants want us to feel special, sure. But they also want us to order more food. And creating a party atmosphere inspires us to throw caution to the wind. In fact, a 2008 study in the *International Food Research Journal* found that people are less likely to make healthy restaurant choices when they feel they're dining out for a special occasion.

In theory, it's great: Go out to celebrate, indulge for the night, and then go back to normal life. But sitting in a restaurant is normal life for most people: In fact, 1 in 10 Americans eats out almost every single day. That means that your "special occasion" is about as special as taking a shower.

In this chapter, you'll discover exactly how not-so-special some of your restaurant favorites really are, and some easy ways to make sure the terrific spread at the buffet doesn't turn into a terrific spread at your waistline. See, most of your favorite eating establishments have great options on the menu; you just need to know how to spot them.

But it's not just about knowing the right foods to eat: Restaurants have their own special challenges, too. So while you're perusing the menu, keep these points in mind:

➡ ***Don't assume that slow food is healthier food.*** The idea that fast food is bad for us has been beaten into our heads for a generation. But just because you're sitting down and being waited on by an aspiring musician doesn't mean you're eating healthier. In fact, our analysis of 24 national chains revealed that the average sit-down restaurant entrée boasted a whopping 867 calories, compared with 522 in the typical fast-food-franchise dinner.

➡ ***Don't get up-sold.*** The kids at the drive-thru are like dastardly little mortgage brokers, looking to squeeze you into a great deal that you actually can't afford. Studies show that people are more likely to order the sides or supersize their orders when prompted by the helpful young lass in the paper hat. But it's a bad investment: Indeed, supersizing your meal costs you an average of 67 more cents, but loads you up with 397 more calories. Talk about a balloon payment!

➡ ***Don't order dessert.*** No dessert? Oh, come on! You suck, *Eat This, Not That!* guys! Hey, let us rephrase: An indulgent scoop of chocolate ice cream is one of the true pleasures in life. Of course you should have dessert. But here's an awesome weight-loss trick: Pay for your dinner, leave the restaurant, and then go somewhere else for dessert. The reason? First, a change of scenery may short-circuit your cravings. Second, it takes about 20 minutes for your body to signal that you've had enough to eat. By the time you're on the road to Heidi's House of Hot Fudge, you may discover that you weren't as hungry as you thought. That's calories off your belly—and money in your pocket! (And if you're still hungry when you get there? Then go ahead!)

A&W

D   A&W refuses to banish trans fats from its restaurants, and until it finally does, we're determined to keep this burger and root beer joint in our crosshairs. Although the hazardous oil is sprinkled throughout the menu, it's the side dishes that pack the most punishing wallops. Nearly every other chain in the fast-food industry has ditched the trans fatty oil. What's the holdup, A&W?

SURVIVAL STRATEGY

The best item on the entire menu is the Grilled Chicken Sandwich. Start with that or a small burger, skip the sides and the regular root beer, and finish (if you must have something sweet) with a small sundae or a vanilla cone.

Eat This

Grilled Chicken Sandwich

400 calories
15 g fat
(3 g saturated)
820 mg sodium

> You won't find a better balance of protein, fat, and carbs available at a drive-thru window. Just as impressive is a sodium count well below 1,000 milligrams, a rarity with fast-food chicken sandwiches.

Other Picks

Papa Single Burger	470 calories 25 g fat (8 g saturated, 0.5 g trans) 1,000 mg sodium
Chili	190 calories 6 g fat (2 g saturated) 640 mg sodium
Strawberry Sundae	300 calories 8 g fat (4 g saturated) 140 mg sodium

660 calories

46 g fat
(7.5 g saturated,
2 g trans)

1,290 mg sodium

Not That!

Chicken Strips
with Ranch Dipping Sauce

At most fast-food joints, chicken strips are a fairly safe bet, but these are not only significantly more caloric than your average chicken pieces (see all that breading?), but also pack more than a day's worth of trans fats. If you want chicken at A&W, better make sure the bird hasn't been anywhere near the fryer.

Other Passes

550 calories
25 g fat (4.5 g saturated, 1.5 g trans)
1,130 mg sodium

Crispy Chicken Sandwich

570 calories
40 g fat (21 g saturated, 1 g trans)
1,220 mg sodium

Cheese Curds
(regular)

840 calories
36 g fat (23 g saturated, 2 g trans)
230 mg sodium

Strawberry Shake
(medium)

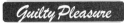

Guilty Pleasure
Corn Dog Nuggets
(8 pieces)

280 calories
13 g fat (3 g saturated,
0.5 g trans)
830 mg sodium

Surprisingly enough, the Corn Dog Nuggets are the best side on A&W's menu. A small order of french fries has 80 fewer calories, but it also comes with 2 full grams of trans fats.

The number of menu items with at least 1 gram of trans fats

SIDESWIPED
French Fries
(Regular)

310 calories
12 g fat
(3 g saturated,
3.5 g trans)
460 mg sodium

As far as fries and calories go, A&W's spuds aren't bad. The problem? One regular order packs 3.5 grams of bad cholesterol–boosting trans fats. That's almost 2 days' worth.

Applebee's

After years of stonewalling health-conscious eaters and *ETNT* authors alike, Applebee's has finally released the nutritional numbers for its entire menu. Unfortunately, we now see why they were so reluctant to relinquish them in the first place: the 1,700-calorie Riblets Basket, the 1,310-calorie Oriental Chicken Salad, and the 2,510-calorie Appetizer Sampler. The one bright spot is the Under 550 Calories menu, despite some serious sodium issues.

SURVIVAL STRATEGY

Skip the meal-wrecking appetizers, pastas, and fajitas, and be very careful with salads, too; half of them pack more than 1,000 calories. Concentrate on the excellent line of lean steak entrées, or anything from the laudable 550-calorie-or-less menu.

Eat This

Spicy Pineapple Glazed Shrimp & Spinach

310 calories
5 g fat
(1 g saturated)
1,690 mg sodium

Shrimp and spinach treated properly. Nearly 60 percent of the calories in the salad to the right come from fat. Here, that number shrinks to 15 percent, allowing lean protein to shoulder more of the load.

Other Picks

Asiago Peppercorn Steak
390 calories
14 g fat (6 g saturated)
1,520 mg sodium

Southern BBQ Classic Wings
660 calories
35 g fat (9 g saturated)
1,070 mg sodium

Grilled Shrimp & Island Rice
370 calories
4.5 g fat (1 g saturated)
1,990 mg sodium

940 calories

62 g fat
(11 g saturated)

2,650 mg sodium

Not That!

Grilled Shrimp 'N Spinach Salad

Classic healthy-eater bait. After all, what could possibly be wrong with shrimp and spinach, two of the world's most nutritious ingredients? Nothing, until you drown them in hot bacon fat. Suddenly, a great lunch option is turned into a certifiable health risk, with more than a day's worth of fat and sodium.

2,342

Average amount of sodium, in milligrams, found in the entrées on Applebee's Under 550 Calories Menu

Other Passes

1,040 calories
65 g fat (22 g saturated, 1 g trans)
3,190 mg sodium

Sizzling Steak and Cheese

1,110 calories
55 g fat (11 g saturated, 0.5 g trans)
2,800 mg sodium

Southern BBQ Boneless Wings

1,190 calories
73 g fat (28 g saturated, 1.5 g trans)
3,120 mg sodium

Cajun Shrimp Pasta

Arby's

Arby's offers a long list of sandwiches with fewer than 500 calories, including a trio of new roast chicken sandwiches. Problem is, there's an even longer list of sandwiches with considerably more than 500 calories. Credit Arby's for nixing the trans fat from their frying oil years ago, but it seems they might be a little too proud of that fact; the restaurant doesn't offer a single side that hasn't had a hot oil bath.

SURVIVAL STRATEGY

You're not doing yourself any favors by ordering off the Market Fresh sandwich menu. You're better off with a regular roast beef or Melt Sandwich, which will save you an average of nearly 300 calories over a Market Fresh sandwich or wrap.

Eat This

Roast Chicken, Bacon & Swiss Sandwich

470 calories

19 g fat
(5 g saturated)

1,310 mg sodium

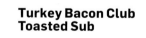

Arby's made its bones selling beef, but the menu has become increasingly chicken and turkey heavy. About half of the white meat entrées are losers, so choose wisely. Thankfully, each of the three roasted chicken sandwiches has fewer than 500 calories.

Other Picks

Turkey Bacon Club Toasted Sub

480 calories
21 g fat (6 g saturated)
1,620 mg sodium

Super Roast Beef Sandwich

440 calories
20 g fat (6 g saturated, 1 g trans)
1,060 mg sodium

Potato Cakes
(small)

260 calories
15 g fat (2 g saturated)
400 mg sodium

Not That!

Chicken Tenders

(large) with Honey Dijon Mustard Dipping Sauce

750 calories

41 g fat
(6 g saturated)

2,070 mg sodium

There are a few guaranteed ways to find yourself in trouble at Arby's. Ordering off the Market Fresh menu is one of them; opting for these terrible tenders is another.

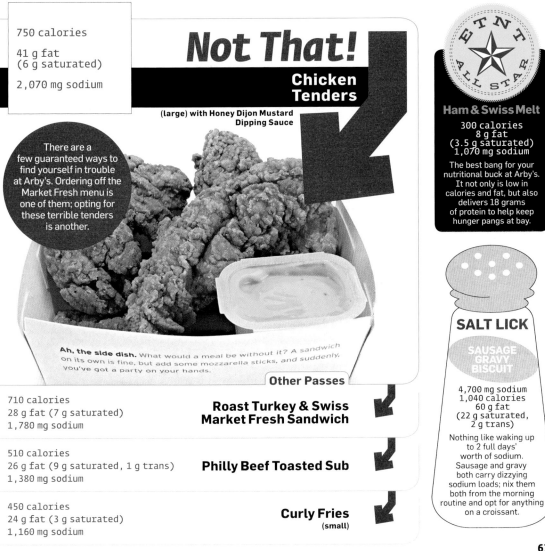

Ah, the side dish. What would a meal be without it? A sandwich on its own is fine, but add some mozzarella sticks, and suddenly you've got a party on your hands.

Other Passes

710 calories
28 g fat (7 g saturated)
1,780 mg sodium

Roast Turkey & Swiss Market Fresh Sandwich

510 calories
26 g fat (9 g saturated, 1 g trans)
1,380 mg sodium

Philly Beef Toasted Sub

450 calories
24 g fat (3 g saturated)
1,160 mg sodium

Curly Fries
(small)

ETNT ALL STAR

Ham & Swiss Melt

300 calories
8 g fat
(3.5 g saturated)
1,070 mg sodium

The best bang for your nutritional buck at Arby's. It not only is low in calories and fat, but also delivers 18 grams of protein to help keep hunger pangs at bay.

SALT LICK

SAUSAGE GRAVY BISCUIT

4,700 mg sodium
1,040 calories
60 g fat
(22 g saturated,
2 g trans)

Nothing like waking up to 2 full days' worth of sodium. Sausage and gravy both carry dizzying sodium loads; nix them both from the morning routine and opt for anything on a croissant.

67

Au Bon Pain

B+

There are plenty of ways you could go wrong here, but Au Bon Pain couples an extensive inventory of healthy items with an unrivaled standard of nutritional transparency. Use the on-site nutritional kiosks to seek out one of dozens of paths to a sensible meal. Or simply opt for one of the excellent soups or salads, or pair two smaller items from the All Portions menu.

SURVIVAL STRATEGY

Banish bagels and baked goods from your breakfast routine and opt for eggs instead. As for lunch, the café sandwiches come in around 650 calories, so make a lean meal instead by combining soup with one of the many low-calorie options on the All Portions menu.

Eat This

Roasted Turkey on Baguette

490 calories

5 g fat (2 g saturated)

1,510 mg sodium

A classic case of how one word can change the entire dynamic of a dish. Opt for roasted over baked and save yourself 260 calories and 23 grams of fat— enough room to tack on a soup or one of ABP's healthy sides.

Other Picks

Roast Beef on Baguette

500 calories
12 g fat (3 g saturated)
1,370 mg sodium

Thai Peanut Chicken Salad
with Thai Peanut Dressing

360 calories
13 g fat (2 g saturated)
1,040 mg sodium

Smoked Salmon and Wasabi on Onion Dill Bagel

430 calories
12 g fat (5 g saturated)
1,090 mg sodium

750 calories

28 g fat
(9 g saturated)

1,990 mg sodium

Not That!

Baked Turkey Sandwich

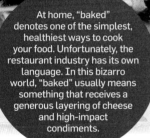

At home, "baked" denotes one of the simplest, healthiest ways to cook your food. Unfortunately, the restaurant industry has its own language. In this bizarro world, "baked" usually means something that receives a generous layering of cheese and high-impact condiments.

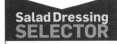

Salad Dressing SELECTOR

Blue Cheese
310 calories
33 g fat (6 g saturated)
460 mg sodium

Caesar
270 calories
28 g fat (5 g saturated)
370 mg sodium

Sesame Ginger
230 calories
20 g fat (3 g saturated)
680 mg sodium

Lite Honey Mustard
170 calories
9 g fat (2 g saturated)
380 mg sodium

Thai Peanut
160 calories
8 g fat (1 g saturated)
740 mg sodium

Balsamic Vinaigrette
120 calories
9 g fat (2 g saturated)
360 mg sodium

Other Passes

810 calories
41 g fat (15 g saturated)
2,220 mg sodium

Regio Sandwich

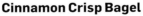

640 calories
51 g fat (14 g saturated)
1,430 mg sodium

Turkey Cobb Salad
with Blue Cheese Dressing

610 calories
23 g fat (14 g saturated, 0.5 g trans)
535 mg sodium

Cinnamon Crisp Bagel
with Honey Pecan Cream Cheese

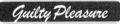

Guilty Pleasure

Chicken Salad Sandwich

490 calories
11 g fat
(2 g saturated)
1,050 mg sodium

Rare is the chicken salad that isn't bogged down by mounds of mayonnaise. Au Bon Pain does it right with a lean version that packs a whopping 30 grams of protein.

Baja Fresh

D Baja Fresh is like communism or friends with benefits: In theory, it sounds great, but in practice, it fails miserably. It's nice that Baja makes all of its menu items fresh on-site, but why can't it make a simple chicken burrito for under 600 calories? And what's up with all of the "naturally occurring" trans fats in their quesadillas and nachos? To minimize damage, turn to the tacos—then turn for the door.

SURVIVAL STRATEGY

Unless you're comfortable stuffing 108 grams of fat into your arteries, avoid the nachos at all costs. In fact, avoid almost everything on this menu. The only safe options are the tacos, the torta, or a salad topped with salsa verde and served without the elephantine tortilla bowl.

Eat This

Chicken Americano Soft Tacos
(2)

460 calories

20 g fat
(9 g saturated)

1,180 mg sodium

Normally a menu item with "Americano" attached to its name is cause for caution, but that's not the case here. Two big tacos stuffed with chicken and cheese for less than half the calories of a chicken burrito? Consider it a Baja bargain.

Other Picks

Grilled Mahi Mahi Tacos (2)

460 calories
18 g fat (3 g saturated)
600 mg sodium

Chicken Baja Ensalada
with Salsa Verde Dressing

325 calories
7 g fat (2 g saturated)
1,590 mg sodium

Chicken Torta
(without chips)

620 calories
23 g fat (6 g saturated)
1,330 mg sodium

Not That!

Chicken, Bean, and Cheese Burrito

970 calories

35 g fat
(18 g saturated,
1 g trans)

2,230 mg sodium

Taco versus burrito? It's a battle that's been waged on the menus of Mexican-American chains for years. Despite the fact that they carry the same fillings, the nod almost always goes to the taco, since two taco tortillas have about half as many calories as a single massive burrito blanket.

Other Passes

Cheese Quesadilla

1,200 calories
78 g fat (37 g saturated, 2.5 g trans)
2,140 mg sodium

Caesar Style Salad Burrito

940 calories
50 g fat (19 g saturated)
1,930 mg sodium

Chicken Tostado Salad

1,140 calories
55 g fat (14 g saturated, 1 g trans)
2,370 mg sodium

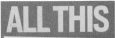

ALL THIS

5 Baja Chicken Tacos,
3 Steak Americano
Soft Tacos, and a
side of Pinto Beans

OR

THAT

Charbroiled Steak Nachos

2,120 calories
118 g fat
(44 g saturated,
4.5 g trans)
2,990 mg sodium

HIDDEN DANGER

Mango Chipotle Chicken Salad

Don't let the healthy-sounding ingredients distract you from the fact that this salad comes in a massive deep-fried tortilla shell. Take the offensive against temptation and ask for your salad in a bowl or on a plate. Keep the Chipotle Vinaigrette, but scrap the Chipotle Glaze for further savings.

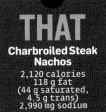

930 calories
52 g fat
(33 g saturated,
2.5 g trans)
1,960 mg sodium

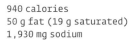

C–

Baskin-Robbins has a long tradition of carrying some of the worst frozen fare in the country, and this year the tradition continues. Sure, they shed their atrocious line of Premium Shakes, but it's going to take a lot more downsizing to earn a higher grade from us. The Premium Sundae line averages 1,135 calories, and even the average small Fruit Blast Smoothie contains 93 grams of sugars.

SURVIVAL STRATEGY

With choices like frozen yogurt, sherbet, and no-sugar-added ice cream, Baskin's lighter menu is the one bright spot in this otherwise dark world. Beyond that, look to the freezer for a Grab-N-Go treat. Stacked next to a shake, sundae, or even a smoothie, these are great bets.

Eat This

Strawberry Cheesecake Ice Cream

(two 2.5-oz scoops) in a Cake Cone

365 calories

18 g fat
(10 g saturated)

38 g sugars

Eating a towering cake cone filled with cheesecake ice cream could be construed as the work of a glutton, but this is gluttony you can afford every so often. Compared to most BR in-house creations, this seems downright prudent.

Other Picks

Reese's Peanut Butter Cup 31° Below Pie (1 slice)

340 calories
18 g fat (8 g saturated)
28 g sugars

Daiquiri Ice
(4-oz scoop)

130 calories
0 g fat
34 g sugars

Jamoca Almond Fudge Ice Cream (4-oz scoop)

270 calories
15 g fat (7 g saturated)
28 g sugars

710 calories

23 g fat
(15 g saturated,
0.5 g trans)

149 g sugars

Not That!

Strawberry Banana 31° Below

(medium)

From the sound of it, this could be a moderately healthy, fruit-based frozen treat. But no fruit we know of contains more sugar than three 12-ounce cans of Coke. Unless it's a slice of frozen pie, avoid all of the special treats concocted by BR.

Other Passes

1,220 calories
80 g fat (32 g saturated, 1 g trans)
92 g sugars

Reese's Peanut Butter Cup Premium Sundae

510 calories
5 g fat (3.5 g saturated)
111 g sugars

Orange Sherbet Freeze
(medium)

330 calories
18 g fat (10 g saturated)
34 g sugars

Icing on the Cake Ice Cream
(4-oz scoop)

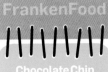

FrankenFood

Chocolate Chip Cookie Dough Shake

1,690 calories
72 g fat
(46 g saturated,
2 g trans)
195 g sugars

We always thought milkshakes were supposed to be made of milk and ice cream, but according to Baskin-Robbins, you need an ingredient list more akin to an inventory sheet for a chemistry lab. There are 45 ingredients in total, some with such appetizing names as sorbitan monostearate and aluminum sulfate.

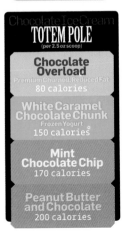

Chocolate Ice Cream

TOTEM POLE
(per 2.5 oz scoop)

Chocolate Overload
Premium Churned, Reduced Fat
80 calories

White Caramel Chocolate Chunk
Frozen Yogurt
150 calories

Mint Chocolate Chip
170 calories

Peanut Butter and Chocolate
200 calories

Ben & Jerry's

C What sets Ben & Jerry's apart from the competition amounts to more than just an affinity for jam bands and hacky sacks. The shop also adheres to a lofty commitment to the quality and sources of its ingredients. All dairy is free from rBGH (recombinant bovine growth hormone) and the chocolate, vanilla, and coffee ingredients are all Fair Trade Certified. From a strictly nutritional standpoint, though, it's still just an ice cream shop.

SURVIVAL STRATEGY

With half of the calories of the ice cream, sorbet makes the healthiest choice on the menu. If you demand dairy, the frozen yogurt can still save you up to 100 calories per scoop.

Eat This

Dave Matthews Band's Magic Brownies Ice Cream

(½ cup)

230 calories

12 g fat
(7 g saturated)

22 g sugars

Despite the drug-addled subtext, Magic Brownies is one of the best of the normal ice creams you'll find from Ben & Jerry's.

BEN & JERRY'S

Other Picks

Berried Treasure Sorbet
(per ½ cup)

110 calories
0 g fat
25 g sugars

Willie Nelson's Country Peach Cobbler (per ½ cup)

220 calories
11 g fat (7 g saturated)
26 g sugars

340 calories

20 g fat
(10 g saturated)

25 g sugars

Not That!

Chubby Hubby Ice Cream

(½ cup)

If the name isn't warning enough, then maybe this is: At 340 calories, this is among the most calorie-dense ice creams in America. Tack on half a day's saturated fat in a meager half-cup serving and you can see why wives might be worried when their husbands want a scoop or two of this stuff.

Other Passes

250 calories
15 g fat (8 g saturated)
25 g sugars

Banana Split Ice Cream
(per ½ cup)

280 calories
14 g fat (9 g saturated)
25 g sugars

Bonnaroo Buzz
(per ½ cup)

ICE CREAM EQUATIONS

SORBET
Water + sugar + fruit puree =
100 calories per serving for any and all flavors

FROZEN YOGURT
Skim milk + water + sugar + flavorings (cookie dough, raspberry puree, and so on) =
130 to 160 calories per serving

NO SUGAR ADDED
Ice cream – sugar + artificial sweetener =
About 180 calories per serving

ICE CREAM
Cream + skim milk + sugar + ingredients =
152 to 276 calories per serving (from Orange and Cream and Coconut Seven Layer Bar, respectively)

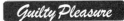

Guilty Pleasure

Red Velvet Cake Ice Cream
(1/2 cup)

250 calories
13 g fat
(8 g saturated)
23 g sugars

If you think this new scoop sounds super-indulgent, that's because it is. Treat yourself for about half the calories of a slice of real red velvet cake.

Blimpie

B-

In the past, we admonished Blimpie for its love of trans fat. Since then, the chain has quietly removed all the dangerous oils from its menu and earned itself a place of honor in our book. But that doesn't mean the menu is free from danger. Blimpie likes to splash oil on just about everything containing deli meat, and there are a handful of sinful subs that top the 1,000-calorie mark.

SURVIVAL STRATEGY

A Bluffin makes a solid breakfast, and the Grilled Chicken Teriyaki Sandwich is one of the best in the business. But skip the wraps and most of the hot sandwiches. And no matter which sandwich you choose, swap out mayo and oil for mustard or light dressing.

Eat This

French Dip Ciabatta Panini Sandwich

430 calories

11 g fat (4.5 g saturated)

1,820 mg sodium

Shavings of fatty prime rib and blankets of cheese usually make French dips menu items to avoid, but a Blimpie dip turns out to be a respectable sandwich. Much of the sodium comes from the side of au jus, so go easy on the dunking.

Other Picks

Club Sandwich on Wheat (6")
410 calories
14 g fat (4.5 g saturated)
1,040 mg sodium

Bacon, Egg & Cheese Bluffin
270 calories
12 g fat (5 g saturated)
890 mg sodium

Blimpie Burger
460 calories
24 g fat (10 g saturated, 1 g trans)
1,280 mg sodium

600 calories

35 g fat
(11 g saturated)

1,410 mg sodium

Not That!

Philly Steak & Onion Sandwich
(6")

This is what we like to call a Top Swap, a painless substitution between two nearly identical menu items that will save you major calories. Both subs here are substantial steak sandwiches, but opting for the cheese-covered French Dip over the Philly will save you 170 calories and cut your fat in third.

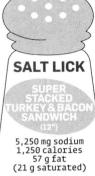

SALT LICK

SUPER STACKED TURKEY & BACON SANDWICH
(12")

5,250 mg sodium
1,250 calories
57 g fat
(21 g saturated)

Blimpie loves the salt shaker, so anything Super Stacked will come at a cost to your blood pressure. This particular sub has more sodium than 138 Saltine Crackers.

Other Passes

590 calories
22 g fat (6 g saturated)   **Sicilian Ciabatta Sandwich**
2,170 mg sodium

800 calories
50 g fat (20 g saturated)   **Sausage, Egg & Cheese Burrito**
2,620 mg sodium

580 calories
31 g fat (13 g saturated)   **Meatball Sandwich** (6")
1,960 mg sodium

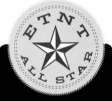

ETNT ALL STAR

Turkey & Cranberry Sandwich
(6")

350 calories
4 g fat
(0.5 g saturated)
1,220 mg sodium

Blimpie is one of the few chains in America to recognize cranberry's potential to cut calories and pack on big flavor.

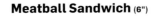

77

Bob Evans

C−

No menu in America is more perplexing than Bob's. On one hand, the Ohio-based chain offers up an array of great entrées and side options, making it easy to cobble together a well-balanced meal. On the other, the menu is littered with land mines like 1,200-calorie multigrain pancakes and 1,000-calorie chicken salads. Until Mr. Evans shows us some consistency, we'll be showing him a lousy report card.

SURVIVAL STRATEGY

Breakfast should consist of staples like oatmeal, eggs, fruit, and yogurt; for lunch and dinner, stick with grilled chicken or fish paired with one of the fruit and non-fried vegetable sides. Or opt for one of Bob's new perfectly portioned Savor Size entrées (just be sure to skip the chicken parm).

Eat This

2 Scrambled Eggs & 2 Slices of Bacon

with Home Fries and Strawberry Banana Mini Fruit and Yogurt Parfait

554 calories
26 g fat
(8 g saturated)
1,316 mg sodium
59 g carbohydrates

The à la carte approach is your best strategy at large breakfast chains like Denny's, IHOP, and Bob Evans. Order two eggs any style and tack on ham or bacon, a starch (preferably whole-wheat toast), and a side of fruits or vegetables.

Other Picks

Seafood Combination Platter
with Shrimp and Flounder, Steamed Broccoli Florets, and Apple Sauce

634 calories
32 g fat (8 g saturated)
1,114 mg sodium

Half-Sandwich Combo
with Turkey Bacon Melt and Garden Salad with Balsamic Vinaigrette

399 calories
16 g fat (5 g saturated)
1,328 mg sodium

Pot Roast Stroganoff
(Savor Size)

425 calories
23 g fat (9 g saturated)
905 mg sodium

1,202 calories

16 g fat
(6 g saturated)

1,537 mg sodium

247 g carbohydrates

Not That!

Multigrain Hotcakes

(3) with Butter and Syrup

It's a sad reality that most people who order these hotcakes do so with the full belief that they're doing their bodies a favor by going the multigrain route. Instead, they end up with more than half a day's worth of both calories and, bizarrely enough, sodium, plus a heap of empty carbs that will send their blood sugar soaring. There's no worse way to start the day.

ATTACK OF THE APPETIZER

County Fair Cheese Bites

952 calories
66 g fat
(33 g saturated,
1 g trans)
1,622 mg sodium

When "County Fair" is in the name, this is what you should expect. Split these deep-fried balls of cheese with three others and you'll still be saddled with nearly half a day's worth of saturated fat.

ALL THIS

**1 Sirloin Steak,
3 Scrambled Eggs,
1 Slice of
Smoked Ham, a Side
of Home Fries, and
a Bowl of Oatmeal**

OR

THAT

**Chicken Country
Biscuit Bowl**

1,154 calories
65 g fat
(25 g saturated)
3,465 mg sodium

Other Passes

1,389 calories
83 g fat
(16 g saturated, 1 g trans)
1,535 mg sodium

Crispy Buttermilk Shrimp, French Fries, and Coleslaw

639 calories
36 g fat (13 g saturated)
1,511 mg sodium

Cranberry Pecan Chicken Salad

835 calories
42 g fat (15 g saturated)
2,201 mg sodium

Chicken Parmesan with Meat Sauce
(Savor Size)

B

With the addition of two new sides containing 7 and 8 grams of saturated fat, Boston Market's menu continues to head in the wrong direction. Healthy combination platters can still be had, but more dietary land mines is not what this menu needs. What it does need? Less butter, less cheese, and makeovers of the Meatloaf, Pastry Top Chicken Pot Pie, and Boston Carver sandwiches.

SURVIVAL STRATEGY

Pair roasted turkey, ham, white-meat chicken, or even beef brisket with a vegetable side or two, and you've got a solid dinner. But avoid calorie-laden dark-meat chicken, meat loaf, potpie, and almost anything served between two pieces of bread, with the possible exception of the Sliders.

Eat This

Roasted Turkey Breast

(large) with Garlic Dill New Potatoes and Mediterranean Green Beans

520 calories

17 g fat
(5.5 g saturated)

1,210 mg sodium

The piecemeal approach is still the best way to go at Boston Market, and there's no better place to start than with turkey breast. A 7-ounce piece contains 54 grams of protein, meaning that an astounding 83 percent of the turkey's 260 calories come from the metabolism-spiking macronutrient.

Other Picks

Beef Brisket (regular) and Fresh Vegetable Stuffing

420 calories
21 g fat (4.5 g saturated)
1,150 mg sodium

BBQ Chicken Sliders (2)

420 calories
10 g fat (2 g saturated)
1,040 mg sodium

1,110 calories

50 g fat
(17 g saturated)

2,500 mg sodium

Not That!

Half Rotisserie Chicken

with Mashed Potatoes and Cornbread

Peel aside the skin on this rotisserie bird and you'll save 200 calories and 21 grams of fat. But if you just can't resist, order a quarter bird instead. More importantly, find some better partners for the bird. The cornbread and mashed potatoes combine for 470 calories and 1,120 milligrams of sodium—and that's before you add gravy.

Other Passes

840 calories
45 g fat (12 g saturated)
1,660 mg sodium

Brisket Dip Carver Sandwich

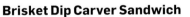

520 calories
28 g fat (5 g saturated)
1,000 mg sodium

Turkey Sliders

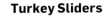

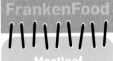

FrankenFood

Meatloaf
(large)

720 calories
45 g fat
(20 g saturated,
3 g trans)
1,635 mg sodium

Meatloaf might be comfort food, but the recipe for Boston Market's loaf boasts a 45-ingredient lineup of additives you won't find in your kitchen. That is, unless your mom's recipe calls for modified starch, maltodextrin, and xantham gum.

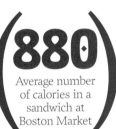

(880)

Average number of calories in a sandwich at Boston Market

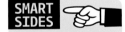

SMART SIDES

For all of the deceptively deleterious sides at Boston Market (see Sweet Potato Casserole, Caesar Salad, et al), three can stand tall among the best in the biz: the Garlic Dill Potatoes, the green beans, and the fresh steamed vegetables.

Burger King

BK's motto has been "Have It Your Way" for 38 years, but how often do you really follow this mantra? Swapping out mayo, tartar sauce, or BK Stacker Sauce for ketchup, mustard, or A.1. is a good start, but also be sure to pile on the produce for no added charge. Pair one of the better sandwiches with a side salad, Apple Fries, or even a four-piece Tenders and you're in business. Now, if only the King would banish trans fats from his kingdom.

SURVIVAL STRATEGY

For breakfast, pick the Ham Omelet Sandwich. For lunch, match the regular hamburger, the Whopper Jr., or the Tendergrill Sandwich with Apple Fries and water, and you'll escape for under 600 calories.

Eat This

Whopper
(without Mayo)

510 calories
22 g fat
(9 g saturated,
0.5 g trans)
840 mg sodium

We've bagged on this burger for years, but that was before we had a simple lightbulb idea: What if we just removed the mayo? The burgermeisters at BK have a heavy hand with the condiments, so this one move alone saves you 160 calories and 18 grams of fat.

Other Picks

Buck Double

360 calories
18 g fat (8 g saturated)
520 mg sodium

Chicken Tenders with BBQ Sauce (8 pieces)

420 calories
22 g fat (4.5 g saturated)
1,000 mg sodium

Bacon, Egg & Cheese Croissan'wich

360 calories
19 g fat (8 g saturated, 0.5 g trans)
840 mg sodium

630 calories

39 g fat
(7 g saturated,
0.5 g trans)

1,390 mg sodium

Not That!
Original Chicken Sandwich

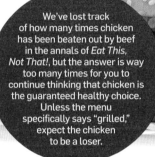

We've lost track of how many times chicken has been beaten out by beef in the annals of *Eat This, Not That!*, but the answer is way too many times for you to continue thinking that chicken is the guaranteed healthy choice. Unless the menu specifically says "grilled," expect the chicken to be a loser.

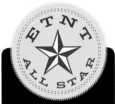

E T N T ALL STAR

Whopper Jr. (without Mayo)

260 calories
10 g fat
(4 g saturated)
460 mg sodium

Sans mayo, the Whopper Jr. is a star beyond just the realm of Burger King. Order it solo for a solid snack or pair it with Chicken Tenders or a side garden salad for a satisfying meal.

Other Passes

770 calories
46 g fat (17 g saturated, 0.5 g trans)
1,380 mg sodium

Steakhouse XT Burger

680 calories
45 g fat (9 g saturated)
1,570 mg sodium

TenderCrisp Garden Salad
with Ken's Honey Mustard Dressing

490 calories
31 g fat (11 g saturated)
1,000 mg sodium

Sausage, Egg & Cheese Croissan'wich

C–

Not much new to report here: The pastas, salads, and entrées are still horrible, and the spaghettini still ruins every meal it touches. The one bright spot on CPK's rather dismal menu is the new-and-improved Small Cravings Menu. Aside from the quesadilla and tacos, all are under 400 calories. This move alone is worth a nudge up from last year's D+, but there's still much work to be done.

SURVIVAL STRATEGY

Either turn a healthier appetizer (like the chicken dumplings, crab cakes, or spring rolls) or something from the new Small Cravings Menu into an entrée, or pair a few slices of Thin Crust Pizza with a cup of Tuscan White Bean Minestrone or Smashed Pea and Barley Soup.

Eat This

Roasted Artichoke & Spinach with Grilled Chicken

Thin Crust Pizza (3 slices) and Tuscan White Bean Minestrone (cup)

526 calories
N/A g fat
(9 g saturated)
1,315 mg sodium

The exact same concept was used to create both the pizza and the pasta—chicken, spinach, starch—but the plate of pasta has more than two times the calories of these three slices of pie.

Other Picks

Blackened Wild Caught Mahi Mahi
with Wok-Stirred Vegetables

591 calories
N/A g fat (4 g saturated)
1,784 mg sodium

White Corn Guacamole & Chips

362 calories
N/A g fat (3 g saturated)
759 mg sodium

Korean BBQ Steak Tacos

454 calories
N/A g fat (3 g saturated)
645 mg sodium

Not That!

Asparagus & Spinach Spaghettini

with Grilled Chicken

1,233 calories

N/A g fat
(11 g saturated)

1,302 mg sodium

California cuisine has a reputation for being healthy fare built around fresh vegetables and lean protein. While CPK's menu certainly speaks the language—with descriptions that read like the very essence of nutritious eating—it fails time and again in its execution. Sadly, 1,200-calorie plates like this are the rule, not the exception.

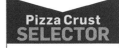

Pizza Crust SELECTOR

Traditional
614 calories
N/A g fat (2 g saturated)
1,115 mg sodium

Honey-Wheat with Whole Grain
594 calories
N/A g fat (1 g saturated)
948 mg sodium

Thin
440 calories
N/A g fat (0 g saturated)
958 mg sodium

MENU MAGIC

Choosing Wok-Stirred Vegetables in lieu of CPK's insidious spaghettini with your entrée will save you between 480 and 658 calories.

Other Passes

785 calories
N/A g fat (8 g saturated)
1,711 mg sodium

Blackened Pan-Sautéed Salmon
with Wok-Stirred Vegetables

873 calories
N/A g fat (15 g saturated)
1,242 mg sodium

Spinach Artichoke Dip

1,172 calories
N/A g fat (19 g saturated)
1,519 mg sodium

Avocado Club Egg Rolls

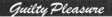

Guilty Pleasure

Frozen Strawberry Lemonade

124 calories
30 g carbohydrates

Restaurants typically load their blended beverages with syrups and other excess sugars, so kudos to CPK. None of the lemonades top 150 calories.

Carl's Jr.

For a place that used to be an unabashed peddler of problematic foods, Carl's Jr. has shown a surprisingly strong desire to right its nutritional wrongs. Now, to balance out a menu still littered with some of the worst burgers and breakfast options in America, Carl's offers a line of grilled chicken sandwiches, salads, and, most impressively, the fast-food industry's first successful line of turkey burgers.

SURVIVAL STRATEGY

There are three clear-cut paths to salvation at Carl's: the Original Grilled Chicken Salad with low-fat balsamic dressing, the Charbroiled BBQ Chicken Sandwich, or any of the three new turkey burgers. Stray from these paths at your own calorie-laden, fat-riddled peril.

Eat This

Teriyaki Turkey Burger

470 calories
14 g fat
(5 g saturated)
1,120 mg sodium

Together, *ETNT* and CKE Restaurants, the parent company of Carl's Jr. and Hardee's, have created a delicious line of charbroiled turkey burgers, all with less than 500 calories! Teriyaki not your thing? Try CJ's Guacamole Turkey Burger. You can't lose.

Other Picks

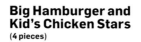

Big Hamburger and Kid's Chicken Stars
(4 pieces)

640 calories
28 g fat (10 g saturated, 0.5 g trans)
1,380 mg sodium

Spicy Chicken Sandwich

420 calories
26 g fat (5 g saturated)
1,260 mg sodium

Hand-Breaded Chicken Tenders
(3 pieces)

340 calories
19 g fat (3.5 g saturated)
1,160 mg sodium

660 calories

39 g fat
(13 g saturated)

1,240 mg sodium

Not That!

Famous Star with Cheese

Dozens of newfangled burgers have come and gone over the years, but the Famous Star has been a staple since the beginning. Truth is, it's better than all but three beef burgers on the Carl's menu (the Big Hamburger, Single Teriyaki Burger, and Low Carb Six Dollar Burger edge it out), but it still packs 65 percent of your daily saturated fat allotment.

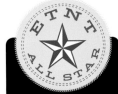

ETNT ALL STAR

Charbroiled BBQ Chicken

390 calories
7 g fat
(1.5 g saturated)
980 mg sodium

As the menu has been bombarded for years with 1,000-calorie burger behemoths, this chicken sandwich has served as a deliciously lean safe haven for discerning eaters.

SIDESWIPED

Chili Cheese Fries

820 calories
46 g fat
(14 g saturated)
1,710 mg sodium

Calling anything with 820 calories a side should be a punishable offense. Pair an order of these fries with a Super Star with Cheese and you'll wind up with a 1,740-calorie meal.

CONDIMENT CATASTROPHE

Santa Fe Sauce
The first ingredient is soybean oil, which is why everything this sauce touches turns to garbage.

Other Passes

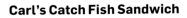

1,320 calories
75 g fat
(24 g saturated, 2 g trans)
2,860 mg sodium

The Original Six Dollar Burger
and Natural-Cut French Fries (medium)

680 calories
37 g fat (6 g saturated)
1,260 mg sodium

Carl's Catch Fish Sandwich

450 calories
29 g fat (5 g saturated)
900 mg sodium

CrissCut Fries

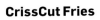

87

The Cheesecake Factory

F With more calories than a county fair concession stand and more sodium than a salt flat, the Cheesecake Factory's menu is in desperate need of an overhaul. But don't expect that to happen anytime soon. This place is unapologetic about its dangerously fat-tastic food. Until we see major changes, we're going to continue to award the Cheesecake Factory the title of Worst Restaurant in America.

SURVIVAL STRATEGY

Your best survival strategy is to turn your car around and head home for a meal cooked in your own kitchen. Failing that, skip Pasta, Specialties, Combos, and Sandwiches at all cost. Split a pizza or a salad, or opt for the surprisingly decent Factory Burger.

Eat This

Seared Tuna Tataki Salad

550 calories
N/A g fat
(4 g saturated)
1,385 mg sodium

A rare moment of brilliance in a sprawling menu of mishaps. When you consider the average normal dinner salad here packs an astounding 1,411 calories, the tuna tataki looks even more impressive—and vital for survival.

Other Picks

Factory Burger
730 calories
N/A g fat (15 g saturated)
1,016 mg sodium

Popcorn Shrimp (½ order)
290 calories
N/A g fat (2.5 g saturated)
463 mg sodium

Shiitake Mushroom, Spinach and Goat Cheese Scramble
570 calories
N/A g fat (16 g saturated)
994 mg sodium

Not That!
Wasabi Crusted Ahi Tuna

1,640 calories

N/A g fat
(48 g saturated)

1,102 mg sodium

> Somehow the twisted minds behind the Cheesecake Factory's fare take the same lean protein and convert it into a dish with more than 2 days' worth of saturated fat and more calories than a 10-pack of Fresco Grilled Steak Soft Tacos from Taco Bell.

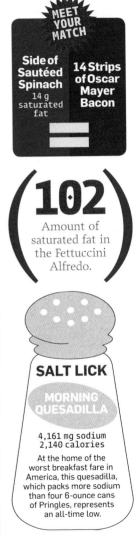

MEET YOUR MATCH

Side of Sautéed Spinach 14 g saturated fat	14 Strips of Oscar Mayer Bacon

102

Amount of saturated fat in the Fettuccini Alfredo.

SALT LICK

MORNING QUESADILLA

4,161 mg sodium
2,140 calories

At the home of the worst breakfast fare in America, this quesadilla, which packs more sodium than four 6-ounce cans of Pringles, represents an all-time low.

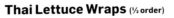
Other Passes

1,440 calories
N/A g fat (28 g saturated)
1,635 mg sodium

Classic Burger

490 calories
N/A g fat (4 g saturated)
1,049 mg sodium

Thai Lettuce Wraps (½ order)

1,050 calories
N/A g fat (32 g saturated)
1,336 mg sodium

California Omelette

Chevys Fresh Mex

D+

We're starting to wonder if Chevys and Baja Fresh are in cahoots. Although Chevys also claims to make most of its food fresh every day, the menu is an instruction manual for putting on pounds. Even the kids aren't safe, with 750-calorie tacos being their best option. Getting a decent entrée here is next to impossible, so stick to the À la Carte menu—preferably crispy tacos or tamales.

SURVIVAL STRATEGY

Forget the combo meals and specials that Chevy's designs. The tamalitos, rice, and beans that come with those plates will ruin your dinner, no matter how healthy the rest of the meal is. Construct your own meal by pairing a taco or two with an enchilada or tamale. Be sure to skip the sides.

90

Eat This

Carnitas Crispy Tacos
(2 from the À la Carte menu, no sides)

540 calories
24 g fat
(8 g saturated)
460 mg sodium

A perfectly fine dinner, assuming you stop here. Carelessly shovel down the default sides of rice and beans that come with most orders and you'll tack on an automatic 460 calories to your meal.

Other Picks

Salsa Chicken Enchilada and Soft Picadillo Beef Taco
(from the À la Carte menu, no sides)

520 calories
26 g fat (10 g saturated)
990 mg sodium

Slow-Roasted Pork Tamale
(from the À la Carte menu)

370 calories
10 g fat (4 g saturated)
450 mg sodium

Sopapillas

550 calories
24 g fat (10 g saturated)
37 g sugars

860 calories

46 g fat
(16 g saturated)

1,660 mg sodium

Not That!

Crispy Chicken Flautas

(2 from the À la Carte menu, no sides)

The concept is the same—crispy tortilla and savory protein filling—but the outcomes are dramatically different. Just think of all the things you could enjoy with the 320 calories you save by swapping the flautas for tacos: an Egg McMuffin, a 6-inch roast beef sandwich from Subway, or maybe two scoops of Breyers All Natural Mint Chocolate Chip ice cream.

Other Passes

950 calories
51 g fat (19 g saturated)
1,690 mg sodium

Chicken Mole Enchiladas

600 calories
35 g fat (14 g saturated)
1,170 mg sodium

Mini Chimichanga
(from the À la Carte menu)

740 calories
23 g fat (12 g saturated)
115 g sugars

Chevys Flan

HIDDEN DANGER

Chevys Healthy Dining Menu

Chevys proudly reels off a list of supposedly nutritious options on its Web site, but read the fine print and you'll see there is trouble afoot. The Mixed Baby Green side salad count doesn't include dressing, the fajita numbers are without tortillas and fixings, and the taco plates don't have sides factored in. When you add up all the numbers, very few of the items on this not-so-special menu make the grade.

1,038 calories
N/A g fat
(11 g saturated)
1,704 mg sodium

(34)

Average grams of saturated fat in Chevys Made-from-Scratch Enchiladas

91

Chick-fil-A

Chick-fil-A ranks among the best of the country's major fast-food establishments, thanks to a line of low-calorie chicken sandwiches and an impressive roster of healthy sides like fruit cups and various salads. But a recent revision to their nutritional information revealed a menu inching ever-upward in the calorie and sodium departments. Any more movement and this A- becomes a B.

SURVIVAL STRATEGY

Instead of nuggets or strips, look to the Chargrilled Chicken Sandwiches, which average only 355 calories apiece. And sub in a healthy side—fruit or soup—for the standard fried fare. Just don't supplement your meal with a shake—none has fewer than 500 calories.

Eat This

Chargrilled Chicken Club Sandwich

410 calories
12 g fat
(5 g saturated)
1,370 mg sodium

Not the best sandwich on the menu (that distinction goes to the 290-calorie Chargrilled Chicken Sandwich), but considering that this one comes cloaked in cheese and crowned with bacon, it sports an impressively low caloric price tag.

Other Picks

Chick-fil-A Chick-n-Strips (3)
with Honey Mustard Dipping Sauce

405 calories
17 g fat (3.5 g saturated)
1,380 mg sodium

Chargrilled Chicken Sandwich

290 calories
4 g fat (1 g saturated)
1,030 mg sodium

Chicken Breakfast Burrito

450 calories
20 g fat (8 g saturated)
990 mg sodium

570 calories

27 g fat
(8 g saturated)

1,810 mg sodium

Not That!

Spicy Chicken Sandwich Deluxe

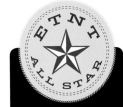

Chick-fil-A Nuggets
(8 pieces)

260 calories
12 g fat
(2.5 g saturated)
990 mg sodium

Chick-fil-A is home to the best nuggets in the fast-food world. Protein accounts for an impressive 43% of the 260 calories. If you're going to dip, make it barbecue or honey mustard.

This year, Chick-fil-A decided to wade into the world of spicy chicken sandwiches, hoping to compete with the likes of Wendy's and Burger King in this increasingly crowded sector of the fast-food world. Unfortunately, the results aren't altogether encouraging: This sandwich is officially the worst on Chick-fil-A's entire menu.

Side SELECTOR
(medium)

Fruit Cup
70 calories

Side Salad
with Reduced Fat Berry Balsamic Vinaigrette
140 calories

Carrot & Raisin Salad
260 calories

Chick-fil-A Waffle Potato Fries
360 calories

Cole Slaw
360 calories

Other Passes

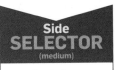

460 calories
15 g fat (6 g saturated)
1,510 mg sodium

Chicken Caesar Cool Wrap

490 calories
22 g fat (6 g saturated)
1,660 mg sodium

Chick-fil-A Chicken Sandwich Deluxe

500 calories
27 g fat (13 g saturated)
1,390 mg sodium

Bacon, Egg & Cheese Biscuit

93

Chili's

D+

From tacos to salads to baby back ribs, Chili's serves up some of the country's saltiest, fattiest fare. Worst among the offenders are the burgers, fajitas, and appetizers, including the 2,100-calorie Texas Cheese Fries. The Guiltless Grill menu is Chili's attempt to offer healthier meals, but with only a handful of options and a sky-high average sodium count, it's a meager attempt at nutritional salvation.

SURVIVAL STRATEGY

There's not too much to choose from after you eliminate the ribs, burgers, fajitas, starters, and salads. You're best bet is the Create Your Own Combo section. Pair a spicy shrimp skewer with Margarita Chicken or sirloin and a side of black beans and salsa.

Eat This

Caribbean Salad with Grilled Chicken

610 calories
25 g fat
(4 g saturated)
800 mg sodium

Only 10 entrées on the menu carry less than 700 calories, and of those only five have 1,500 milligrams or less of sodium. With those stats, it's hard to believe this salad isn't just a mirage.

Other Picks

Grilled Salmon with Garlic and Herbs
with Rice and Seasonal Veggies

620 calories
27 g fat (9 g saturated)
1,480 mg sodium

Southwestern BLT Toasted Sandwich
with Homestyle Fries (Lunch Break)

630 calories
33 g fat (8 g saturated)
1,370 mg sodium

Margarita Grilled Chicken
(served with rice and black beans)

550 calories
14 g fat (4 g saturated)
1,870 mg sodium

970 calories

62 g fat
(19 g saturated)

2,170 mg sodium

Not That!

Grilled BBQ Chicken Salad

This is typical Chili's fare: good on paper, lousy on the plate. Before we began researching these books, we never would have believed that a simple grilled chicken salad could contain almost a full day's allotment of sodium and saturated fat. But after 4 years in the trenches, nothing surprises us anymore.

Other Passes

1,480 calories 81 g fat (38 g saturated) 4,480 mg sodium	**Cajun Pasta with Grilled Shrimp**
1,070 calories 67 g fat (21 g saturated) 2,480 mg sodium	**Bacon Ranch Chicken Quesadillas** with Homestyle Fries (Lunch Break)
1,260 calories 60 g fat (18 g saturated) 4,320 mg sodium	**Chicken Club Tacos** (served with rice and black beans)

MEET YOUR MATCH

Brownie Sundae 1,290 calories	**1 pint of Ben & Jerry's Brownie Batter Ice Cream**

=

1,786
Average number of calories in a burger entrée with fries

ATTACK OF THE APPETIZER

Skillet Queso with Chips

1,710 calories
101 g fat
(37 g saturated)
3,490 mg sodium

So you think you're doing the smart thing by skipping the nachos and going with something a bit lighter? Not so fast. Chili's Skillet Queso is just cheese dip mixed with ground beef and a pile of fried chips—i.e., a deconstructed plate of nachos.

95

Chipotle Mexican Grill

We've always commended Chipotle for the integrity of its ingredients and the flexibility of its menu. But this burrito bar could still do a lot better. After years of telling people to avoid the meal-wrecking chips (570 calories), flour burrito tortillas (290 calories), and vinaigrette (260 calories), we have a challenge for Chipotle founder and CEO Steve Ells: Offer a smaller-size version of your belly-busting burrito.

SURVIVAL STRATEGY

Chipotle assures us that they'll make anything a customer wants, as long as they have the ingredients. With fresh salsa, beans, lettuce, and grilled vegetables, you can do plenty of good. Skip the 13-inch tortillas, white rice, and sour cream and you'll do well.

Eat This

Chicken Crispy Tacos

(3) with Black Beans, Fresh Tomato Salsa, Fajita Vegetables, and Lettuce

535 calories

14 g fat (3.5 g saturated)

1,290 mg sodium

Salvation lies in the crispy arms of the Chipotle hard-shell taco. Tack on black beans and Fajita Vegetables and you end up with a hugely satisfying meal complete with 43 grams of protein and 13 grams of fiber.

Other Picks

Salad with Steak, Black Beans, Cheese, and Fresh Tomato Salsa

440 calories
16 g fat (7 g saturated)
1,225 mg sodium

Burrito Bowl
with Barbacoa Beef, Black Beans, Cheese, Lettuce, and Fresh Tomato Salsa

545 calories
19.5 g fat (8 g saturated)
1,560 mg sodium

Guacamole (side) with Crispy Taco Shells (3)

330 calories
19 g fat (3.5 g saturated)
220 mg sodium

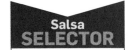

Not That!

Chicken Burrito

**with Cilantro-Lime Rice, Black Beans,
Corn Salsa, Cheese, Sour Cream, and Lettuce**

1,035 calories

39.5 g fat
(17.5 g saturated)

2,340 mg sodium

Unless you're willing to go the minimalist route with black beans and salsa only, there's just no way to create a burrito at Chipotle that doesn't pack more than 700 calories and 1,500 milligrams of sodium.

Salsa SELECTOR

Green Tomatillo
(2 oz)
15 calories
230 mg sodium

Fresh Tomato
(3.5 oz)
20 calories
470 mg sodium

Red Tomatillo
(2 oz)
40 calories
510 mg sodium

Roasted Chili-Corn
(3.5 oz)
80 calories
410 mg sodium

Other Passes

680 calories
40.5 g fat
(11 g saturated)
1,505 mg sodium

Salad with Chicken, Black Beans, Cheese, and Vinaigrette

705 calories
25 g fat (10.5 g saturated)
2,040 mg sodium

Soft Tacos (3)
with Pork Carnitas, Black Beans, Cheese, Lettuce, and Fresh Tomato Salsa

590 calories
27 g fat (3.5 g saturated)
890 mg sodium

Chips with Fresh Tomato Salsa

CONDIMENT CATASTROPHE

Vinaigrette
(2 fl oz)
260 calories
24.5 g fat
(4 g saturated)
700 mg sodium

Vinaigrettes are traditionally 3 parts oil to one part vinegar, so calories add up quick. Opt for a salsa instead and save yourself up to 245 calories.

C-

What makes Cold Stone novel is also what makes it so dangerous. The regular ice cream is fatty enough, but calorie counts quickly escalate when the mix-ins and toppings come into play. Small shakes average more than 1,000 calories and cakes and plated desserts don't fare much better. Either stick to sorbet, frozen yogurt, and Sinless Sans Fat ice cream, or save this spot for (very) special occasions.

SURVIVAL STRATEGY

Keep your intake under 400 calories by filling a 6-ounce Like It–size cup with one of the lighter scoops, and then sprinkle fresh fruit on top. Or opt for one of the creamery's 16-ounce real-fruit smoothies, which average just 252 calories apiece.

Eat This

Double Chocolate Devotion Cupcake

360 calories
19 g fat
(13 g saturated)
40 g sugars

It's a sure sign that a menu is serious trouble when a big, choco-tastic cupcake emerges on the Eat This side of the page. Beyond the sorbets and Sinless Sans Fat ice creams, you won't find many items with fewer than 360 calories.

Other Picks

Chocolate Dipped Strawberry with Reddi-wip (Like It size)

355 calories
21.5 g fat
(13 g saturated, 0.5 g trans)
31 g sugars

Butter Pecan Ice Cream with Cinnamon (Like It size)

320 calories
19 g fat (12 g saturated, 0.5 g trans)
28 g sugars

Raspberry Truffle Mocha Latte Lite Blended Coffee (Like It size)

170 calories
2 g fat (2 g saturated)
28 g sugars

Not That!

Brownie a La Cold Stone

810 calories

55 g fat
(40 g saturated,
0.5 g trans)

75 g sugars

We've rarely seen a brownie that can earn our approval, much less a brownie smothered in hot fudge, caramel, and whipped cream that can. The net result of this concoction delivers more saturated fat than you'd find in a full cup of mayonnaise. Why do the damage when you can satisfy your chocolate craving for so much less?

Other Passes

740 calories
33 g fat (21 g saturated, 0.5 g trans)
62 g sugars

No Fair Funnel Cake

480 calories
32 g fat (13 g saturated, 0.5 g trans)
37 g sugars

Fudge Brownie Batter Ice Cream with Walnuts
(Like It size)

280 calories
12 g fat (8 g saturated)
35 g sugars

Vanilla Crème Latte
(Like It size)

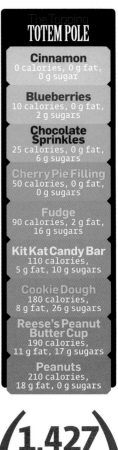

The Topping
TOTEM POLE

Cinnamon
0 calories, 0 g fat, 0 g sugar

Blueberries
10 calories, 0 g fat, 2 g sugars

Chocolate Sprinkles
25 calories, 0 g fat, 6 g sugars

Cherry Pie Filling
50 calories, 0 g fat, 0 g sugars

Fudge
90 calories, 2 g fat, 16 g sugars

Kit Kat Candy Bar
110 calories, 5 g fat, 10 g sugars

Cookie Dough
180 calories, 8 g fat, 26 g sugars

Reese's Peanut Butter Cup
190 calories, 11 g fat, 17 g sugars

Peanuts
210 calories, 18 g fat, 0 g sugars

1,427
The average number of calories in one of Cold Stone Creamery's Love It size milk shakes

99

Così

B

It's unfortunate that some of Così's best fare is available only during certain seasons. The year-round items aren't horrible compared with the industry status quo, but the majority could stand to shed a couple hundred calories. This includes a handful of sandwiches and salads; all of the melts, omelette sandwiches, muffins, and scones; and especially the flatbread pizzas, which average 833 calories per pie.

SURVIVAL STRATEGY

Only two items on Così's Lighter Side menu top the 500-calorie mark: the Così Cobb Light Salad and the Chicken TBM Light. The remaining five items are your best bet for a low-calorie lunch or dinner. As for breakfast, oatmeal, parfaits, and wraps are all sound starts to your day.

Eat This
Tandoori Chicken Sandwich

533 calories
22 g fat
(2 g saturated)
816 mg sodium

We love that Così shows a willingness to play around with interesting flavor combinations. Sometimes the results are brilliant (see below), and sometimes they're downright depressing (see right).

Other Picks

Così Club Sandwich
455 calories
7 g fat (4 g saturated)
964 mg sodium

Bombay Chicken Salad
461 calories
32 g fat (5 g saturated)
1,015 mg sodium

Roasted Veggie and Egg White Wrap
264 calories
12 g fat (4 g saturated)
683 mg sodium

913 calories

22 g fat
(11 g saturated)

1,455 mg sodium

Not That!

Smoky BBQ Chicken Flatbread

The worst item in the worst section of Così's menu. Not only does this pie pack nearly 1,000 calories, it also delivers 124 grams of quick-burning carbohydrates and 33 grams of sugar—more than you'd find in two servings of Cocoa Krispies.

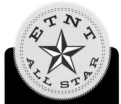

Spinach Florentine Breakfast Wrap

377 calories
25 g fat
(9 g saturated)
624 mg sodium

With 11 grams of fiber and 27 metabolism-revving grams of protein, this handheld Così creation is one of the best breakfasts in America. You won't find a better way to spend 377 calories anywhere else in the world of chain restaunts.

CONDIMENT CATASTROPHE

Balsamic Vinaigrette
(2oz)

357 calories
39 g fat
(3 g saturated)
169 mg sodium

Così's balsamic vinaigrette has more calories than any other salad dressing on the menu, including the Parmesan peppercorn ranch dressing. Opt for a fat-free dressing instead and you'll save more than 300 calories.

Other Passes

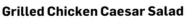

778 calories
42 g fat (16 g saturated)
2,455 mg sodium

Italiano Sandwich

603 calories
43 g fat (9 g saturated)
1,543 mg sodium

Grilled Chicken Caesar Salad

447 calories
31 g fat (17 g saturated)
466 mg sodium

Veggie Quiche

Dairy Queen

C-

With the addition of the 7-ounce Mini Blizzard—a perfect size for killing cravings—Dairy Queen earned its first C ever last year. Still, a wide array of bad burgers, bulging chicken baskets, and blindingly sweet concoctions leave plenty of room for error. Here's a look at one hypothetical meal: a Mushroom Swiss Burger with regular onion rings and a small Snickers Blizzard—a shocking 1,650-calorie meal.

SURVIVAL STRATEGY

Your best offense is a solid defense: Skip elaborate burgers, fried sides, and specialty ice cream concoctions. Order a Grilled Chicken Sandwich or an Original Burger, and if you must have a treat, stick to a soft-serve cone or a small sundae.

Eat This

Banana Sundae
(medium)

330 calories

10 g fat
(6 g saturated,
0.5 g trans)

42 g sugars

Think of this as a mini banana split. Topped with fresh fruit and a mountain of whipped cream, it feels like a steal at 330 calories.

Other Picks

Grilled Chicken Wrap and French Fries (regular)

510 calories
26 g fat (5.5 g saturated)
1,090 mg sodium

Original Cheeseburger

400 calories
18 g fat (9 g saturated, 0.5 g trans)
920 mg sodium

Cherry Dilly Bar

210 calories
12 g fat (8 g saturated)
20 g sugars

620 calories

23 g fat
(17 g saturated,
1 g trans)

70 g sugars

Not That!

Banana Shake
(medium)

This is a perfect illustration of the dangers of the sippable dessert. While we've found dozens of cones and sundaes to celebrate around the country, to this day we have yet to uncover a single milk shake worth tussling with. Consider that next time you're faced with the option.

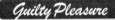

(837)
The average number of calories in a medium Dairy Queen Blizzard

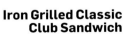

Other Passes

610 calories
31 g fat (5.5 g saturated)
1,260 mg sodium

Crispy Chicken Sandwich with Cheese

580 calories
29 g fat (9 g saturated)
1,750 mg sodium

Iron Grilled Classic Club Sandwich

790 calories
49 g fat (44 g saturated, 0.5 g trans)
61 g sugars

Cherry Dipped Cone
(medium)

Denny's

It's been a busy year for Denny's. First came its $4 Fried Cheese Melt with four fried cheese sticks tucked inside a grilled cheese sandwich. Then came Baconalia, Denny's perverse seven-dish celebration of all things bacon. Just as it appeared the diner had hit rock bottom, it bounced back with a newly expanded line of first-rate Fit Fare entrées. It's just enough for Denny's to salvage a C-.

SURVIVAL STRATEGY

Look for the Fit Fare menu, which gathers together all the healthiest options at Denny's. Outside of that, stick to the shrimp skewers, grilled chicken, or soups. For breakfast, order a Veggie Cheese Omelette or create your own meal from à la carte options.

Eat This

Tilapia Ranchero

with Smoked Cheddar Mashed Potatoes and Garlic Dinner Bread

450 calories
15 g fat
(5 g saturated)
1,020 mg sodium

Every once in a while, Denny's delivers on a truly lean dish that's still appetizing enough to draw in people not looking for bland diet fare. Garlic bread and cheesy potatoes aren't the types of sides you'd normally find on the left side of this book, so embrace it.

Other Picks

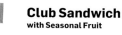

Club Sandwich
with Seasonal Fruit

620 calories
32 g fat (5 g saturated)
1,537 mg sodium

Bacon Chipotle Skillet
with Green Beans & Red Potatoes

540 calories
24 g fat (8 g saturated)
1,310 mg sodium

Fit Slam

390 calories
12 g fat (4 g saturated)
850 mg sodium

1,330 calories

81 g fat
(14 g saturated,
1 g trans)

2,100 mg sodium

Not That!

Haddock Fillet

with Wavy-Cut French Fries, Coleslaw, Tartar Sauce, and Garlic Dinner Bread

> If you ever happen across haddock on a menu, divert your attention elsewhere. That's because haddock is a fish whose ultimate destiny is invariably a dip in batter and a bath in hot oil. Fatty tartar sauce and fried potatoes are never far behind.

FrankenFood

Fried Cheese Melt
with Marinara Sauce

830 calories
40 g fat
(17 g saturated,
1 g trans)
2,920 mg sodium

Denny's received a lot of attention in 2010 when it released this cheesy creation. We're not sure what's worse: The fact that it's a grilled cheese sandwich stuffed with deep-fried mozzarella cheese sticks, or that the meal only costs $4.

ATTACK OF THE APPETIZER

Sampler
(without sauce)
with Ranch
Dipping Sauce

1,510 calories
85 g fat
(9 g saturated, 5 g trans)
3,910 mg sodium

With so many brown, greasy foods gathered together, it's a shock they don't deep-fry the plate as well. Opt for the Sweet and Tangy BBQ Chicken Wings instead and save 1,060 calories.

Other Passes

1,020 calories
60 g fat (14 g saturated)
1,530 mg sodium

Hickory Grilled Chicken Sandwich (without sides)

900 calories
33 g fat (9 g saturated)
1,790 mg sodium

Sweet & Tangy BBQ Chicken (with bread and veggies)

530 calories
11 g fat (5 g saturated)
600 mg sodium

Harvest Oatmeal Breakfast

Domino's

B-

Sales have been great for Domino's since the company decided to roll out a bolder sauce and better-seasoned dough, but from a nutritional standpoint, the concerns are exactly the same: fatty meats and oversized pies. Thankfully Domino's Crunchy Thin Crust cheese pizza is still one of the lowest-calorie pies in America. Just avoid the breadsticks and Domino's appalling line of pasta bread bowls and oven-baked sandwiches.

SURVIVAL STRATEGY

The more loaded a pie is at Domino's, the fewer calories it tends to pack. That's because more vegetables and lean meats mean less space for cheese. It doesn't hold true for greasy meats, so choose wisely.

Eat This

Brooklyn Style Crust Chorizo, Mushroom, Onion, and Roasted Red Pepper Pizza

(2 slices, large pie)

520 calories
22 g fat
(10 g saturated)
1,290 mg sodium

We're impressed that Domino's carries chorizo, a spicy Spanish-style hybrid of pepperoni and Italian sausage. Add it to a large pizza for a bit more than a quarter of the caloric cost of regular sausage, then pile on a variety of veggies.

Other Picks

Brooklyn Style Crust Chicken, Ham, Pineapple, Hot Banana Peppers, and Onions Pizza (2 slices, large pie)

560 calories
23 g fat
(10 g saturated)
1,640 mg sodium

Crunchy Thin Crust Pacific Veggie Pizza
(2 slices, large pie)

460 calories
25 g fat (11 g saturated)
900 mg sodium

106

660 calories

36 g fat
(15 g saturated)

1,660 mg sodium

Not That!

Brooklyn Style Crust
Sausage Pizza

(2 slices, large pie)

Surprisingly enough, the Brooklyn Style crust is the lightest of all of Domino's pizza base options, beating out the Crunchy Thin crust by 170 calories and 25 grams of fat per large pizza. The worst of them all, unsurprisingly, is Domino's Deep Dish, with more than twice the calories and nearly five times the fat per slice.

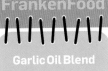

FrankenFood

Garlic Oil Blend

250 calories
8 g fat
(5 g saturated)
160 mg sodium

It's a blend, all right—a blend of 44 freaky ingredients such as "enzyme-modified butter oil" and "FD&C Yellow #5 Lake." We'd be shocked if there were more than 100 people on this planet who know what these are. Until Domino's dumbs down its ingredients list, ask for marinara.

ALL THIS

9 pieces Boneless Chicken, 1 slice medium Crunchy Thin Crust Ham and Pineapple Pizza, 1 Garden Fresh Salad with Light Italian dressing

OR

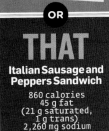

THAT

Italian Sausage and Peppers Sandwich

860 calories
45 g fat
(21 g saturated,
1 g trans)
2,260 mg sodium

Other Passes

720 calories
30 g fat
(15 g saturated)
1,360 mg sodium

Hand Tossed Crust
Memphis BBQ Chicken Pizza
(2 slices, large pie)

680 calories
29 g fat (17 g saturated, 1 g trans)
2,050 mg sodium

Mediterranean
Veggie Sandwich

Dunkin' Donuts

B+

The doughnut king cast out the trans fat in 2007, and they've been pushing the menu toward healthier options ever since—including the DDSmart Menu, which emphasizes the menu's nutritional champions and introduces the low-fat and protein-packed flatbread sandwiches. Now there's no excuse to settle for bagels, muffins, or doughnuts, which are as bad as ever.

SURVIVAL STRATEGY

Use the DDSmart Menu as a starting point, then stick to the sandwiches served on flatbread or English muffins. Beware: Beverages like Coolattas and souped-up coffee drinks can do even more damage than the food here, so keep your joe as plain as possible.

Eat This

Bacon, Egg & Cheese Wake-Up Wraps (2)

420 calories

24 g fat (10 g saturated)

1,160 mg sodium

> These little Wake-Up wonders are one of the reasons Dunkin's breakfast sandwich menu is one of the best in the country. Make sure you grab two, lest your appetite get the best of you before the noon hour.

Other Picks

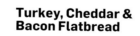

Turkey, Cheddar & Bacon Flatbread

410 calories
20 g fat (7 g saturated)
1,140 mg sodium

Egg and Cheese on English Muffin

320 calories
15 g fat (5 g saturated)
820 mg sodium

Strawberry Frosted Donut

280 calories
15 g fat (7 g saturated)
14 g sugars

580 calories

35 g fat
(11 g saturated)

1,370 mg sodium

Not That!

Big N' Toasty
Breakfast Sandwich

By our count, there are nine excellent breakfast sandwich options at Dunkin', but the Big N' Toasty isn't one of them. Neither is anything served on a biscuit, bagel, or croissant. That leaves wraps and English muffins to chose from as your base.

Other Passes

560 calories
37 g fat (10 g saturated)
890 mg sodium

**Chicken Salad Sandwich
on a Croissant**

400 calories
9 g fat (4.5 g saturated)
800 mg sodium

Cheddar Cheese Bagel Twist

500 calories
18 g fat (9 g saturated)
52 g sugars

Blueberry Crumb Donut

Munchkin
SELECTOR

Cocoa Glazed
35 calories
1 g fat (0 g saturated)
3 g sugars

**Double Cocoa
Kreme Puff**
50 calories
2.5 g fat
(1 g saturated)
4 g sugars

Cinnamon Cake
60 calories
3.5 g fat
(1.5 g saturated)
3 g sugars

Glazed Cake
70 calories
3.5 g fat
(1.5 g saturated)
4 g sugars

Jelly Filled
80 calories
4 g fat (2 g saturated)
2 g sugars

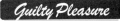

Guilty Pleasure

**Cheeseburger
Stuffed Breadsticks**
(2 breadsticks)

400 calories
12 g fat
(5 g saturated)
800 mg sodium

Sounds like another disgusting food hybrid, but these beefy sticks pack 18 grams of protein with surprisingly little fat. Have one for a snack or two for a light lunch.

Five Guys

Without much more than burgers, hot dogs, and french fries on the menu, it's difficult to find anything nutritionally redeeming about Five Guys. The only option geared toward health-conscious consumers is the Veggie Sandwich. The burgers range from 480 to 920 calories, so how you order can make a big difference to your waistline. Keep your burgers small, choose your topping wisely, and skip the fries.

SURVIVAL STRATEGY

The regular hamburger is actually a double, so order a Little Hamburger and load up on the vegetation. Or skip the patty entirely and play around with the huge variety of toppings —it's not hard to create a solid sandwich.

Eat This

BLT

(Roll, 4 Slices of Bacon, Lettuce, Tomato, and Mustard)

433 calories

23 g fat (9.5 g saturated)

911 mg sodium

Nothing on the menu (not even the Veggie Sandwich) can beat this BLT. It's not technically on the menu, but when your options are as limited as they are at Five Guys, eating well is all about creativity.

Other Picks

Little Bacon Burger
with Grilled Mushrooms, Grilled Onions, and A.1. Sauce

595 calories
33 g fat (14.5 g saturated)
1,021 mg sodium

Grilled Cheese Sandwich
with Jalapeño Peppers, Tomatoes, and Grilled Onions

492 calories
26 g fat (9 g saturated)
903 mg sodium

678 calories

43 g fat
(17 g saturated)

961 mg sodium

Not That!

Little Cheeseburger

with Lettuce, Tomato, Ketchup, and Mayo

MENU MAGIC

Piling veggies on a little hamburger is always a wise choice, but for something a little different, try loading a Grilled Cheese Sandwich with grilled mushrooms, green peppers, grilled onions, and jalapeño peppers for a spicy veggie melt with fewer than 500 calories and 10 grams of saturated fat.

The idea of going to Five Guys and not eating a burger might sound crazy, but it's less crazy than eating a "Little" Cheeseburger that has 75 percent of your day's saturated fat allotment.

The Topping
TOTEM POLE

Mustard
0 calories, 0 g fat, 55 mg sodium

Mushrooms
10 calories, 0 g fat, 100 mg sodium

Ketchup
15 calories, 0 g fat, 190 mg sodium

A1 Steak Sauce
15 calories, 0 g fat, 280 mg sodium

BBQ Sauce
60 calories, 0 g fat, 400 mg sodium

Cheese
70 calories, 6 g fat, 310 mg sodium

Bacon
80 calories, 7 g fat, 260 mg sodium

Mayonnaise
100 calories, 11 g fat, 75 mg sodium

Other Passes

840 calories
55 g fat (26.5 g saturated)
1,050 mg sodium

Cheeseburger

620 calories
30 g fat (6 g saturated)
90 mg sodium

Regular Fries

Friendly's

D For the health-conscious eater, there's nothing particularly friendly about this joint. Breakfast is a sordid affair of fat and refined carbs, while lunch and dinner are headlined by a roster of hyper-caloric sandwiches, salads, and chicken dishes. Even the Under 555 Calories menu, the only bastion of decent eating, is temporary. The best thing we can say about Friendly's is they have good sides.

SURVIVAL STRATEGY

Take advantage of Friendly's massive menu by honing in on the few relatively safe zones. For breakfast, that means eggs à la carte with a side of bacon or ham. For lunch and dinner, turn to the Under 555 Calories menu, or combine a cup of soup with a small salad or a few sides.

Eat This

Cake Cone

with Chocolate Almond Chip and Coffee Ice Cream (1 scoop each)

260 calories
13 g fat
(8 g saturated)
21 g sugars
15 mg sodium

There aren't many places in America where you can pile two scoops of decadent ice cream onto a cone for under 300 calories. Friendly's, for all its faults, can build a decent dessert.

Other Picks

Apple Harvest Chicken Salad
with Salsa Ranch

560 calories
35 g fat (10 g saturated)
1,760 mg sodium

Sweet & Spicy Grilled Shrimp

490 calories
9 g fat (0 g saturated)
1,660 mg sodium

Minestrone (bowl)

170 calories
3 g fat (0 g saturated)
1,230 mg sodium

700 calories

33 g fat
(20 g saturated)

54 g sugars

280 mg sodium

Not That!

Caramel Cone Crunch Sundae

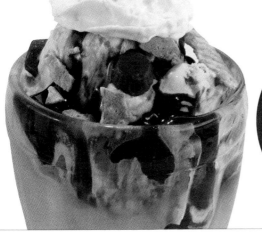

Just another example of why you can't let the establishment dictate the terms of your indulgence. Whether at Cold Stone, Dairy Queen, Baskin-Robbins, or here, the house specialties inevitably pack two to three times the amount of calories you'll find in your own custom creation. Take control.

Other Passes

1,030 calories
84 g fat (16 g saturated)
2,010 mg sodium

Chicken Caesar Salad

1,090 calories
60 g fat (7 g saturated)
3,290 mg sodium

Shrimp Basket

560 calories
18 g fat (6 g saturated)
3,940 mg sodium

Chunky Chicken Noodle (bowl)

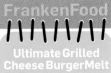

FrankenFood

Ultimate Grilled Cheese BurgerMelt

1,500 calories
97 g fat
(38 g saturated)
2,090 mg sodium

The food scientists have gone mad! Two buttered grilled cheeses have been reimagined as buns for sandwiching a burger. The result is a freakish sandwich with as much fat as 10 McDonald's Hamburgers.

1,190

The number of calories in a kid's Mac & Cheese Quesadilla with Friendly Frank

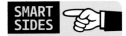

SMART SIDES

For a restaurant with as many choices above 1,000 calories as below, Friendly's has a surprising six side items for 110 calories or fewer. Trade in the standard fries for mixed vegetables, mandarin oranges, or carrot and celery sticks with ranch dressing.

Hardee's

While Hardee's earns its reputation as one of the most perilous fast-food chains by continuing to sire one crazily caloric burger after the next (and by failing to offer any impressive breakfast options), this past year has brought encouraging changes to its menu. Most notably, the creation of a trio of lean turkey burgers now provides diners with a way to squash their hunger without breaking the caloric bank.

SURVIVAL STRATEGY

The Sunrise Croissant and the Frisco Breakfast Sandwich are your only viable options in the early hours. For lunch, look to the roast beef, the Hot Ham 'N' Cheese, or the BBQ Chicken Sandwich. Or seek salvation in a turkey burger, all of which are under 500 calories.

Eat This

Mushroom & Swiss Turkey Burger

480 calories
17 g fat
(7 g saturated)
1,380 mg sodium

Our goal when we teamed up with Carl's Jr. and Hardee's was to help them produce a line of burgers that spoke to the big appetites of their regular clientele, but did so for a fraction of the calories, fat, and sodium of their normal sandwiches. We like to think we did just that.

Other Picks

Hamburger (small) with Hand Breaded Chicken Tenders (3 pieces) with Sweet Baby Ray's BBQ Sauce

630 calories
28 g fat (6.5 g saturated)
1,540 mg sodium

Double Cheeseburger

530 calories
32 g fat (6 g saturated)
1,070 mg sodium

Big Roast Beef

400 calories
21 g fat (7 g saturated)
1,180 mg sodium

Not That!

The Six Dollar Thickburger

930 calories

59 g fat
(21 g saturated)

1,960 mg sodium

The hook for this burger used to be that it was as good as those two-fisted ones you normally plopped down $6 for. Years later, the burger's price tag continues to inch closer to its name and the nutrition numbers are as bad as ever. There's nothing cheap about a burger that packs more salt than a pound of peanuts.

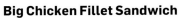

Other Passes

710 calories
38 g fat (7 g saturated)
1,610 mg sodium

Big Chicken Fillet Sandwich

930 calories
64 g fat (21 g saturated)
1,840 mg sodium

⅓ lb. Frisco Thickburger

660 calories
46 g fat (13 g saturated)
930 mg sodium

Big Shef

WEAPON OF MASS DESTRUCTION
Monster Biscuit

770 calories
55 g fat
(18 g saturated)
2,310 mg sodium

A quintuple-stacked tower of terror, this staggering biscuit houses eggs, sausage, bacon, ham, and cheese, all of which combine to attack an entire day's worth of sodium and saturated fat.

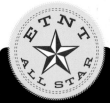

E T N T
ALL STAR

Charbroiled BBQ Chicken Sandwich

400 calories
6 g fat
(1 g saturated)
1,370 mg sodium

Once and always a bouyant life preserver in the choppy Hardee's waters. The 27 grams of hunger-crushing protein help to offset the high sodium count.

IHOP

We knew IHOP was up to no good when it refused to reveal its nutritional information back when we first asked in 2007. But we were shocked when a New York City law forced them to post calorie counts: 1,000-calorie crepes, 1,200-calorie breakfast combos, and 1,700-calorie burgers. The F is for its closed-door policy, but IHOP might not score much better even if we ran the numbers.

SURVIVAL STRATEGY

You'll have a hard time finding a regular breakfast with fewer than 700 calories and a lunch or dinner with fewer than 1,000 calories. Your only safe bet is to stick to the IHOP for Me menu, where you'll find the nutritional content for a small selection of healthier items.

Eat This

Belgian Waffle
with Cinnamon Apple Compote and Whipped Topping and Bacon Strips (2)

580 calories
23.5 g fat
(12 g saturated,
0.5 g trans)

955 mg sodium

Between the whipped cream and the crispy bacon, it's a decadent breakfast, but when stacked against IHOP's frightening lineup of nutrition losers, it's also a prudent breakfast.

Other Picks

Simple & Fit Turkey Bacon Omelette
with Fresh Fruit

420 calories
21 g fat (10 g saturated, 0.5 g trans)
730 mg sodium

Simple & Fit Grilled Tilapia

490 calories
23 g fat (4 g saturated)
1,270 mg sodium

Take Two Combo
with Half Turkey Sandwich and House Salad with Reduced-Fat Italian Dressing

395 calories
22 g fat (4.5 g saturated)
1,445 mg sodium

1,120 calories

54 g fat
(16 g saturated,
1 g trans)

1,190 mg sodium

Not That!
Cinn-A-Stack French Toast

The slabs of soggy bread sport the same flavor profile as the big Belgian waffle, but they also come at a 100 percent caloric markup. Take our advice and avoid any French toast or pancake platters that come with bells and whistles. They're guaranteed to do damage.

WEAPON OF MASS DESTRUCTION
Big Country Breakfast
with Country Fried Steak & Sausage Gravy

2,490 calories
149 g fat
(57 g saturated,
3 g trans)
5,690 mg sodium

IHOP's various breakfast combos are easily the most dangerous meals on the menu. This Big Country Breakfast bomb isn't just the worst of the bunch, it's the worst breakfast in all of North America.

HIDDEN DANGER

Chicken & Spinach Salad

This is how grave the situation has gotten at IHOP. These numbers are abysmal no matter the meal, but 1,600 calories for a spinach and chicken salad? That's embarassing.

1,600 calories
118 g fat
(32 g saturated,
0.5 g trans)
2,340 mg sodium

Other Passes

950 calories
60 g fat (25 g saturated)
2,270 mg sodium

Hearty Ham & Cheese Omelette
with Fresh Fruit

1,310 calories
75 g fat (16 g saturated, 0.5 g trans)
2,690 mg sodium

Maui-Style Crunchy Shrimp
with Caesar Salad and Garlic Bread

1,260 calories
90 g fat (25 g saturated)
2,430 mg sodium

Crispy Chicken Salad
with Grilled Chicken

In-N-Out Burger

B+

In-N-Out has the most pared down menu in America. Wander in and you'll find nothing more than burgers, fries, shakes, and sodas. While that's certainly nothing to build a healthy diet on, In-N-Out earns points for offering plenty of calorie-saving menu tweaks, like the Protein-Style Burger, which replaces the bun with lettuce and saves you 150 calories.

SURVIVAL STRATEGY

A single cheeseburger and a glass of iced tea or H$_2$O make for a reasonable lunch, while the formidable Double-Double should be reserved for an occasional splurge (especially if you use a few of the calorie-lowering secret menu options). But flirt with the fries or the milk shake at your own peril.

Eat This

Double-Single
with Onion, Mustard, and Ketchup

480 calories

24 g fat
(12 g saturated,
0.5 g trans)

1,170 mg sodium

The key to In-N-Out is customization. In this case, we've taken the typical Double-Double, swapped out the spread for mustard and ketchup, and nixed a slice of cheese (do you really need two?). All told, you save 190 calories, 17 grams of fat, and 270 milligrams of sodium—and you still get to eat a bilevel burger.

Other Picks

Hamburger with Grilled Onion, Lettuce, Tomato, Ketchup, and Mustard

310 calories
10 g fat (4 g saturated)
730 mg sodium

Minute Maid Light Lemondae (16 fl oz)

8 calories
0 g fat
0 g sugars

875 calories

45 g fat
(15 g saturated,
0.5 g trans)

1,245 mg sodium

Not That!

Cheeseburger

with Onion and French Fries

An all-too-typical order for a moderately hungry West Coaster pulling into the drive-thru for a quick bite. The real culprit here is the fries, which pack 395 calories per serving and offer absolutely nothing but empty carbs and fat in return. (At least with the burger you get protein—and produce.)

Other Passes

395 calories
18 g fat (5 g saturated)
245 mg sodium

French Fries

195 calories
0 g fat
54 g sugars

Coca-Cola (16 fl oz)

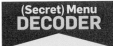

(Secret) Menu DECODER

These are the most popular of **In-N-Out's** *many off-menu items.*

Flying Dutchman
Beef patty (or patties) with double cheese served with no vegetables or bun.

Veggie Burger
All the veggie toppings on a bun, without meat or cheese.

A x B
As many beef patties (A) with as many cheese slices (B) as you want.

Animal Style
Mustard-slathered patty, topped with grilled onions, plus extra pickles and secret sauce. Also offered on fries.

Protein Style
A regular burger wrapped in lettuce, instead of on a bun. Saves 130 calories.

Well-Done Fries
Fries cooked for an extra minute for extra crispiness.

Jack In The Box

Jack in the Box's menu has come a long way in the past few years, but a few major changes still need to be made: Banishing anything in a bowl or burrito, offering more than three burgers with less than 500 calories, and eliminating all partially hydrogenated oils once and for all. Jack might have taken the harmful oils out of the fryer, but they still can be found all over the ingredients lists, including in the sirloin beef patty seasoning.

SURVIVAL STRATEGY

Keep your burger small, or order a Whole Grain Chicken Fajita Pita with a fruit cup on the side. For breakfast, order any Breakfast Jack without sausage. Whatever you do, don't touch the fried foods.

Eat This

Jumbo Jack
(without sauce)

452 calories
22 g fat
(10 g saturated,
1 g trans)
733 mg sodium

The burgers lineup at Jack's is pretty bleak, riddled as it is with seven burgers that pack 800 or more calories. But if it's beef you seek, you won't find a better substantial burger on the menu than this.

Other Picks

Chicken Club Salad
with Grilled Chicken Strips and
Low-Fat Balsamic Vinaigrette Dressing

404 calories
21 g fat (8 g saturated)
1,203 mg sodium

Grilled Chicken Strips

240 calories
6 g fat (1 g saturated)
1,060 mg sodium

Sourdough Breakfast Sandwich

409 calories
21 g fat (8 g saturated)
1,009 mg sodium

Not That!

Mini Sirloin Burgers

748 calories

29 g fat
(12 g saturated,
1 g trans)

1,379 mg sodium

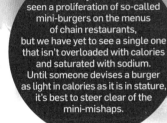

Recent years have seen a proliferation of so-called mini-burgers on the menus of chain restaurants, but we have yet to see a single one that isn't overloaded with calories and saturated with sodium. Until someone devises a burger as light in calories as it is in stature, it's best to steer clear of the mini-mishaps.

Other Passes

Chicken Teriyaki Bowl

692 calories
6 g fat (1 g saturated)
1,703 mg sodium

Crispy Chicken Pita Snack

407 calories
19 g fat (4 g saturated)
864 mg sodium

Grilled Breakfast Sandwich

599 calories
28 g fat (9 g saturated)
1,772 mg sodium

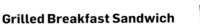

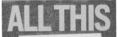

ALL THIS

A Hamburger
with Cheese,
a Chicken Fajita Pita,
a Regular Beef Taco,
and a slice of
Chocolate Overload
Cake

OR

THAT

A Large Oreo Shake
with Whipped
Topping

1,170 calories

ETNT ALL STAR

Chicken Fajita Pita
(with salsa)

326 calories
10 g fat
(6 g saturated)
987 mg sodium

Count this among the best entrées in the entire fast-food universe. Low in calories, packed with protein, and laying claim to 3 grams of fiber, this one would be hard to top in your own kitchen.

121

Jamba Juice

A−

Jamba Juice makes more than a few faux-fruit blends, beverages unnecessarily weighed down with sherbet, sorbet, and other added sugars, but their menu has a ton of real-deal smoothies, as well. This past year saw the addition of an incredible new line of Fruit & Veggie smoothies, as well as new additions to their low-calorie food menu. All in all, Jamba still sits at the top of totem pole.

SURVIVAL STRATEGY

For a perfectly guilt-free treat, opt for a Jamba Light or an All Fruit Smoothie in a 16-ounce cup. And unless you're looking to put on weight for your latest movie role, don't touch the Peanut Butter Moo'd or any of the other Creamy Treats.

Eat This

Orange Carrot Karma Fruit & Veggie Smoothie
(Original size, 24 fl oz)

270 calories
1 g fat
(0 g saturated)
57 g sugars

Jamba's new line of Fruit & Veggie Smoothies is an impressive addition to a menu already abundant with excellent options. Each one packs two full servings of fruit and a serving of vegetables, which means you can sip half of your daily produce requirement through a straw for fewer than 300 calories.

Other Picks

Fresh Banana Oatmeal
(oatmeal, bananas, brown sugar crumble)

370 calories
5 g fat (1 g saturated)
41 g sugars

Original Spiced Chai
(16 fl oz, with 2% milk)

240 calories
5 g fat (3 g saturated)
35 g sugars

Cheddar Tomato Twist

240 calories
4.5 g fat (1.5 g saturated)
430 mg sodium

400 calories

1.5 g fat
(0.5 g saturated)

85 g sugars

Not That!

Mango-a-go-go Smoothie

(Original size, 24 fl oz)

After all these years, our stance remains unchanged: If a "smoothie" starts with a scoop of ice cream (in this case, pineapple sherbet), it isn't a smoothie—it's a milk shake. Save yourself from the glut of added sugars by sticking to Jamba's robust line of all-fruit beverages.

Other Passes

590 calories
18 g fat (3 g saturated)
55 g sugars

Ideal Meal Chunky Strawberry
(16 oz)

390 calories
8 g fat (4.5 g saturated)
53 g sugars

Mocha Marvel
(16 fl oz, with 2% milk)

410 calories
10 g fat (2 g saturated)
640 mg sodium

Sourdough Parmesan Pretzel

WEAPON OF MASS DESTRUCTION
Peanut Butter Moo'd
(Original size, 24 fl oz)

770 calories
20 g fat
(4.5 g saturated)
109 g sugar

The sugar—more than you'd find in nine bowls of Froot Loops—comes almost entirely from the frozen yogurt and chocolate in this concoction. Unless you're a bodybuilder or a Hollywood star trying to pack on the pounds for a new role, make this the last item on your Jamba wish list.

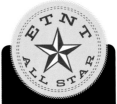

All Fruit Smoothies
This has long been our favorite smoothie line for the simple fact that these are the purest, most fruit-packed creations at Jamba. No added sugars, no funky mixes, and not a single 16-ounce serving has more than 240 calories.

123

KFC

B+

Hold on a second! KFC gets a B+? Surprisingly enough, KFC has more than a few things going for it. The menu's crispy bird bits are offset by skinless chicken pieces, low-calorie sandwich options, and a host of sides that come from beyond the fryer. Plus, they recently introduced grilled chicken to the menu, which shows that they're determined to cast aside the Kentucky fried nutritional demons of their past.

SURVIVAL STRATEGY

Avoid the bowls, pot pies, and fried chicken combos. Look instead to the grilled chicken, Toasted Wrap, or Snackers. Then adorn your plate with one of the Colonel's healthy sides. If you want fried chicken, make sure you order the strips.

124

Eat This

Doublicious
with Grilled Filet

380 calories
11 g fat
(4 g saturated)
950 mg sodium

After 2010's Double Down debacle, we're happy to see the Colonel exploring more sober sandwich conceits. That's not to say that the Doublicious isn't without its indulgences (it does carry bacon and cheese, after all), but it does so for fewer than 400 calories.

Other Picks

Grilled Drumstick and Thigh,
Mashed Potatoes & Gravy, and Corn on the Cob (3")

430 calories
24 g fat (5.5 g saturated)
1,180 mg sodium

Hot Wings (5)

350 calories
20 g fat (2.5 g saturated)
700 mg sodium

Original Recipe Drumstick Value Box

420 calories
25 g fat (4.5 g saturated)
1,180 mg sodium

510 calories

33 g fat
(7 g saturated)

1,010 mg sodium

Not That!

Extra Crispy Breast

Of course, you'd never order just a single fried chicken breast for lunch, but this lonely piece of chicken is here to underscore how much worse it is to go the fried chicken route, especially Extra Crispy, which comes with a 150-calorie surplus breading tax. Tack on a biscuit and Potato Wedges and you're looking at a 1,000-calorie meal.

Other Passes

790 calories
45 g fat (37 g saturated)
1,970 mg sodium

Chicken Pot Pie

500 calories
12 g fat (3 g saturated)
1,540 mg sodium

KFC Buffalo Crispy Strip Snackers (2)

690 calories
45 g fat (9 g saturated)
1,770 mg sodium

Extra Crispy Thigh Value Box

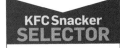

KFC Snacker SELECTOR

KFC Honey BBQ Snacker
210 calories
3 g fat (1 g saturated)
470 mg sodium

KFC Buffalo Crispy Strip Snacker
250 calories
6 g fat (1.5 g saturated)
770 mg sodium

KFC Ultimate Cheese Crispy Strip Snacker
270 calories
8 g fat (2.5 g saturated)
750 mg sodium

KFC Crispy Strip Snacker
290 calories
11 g fat (2.5 g saturated)
730 mg sodium

CONDIMENT CATASTROPHE

KFC Creamy Parmesan Caesar Dressing
260 calories
26 g fat
(5 g saturated)
540 mg sodium

With the 260 calories in this tiny container of this dressing, you could eat an entire order of KFC Gizzards, an Apple Turnover, or 8 packages of the Colonel's Buttery Spread. Skip all of these and order a Honey BBQ Snacker instead.

125

Krispy Krem

The good news is that Krispy Kreme has finally expanded its food menu beyond doughnuts. The bad news is that the new additions are limited to bagels, muffins, and sweet rolls—the same type of nutrient-devoid, carb-heavy fare that it's always specialized in. That being said, its bagels are considerably better than most, and combined with a low-calorie coffee drink, make for a stronger beginning to your day than, say, a cream-filled doughnut.

SURVIVAL STRATEGY

To stay under 500 calories, you'll need to cap your sweet tooth at one filled or specialty doughnut or, worst-case scenario, two original glazed doughnuts.

Eat This

Glazed Cruller and Latte

(12 fl oz)

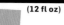

350 calories
17 g fat
(8 g saturated)
27 g sugars

Eating at a doughnut shop is all about damage mitigation. In this case, the Chocolate Iced Glazed, at 240 calories and 11 grams of fat, is one of the lightest doughnuts on the menu, and the Latte comes in at a respectable 130 calories.

Other Picks

Chocolate Iced Glaze

240 calories
11 g fat (5 g saturated)
21 g sugars

Chocolate Iced Chocolate Filled Éclair
with Chocolate Drizzle

290 calories
16 g fat (7 g saturated)
23 g sugars

Blueberry Bagel
with Plain Cream Cheese

350 calories
9 g fat (5 g saturated)
7 g sugars

Not That!
Glazed Kreme Filled Doughnut and Mocha
(12 fl oz)

600 calories

25 g fat
(12 g saturated)

66 g sugars

Few doughnuts on the Krispy Kreme menu are more sugar-dense than the Glazed Kreme Filled, and few drinks on the planet are more syrupy-sweet than a mocha. Together, they make a troubling combination, one guaranteed to hijack your blood sugar level for the duration of the a.m. hours.

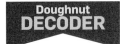

WEAPON OF MASS DESTRUCTION
Arctic Avalanche Chocolate Chip Cookie Dough
(20 fl oz)

1,050 calories
38 g fat
(17 g saturated,
9 g trans)
116 g sugars

Crammed with almost 5 days' worth of trans fats, this dangerous soft-serve deluge is an all-time low for Krispy Kreme. If you're in the mood for a sweet treat, opt for a 12-ounce Orange You Glad or Very Berry Chiller.

Doughnut
DECODER

Original and Sugar Doughnut
200 calories, 12 g fat

Cinnamon Doughnut
210 to 290 calories, as much as 16 g fat

Cake Doughnut
230 to 290 calories, as much as 14 g fat

Iced (but not filled) Doughnut
240 to 280 calories, as much as 14 g fat

Filled Doughnut
290 to 350 calories, as much as 20 g fat

Other Passes

330 calories
19 g fat (9 g saturated)
20 g sugars

Cinnamon Roll Lite

360 calories
21 g fat (10 g saturated)
23 g sugars

Chocolate Iced Kreme Filled Doughnut

380 calories
19 g fat (3.5 g saturated)
26 g sugars

Blueberry Muffin

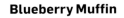

127

Long John Silver's

D+

When we first started handing out grades, many major restaurants still featured trans fats prominently on their menus. But as food scientists uncovered healthier alternatives, most of those establishments switched to trans fat-free frying oils. Now, if only LJS followed suit, it would instantly be one of the healthiest fast-food chains in the country, but until it does, it's one of the absolute worst.

SURVIVAL STRATEGY

The only fish that avoid the trans fat oils are those that are grilled or baked. Beyond that, the commendable Garlic Shrimp Scampi is your safest bet. Pair one of those options with a healthy side. If you need to dip, choose cocktail sauce or malt vinegar instead of tartar sauce.

Eat This

Freshside Grille Grilled Tilapia Entrée

with Rice and Vegetable Medley (without Corn Cobbette and breadstick)

230 calories
3 g fat
(1 g saturated)
830 mg sodium

No restaurant lays claim to a wider variety of nutrition options, from the very worst food in the country (the Breaded Clam Strips, which have 7 grams of trans fats) to some of the best (all of the Freshside Grille menu). Make sure you end up on the right side of the spectrum.

Other Picks

Langostino Lobster Stuffed Crab Cakes (2)

340 calories
18 g fat (4 g saturated)
780 mg sodium

Grilled Pacific Salmon (2 fillets) with Corn Cobbette (without Butter Oil)

240 calories
8 g fat (1.5 g saturated)
440 mg sodium

Breaded Mozzarella Sticks

150 calories
9 g fat (3.5 g saturated)
350 mg sodium

Not That!

Baja Fish Taco

560 calories

38 g fat
(7 g saturated,
3.5 g trans)

1,150 mg sodium

Sure, it's pretty pathetic that a tiny taco like this could pack 130 calories more than a full plate of grilled tilapia and sides, but the more disturbing issue is that in a matter of four bites you'll have chewed through nearly 2 full days' worth of trans fat.

Other Passes

470 calories
23 g fat (5 g saturated, 4.5 g trans)
1,180 mg sodium

Classic Alaskan Pollock Sandwich (1 fillet)

590 calories
30 g fat (7.5 g saturated, 8.5 g trans)
1,420 mg sodium

2-piece Chicken Strip Basket Combo

240 calories
14 g fat (5 g saturated, 4 g trans)
730 mg sodium

Jalapeño Cheddar Bites

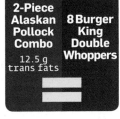

MEET YOUR MATCH

2-Piece Alaskan Pollock Combo

12.5 g trans fats

8 Burger King Double Whoppers

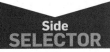

Side SELECTOR

Vegetable Medley
50 calories
2 g fat (0.5 g saturated)
360 mg sodium

Corn Cobbette
(without Butter Oil)
90 calories
3 g fat (0.5 g saturated)
0 mg sodium

Rice
180 calories
1 g fat (0.5 g saturated)
470 mg sodium

Crumblies
170 calories
12 g fat (2.5 g saturated, 4 g trans)
410 mg sodium

Cole Slaw
200 calories
15 g fat (2.5 g saturated)
340 mg sodium

Fries
(platter portion)
230 calories
10 g fat (2.5 g saturated, 3 g trans)
350 mg sodium

McDonald's

The world-famous burger baron has come a long way since the publication of *Fast Food Nation*—at least nutritionally speaking. The trans fat is mostly gone, the number of calorie bombs reduced, and there are more healthy options, such as salads and yogurt parfaits, than ever. Still, too many of the breakfast and lunch items still top the 500-calorie mark, and the dessert menu is a total mess.

SURVIVAL STRATEGY

At breakfast, look no further than the Egg McMuffin—it remains one of the best ways to start your day in the fast-food world. Grilled chicken and Snack Wraps make for a sound lunch. Splurge on a Big Mac or Quarter Pounder, but only if you skip the fries and soda.

Eat This

Cheeseburger and Chicken McNuggets
(4, with barbecue sauce)

540 calories

24 g fat
(8 g saturated,
0.5 g trans)

1,410 mg sodium

The "healthiest" regular Extra Value Meal lunch option at McDonald's, the Premium Grilled Chicken Classic, contains 800 calories and 29 grams of fat—without a drink. Create your own combo by subbing the more substantial McNuggets for standard fries.

Other Picks

McRib

500 calories
26 g fat (10 g saturated)
980 mg sodium

McDouble

390 calories
19 g fat (8 g saturated, 1 g trans)
920 mg sodium

Southern Style Chicken Biscuit

410 calories
20 g fat (8 g saturated)
1,180 mg sodium

710 calories

23 g fat
(15 g saturated,
0.5 g trans)

1,080 mg sodium

Not That!

Crispy Chipotle BBQ Snack Wrap

and French Fries (medium)

A medium order of fries packs 380 calories on its own, which means that unless you pair it with a cup of fruit, you'll have a pretty lousy meal on your hands. The Crispy Chipotle BBQ wrap, one of the worst options from the popular Snack Wrap line, only adds insult to injury.

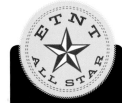

Egg McMuffin

300 calories
12 g fat
(5 g saturated)
820 mg sodium

Other breakfast sandwiches come and go, but the McMuffin never fails to deliver a crucial punch of protein during the most clutch time of all—the early morning hours. Given its status as one of the battle-tested veterans of the industry, the Egg McMuffin would make our starting lineup in the Fast-Food All-Star Game.

Other Passes

770 calories
40 g fat (17 g saturated, 2 g trans)
1,170 mg sodium

Angus Mushroom & Swiss

530 calories
17 g fat (6 g saturated)
1,410 calories

Premium Grilled Chicken Club Sandwich

560 calories
27 g fat (9 g saturated)
1,300 mg sodium

Bacon, Egg & Cheese Bagel

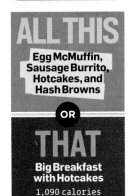

ALL THIS

Egg McMuffin, Sausage Burrito, Hotcakes, and Hash Browns

OR

THAT

Big Breakfast with Hotcakes

1,090 calories

131

Olive Garden

Olive Garden is in desperate need of a menu makeover. The chicken and beef entrées are a mess, the seafood is swimming in sodium, and the average dinner-size plate of pasta packs 976 calories. All of this is before you tack on the breadsticks and salad. Olive Garden cooks need to learn to lay off the oil and the salt, then maybe we'll bump them up to a C.

SURVIVAL STRATEGY

Most pasta dishes are burdened with at least a day's worth of sodium and more than 1,000 calories, so stick to the mushroom or cheese ravioli. As for chicken and seafood, stick with the Herb-Grilled Salmon, or Parmesan Crusted Tilapia. And lay off the breadsticks!

Eat This

Steak Toscano

590 calories
20 g fat
(4.5 g saturated)
1,460 mg sodium

This 12-ounce strip is not only a huge improvement over the braised beef alternative, but also manages to beat out every other entrée on the menu, save the Venetian Apricot Chicken, the Herb-Grilled Salmon, and the Seafood Brodetto.

Other Picks

Stuffed Mushrooms
280 calories
19 g fat (5 g saturated)
720 mg sodium

Herb-Grilled Salmon
520 calories
26 g fat (6 g saturated)
760 mg sodium

Spaghetti with Meat Sauce
710 calories
22 g fat (8 g saturated)
1,340 mg sodium

1,060 calories

58 g fat
(26 g saturated)

2,970 mg sodium

Not That!
Chianti Braised Short Ribs

These ribs pack more calories than five Krispy Kreme Original Glazed Doughnuts, more saturated fat than 43 Chicken Nuggets from Wendy's, and more sodium than 17 small bags of plain Lays potato chips. Do you really need another reason not to order them?

Other Passes

1,030 calories
63 g fat (21 g saturated)
1,590 mg sodium

Lasagna Fritta

900 calories
40 g fat (17 g saturated)
3,490 mg sodium

Grilled Shrimp Caprese

1,110 calories
50 g fat (20 g saturated)
2,180 mg sodium

Spaghetti & Meatballs

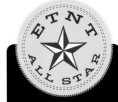

ETNT ALL STAR

Venetian Apricot Chicken

380 calories
4 g fat
(1.5 g saturated)
1,420 mg sodium

On a menu flush with fatty dishes, this fruity entrée is a welcome exception. Just to show you how special it is, the next best chicken dish, the Chicken Marsala, packs 770 calories and 37 grams of fat.

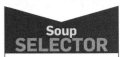

Soup SELECTOR

Minestrone
100 calories
1 g fat (0 g saturated)
1,020 mg sodium

Pasta e Fagioli
130 calories
2.5 g fat (1 g saturated)
680 mg sodium

Zuppa Toscana
170 calories
4 g fat (2 g saturated)
960 mg sodium

Chicken & Gnocchi
250 calories
8 g fat (3 g saturated)
1,180 mg sodium

On the Border

On the Border is a subsidiary of Brinker International, the same parent company that owns Chili's. It should come as no surprise then that its food is a mess, just like its corporate cousin's. The massive menu suffers from appetizers with 134 grams of fat, salads with a full day's worth of sodium, and fish taco entrées with up to 2,240 calories. A la carte items offer the only real hope here.

SURVIVAL STRATEGY

The Border Smart Menu highlights just three items with fewer than 600 calories and 25 grams of fat each (and an average of 1,490 milligrams of sodium apiece). Create your own combo plate with two individual items, but be sure to pass on the sides.

Eat This

Create Your Own Combo

with Chicken Enchilada with Sour Cream Sauce and Crispy Chicken Taco

470 calories
23 g fat
(9 g saturated)
990 mg sodium

Surviving the Border's long, tortured menu of missteps means ignoring the regular entrées and opting to go à la carte. That's the only way to construct a meal with fewer than 500 calories that will still fill your belly.

Other Picks

Chicken Flautas
with Chili con Queso and Black Beans

550 calories
29 g fat (9 g saturated)
1,670 mg sodium

Jalapeño-BBQ Salmon

590 calories
21 g fat (6 g saturated)
1,220 mg sodium

Chicken Tortilla Soup
(cup) and house salad with Fat-Free Mango Citrus Vinaigrette

575 calories
30 g fat (11 g saturated)
1,230 mg sodium

1,050 calories

48 g fat
(18 g saturated)

2,990 mg sodium

Not That!

Grilled Pepper Jack Chicken Enchilada

and Rice

Only two dinner entrées have fewer than 600 calories and 2,000 milligrams of sodium—and one's a salad. Sadly enough, these enchiladas are an average dish at On the Border.

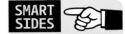
SMART SIDES

Pico de Gallo
15 calories
1 g fat (0 g saturated)
55 mg sodium

Guacamole
50 calories
5 g fat (1 g saturated)
90 mg sodium

Grilled Vegetables
80 calories
1 g fat (0 g saturated)
75 mg sodium

Black Beans
180 calories
3 g fat (1 g saturated)
830 mg sodium

3,153

The average amount of sodium in On the Border's burrito and chimi meals

MENU MAGIC

The real trouble at Mexican restaurants is found in the condiments and sides. Sub grilled vegetables for the Mexican rice to save up to 210 calories and 570 milligrams of sodium. Strip away another few hundred calories by skipping cheese and sour cream.

Other Passes

840 calories
55 g fat (20 g saturated)
1,530 mg sodium

Beef Empanadas
with Chili con Queso and Refried Beans

2,150 calories
144 g fat (31 g saturated)
3,740 mg sodium

Dos XX Fish Tacos

1,680 calories
124 g fat (38 g saturated)
2,610 mg sodium

Grande Taco Salad
with Seasoned Ground Beef and Chipotle Honey Mustard Dressing

Outback Steakhouse

Rejoice! Outback.com is now home to one of the finest nutritional tools we've seen. Go online and take a spin, but be prepared, because the numbers are bound to shock. Appetizers lurk in the 1,000 to 2,000 range, steaks and other cuts of meat routinely carry more than 800 calories, and the average side dish has more than 350 calories. Trouble abounds.

SURVIVAL STRATEGY

Curb your desire to order the 14-ounce rib eye (1,193 calories) by starting with the Seared Ahi Tuna. Then move on to one of the leaner cuts of meat: the petite fillet, the Outback Special, or the pork tenderloin. If you skip the bread and house salad (590 calories) and choose steamed veggies as your side, you can escape for less than 1,000 calories.

Eat This

Outback Special Steak
(9 oz, cooked without butter) and Grilled Shrimp Add-On Mates

500 calories
21 g fat (8 g saturated)
1,108 mg sodium

The Outback Special is nothing but a sirloin steak, which is fine in our book, given its status as one of the leanest cuts of beef. You'll find no better sidekick than grilled shrimp, which contain fewer than half the calories of the scallops.

Other Picks

Grilled Chicken on the Barbie
with Fresh Seasonal Veggies

633 calories
27 g fat (12 g saturated)
1,152 mg sodium

Fresh Tilapia
with Pure Lump Crab Meat and Fresh Seasonal Veggies (without butter)

588 calories
32 g fat (14 g saturated)
834 mg sodium

Classic Blue Cheese Wedge Salad

357 calories
24 g fat (8 g saturated)
1,159 mg sodium

1,118 calories

85 g fat
(36.5 g saturated)

4,768 mg sodium

Not That!

Chargrilled Ribeye Steak

**(10 oz) and Grilled Scallops
Add-On Mates**

Rib eyes are at the bottom of the steak totem pole. That's because they tend to be heavily marbled and invariably fringed with a thick layer of external fat. Tack on a small order of scallops, which by itself contains a staggering 2,379 milligrams of sodium, and you've created a Surf 'n' Turf capable of sinking even the sturdiest vessel.

Other Passes

1,104 calories
58 g fat (22.5 g saturated)
1,482 mg sodium

Grilled Chicken & Swiss Sandwich
and Aussie Fries

1,186 calories
55 g fat (29 g saturated)
2,784 mg sodium

Shrimp en Fuego Fettuccine

523 calories
36 g fat (9 g saturated)
892 mg sodium

Blue Cheese Pecan Chopped Salad

Panda Express

Oddly enough, it's not the wok-fried meat or the viscous sauces that do the most harm on this menu—it's the more than 400 calories of rice and noodles that form the foundation of each meal. Scrape these starches from the plate, and Panda Express starts to look a lot healthier. Only one entrée item has more than 500 calories, and there's hardly a trans fat on the menu. Problems arise when multiple entrées and sides start piling up on one plate, though, so bring your self-restraint to the table.

SURVIVAL STRATEGY

Avoid these entrées: Orange Chicken, Sweet & Sour Chicken, Beijing Beef, and anything with pork. Then swap in Mixed Veggies for the scoop of rice.

Eat This

Potato Chicken Entrée and Veggie Spring Rolls

380 calories
18 g fat (3 g saturated)
1,350 mg sodium

Want something starchy to go with your stir-fry? Two of these crispy spring rolls will only set you back 160 calories, 260 fewer than a single scoop of white rice.

Other Picks

Kobari Beef
210 calories
7 g fat (1.5 g saturated)
840 mg sodium

Crispy Shrimp
260 calories
13 g fat (2.5 g saturated)
810 mg sodium

Black Pepper Chicken and Mixed Veggies
320 calories
14.5 g fat (3 g saturated)
1,510 mg sodium

660 calories

29 g fat
(6 g saturated)

650 mg sodium

Not That!

SweetFire Chicken Breast Entrée

and Chicken Potstickers (3)

Panda's line of chicken breast entrées may look appealing on paper, but two of the three options pack at least 390 calories, with the String Bean Chicken Breast being the only truly sound pick.

Other Passes

690 calories
41 g fat (8 g saturated, 0.5 g trans)
930 mg sodium

Beijing Beef

390 calories
19 g fat (3 g saturated)
500 mg sodium

Golden Treasure Shrimp

790 calories
29 g fat (5 g saturated)
1,410 mg sodium

Sweet & Sour Chicken Breast and Chow Mein

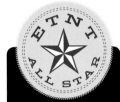

ETNT ALL STAR

Broccoli Beef

150 calories
6 g fat
(1.5 g saturated)
720 mg sodium

The lowest-calorie entrée on Panda's menu, Broccoli Beef is a standout for its sheer versatility. Pair an order with another low-cal entrée, veggies, or even an appetizer and you'll have a satisfying meal for a scant amount of calories. PF Chang's version, by comparison, packs 870 calories and more than 4,500 milligrams of sodium.

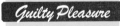

Guilty Pleasure

Kung Pao Chicken

300 calories
19 g fat
(3.5 g saturated)
880 mg sodium

Kung Pao Chicken is one of those Chinese favorites that can be really reasonable or insanely caloric depending on the venue. Panda's version is the former, and the sprinkling of nutrient-rich peanuts is a crunchy bonus.

Panera Bread

B-

For every step forward, Panera Bread takes a step back. In 2009, they gave us the Breakfast Power Sandwich, a bright spot on a disappointing morning menu. This year? Both new breakfast sandwiches clear 650 calories and contain at least 10 grams of saturated fat. Calorie counts for their other sandwich lines have inched down, but only 4 out of 17 have 600 calories or fewer. Until we see real progress, this B- won't budge.

SURVIVAL STRATEGY

For breakfast, choose between the Egg & Cheese breakfast sandwich and 280-calorie granola parfait. Skip the stand-alone sandwich lunch. Instead, pair soup and a salad, or order the soup and half-sandwich combo.

Eat This

Half Smoked Turkey Breast Sandwich on Country Miche

and Steak Chili (small, without cornbread)

470 calories
14 g fat
(5 g saturated)
1,570 mg sodium

Not technically part of Panera's admirable You Pick Two meal option, but sometimes you have to bend the rules to win. Pay the extra charge to make Panera's new Steak Chili part of your meal: For 260 calories, you get 18 grams of protein, and 4 grams of fiber.

Other Picks

You Pick Two Half Smokehouse Turkey Panini on Three Cheese Miche
and Half Classic Café Salad

430 calories
18 g fat
(7 g saturated)
1,310 mg sodium

Thai Chopped Chicken Salad

390 calories
15 g fat (2.5 g saturated)
1,330 mg sodium

Egg & Cheese on Ciabatta Breakfast Sandwich

390 calories
15 g fat (7 g saturated)
710 mg sodium

Not That!

Full Frontega Chicken Panini on Focaccia

840 calories

38 g fat
(9 g saturated,
0.5 g trans)

1,910 mg sodium

Only three full-size sandwiches at Panera have fewer than 600 calories, and all of those are found on the Café Sandwich menu. The average sub among the Hot Paninis and Signature Sandwiches packs a walloping 798 calories.

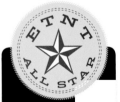

WEAPON OF MASS DESTRUCTION
Signature Mac & Cheese
(large)

980 calories
61 g fat
(26 g saturated,
1 g trans)
2,030 mg sodium

For accuracy's sake, Panera should rename this meal Cheese & Mac. Into only 2 cups of pasta they've managed to dump enough cheese to account for more fat than you'll find in a Wendy's Baconator Double.

ETNT ALL STAR

Breakfast Power Sandwich

340 calories
14 g fat
(7 g saturated)
820 mg sodium

What's not to love? It's a hearty helping of ham, egg, and cheese on whole-grain bread that delivers 23 grams of hunger-staving protein and 4 grams of fiber in a measly 340 calories.

Other Passes

630 calories
33 g fat
(11 g saturated, 1 g trans)
1,490 mg sodium

You Pick Two Half Italian Combo on Ciabatta
and Half Caesar Salad

500 calories
36 g fat (9 g saturated, 0.5 g trans)
1,130 mg sodium

Chopped Chicken Cobb Salad

540 calories
34 g fat (19 g saturated, 0.5 g trans)
910 mg sodium

Spinach & Artichoke Baked Egg Soufflé

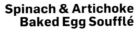

141

Papa John's

C

We're glad that Papa John's struck its disastrous pan crust pizza from the menu, but with it also went its whole-wheat crust option. Now, very little separates Papa from the rest of the pizza competition. It still has some high-quality toppings, but they're nothing you can't get elsewhere. What hasn't changed? The breadsticks still deliver far too many calories and the Special Garlic sauce can wreck even the healthiest slice.

SURVIVAL STRATEGY

As with any other pizza place, it's best to start with a thin base, ask for light cheese, and cover it with anything other than sausage, pepperoni, or bacon.

Eat This

Tuscan Six Cheese Original Crust Pizza
(1 slice, medium pie) and Chickenstrips (4)

590 calories
18 g fat
(5.5 g saturated)
1,440 mg sodium

Don't hold yourself hostage to just cheese and bread. Four of Papa's Chickenstrips only carry 260 calories and deliver 24 grams of hunger-slaying protein. That's fewer calories and more protein than any large specialty slice.

Other Picks

Garden Fresh Thin Crust Pizza
(2 slices, large pie)

440 calories
22 g fat (8 g saturated)
720 mg sodium

Pepperoni Original Crust Pizza
(2 slices, medium pie)

460 calories
20 g fat (8 g saturated)
1,220 mg sodium

The Works
(2 slices, 12-inch original crust)

460 calories
18 g fat (8 g saturated)
1,300 mg sodium

810 calories

48 g fat
(16 g saturated)

1,920 mg sodium

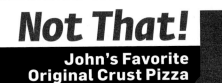

Not That!

John's Favorite
Original Crust Pizza

(1 slice, medium pie) and Cheesesticks (4)
with Special Garlic Dipping Sauce

We hope John also has a favorite gym. Each one of his favorite slices contains a disturbing 6 grams of saturated fat thanks to generous portions of pepperoni, sausage, and six different cheeses.

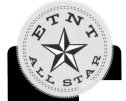

Spinach Al*
Original Crust Pizza
(1 slice, large)

280 calories
10 g fat
(4.5 g saturated)
690 mg sodium

We know what you're thinking: Alfredo, an All Star? The word might always denote danger with pasta, but at Papa John's it represents one of the leanest slices in America.

HIDDEN DANGER

Parmesan
Breadsticks
(2 breadsticks)
Just how dangerous is John's Special Garlic Sauce? Well, each of these doughy logs gets basted with the stuff, and they're the most caloric stick the menu

340 calories
10 g fat
(1.5 g saturated)
720 mg sodium

Other Passes

540 calories
30 g fat (12 g saturated)
1,180 mg sodium

The Works Thin Crust Pizza
(2 slices, large pie)

580 calories
32 g fat (14 g saturated)
1,600 mg sodium

Chicken Cordon Bleu
Thin Crust Pizza
(2 slices, large pie)

580 calories
26 g fat (10 g saturated)
1,560 mg sodium

Hawaiian BBQ Chicken Pizza
(2 slices, 14-inch thin crust)

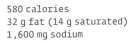

Perkins

D Of the more than 90 dishes at Perkins, only five qualify for the "Calorie Counter" menu. Outside of that you'll find entrées with more than 4,000 milligrams of sodium, pasta plates with more than 100 grams of fat, and an all-day omelet menu that averages more than 1,500 calories per order. Currently the chain has stores in 34 states. Hopefully it cleans up before it hits the other 16.

SURVIVAL STRATEGY

Stick with the sirloin pictured here or choose something off the Calorie Counter menu. Stray from that and your chances of nutritional survival take a nose dive. Even the Grilled Salmon with broccoli, a dish that seems impossible to screw up, packs 1,150 calories.

Eat This

Top Sirloin Steak Dinner

with Baked Potato with Whipped Butter Blend and Butter-Steamed Broccoli

650 calories
32 g fat
(12 g saturated,
0.5 g trans)
380 mg sodium

The fat's a bit high, but this 7-ounce steak dinner is about as good as it gets at problem-riddled Perkins. Scrap the dinner roll, or you'll add on another 120 calories.

Other Picks

Energizer Wrap with Salsa and Fruit
680 calories
19 g fat (7 g saturated)
2,560 mg sodium

Florentine Benedict
420 calories
11 g fat (4.5 g saturated)
1,250 mg sodium

Green Beans with Bacon
120 calories
10 g fat (3 g saturated)
470 mg sodium

840 calories

54 g fat
(23 g saturated,
2 g trans)

2,340 mg sodium

Not That!

Down Home Meatloaf

**with Mashed Potatoes with Brown Gravy
and Butter-Steamed Broccoli**

Perkins's menu is littered with comfort foods that have uncomfortably high amounts of calories, fat, and sodium. Temper the damage with some of the healthier vegetable sides, but be sure to ask for them without butter or oil.

Other Passes

1,430 calories
112 g fat (25.5 g saturated)
3,930 mg sodium

Chef Wrap and Side Salad with Ranch

1,160 calories
51 g fat (19 g saturated, 0.5 g trans)
3,450 mg sodium

Classic Eggs Benedict

440 calories
8 g fat (2 g saturated)
1,290 mg sodium

Herb Rice

SALT LICK

SOUTHERN FRIED CHICKEN BISCUIT PLATTER

6,680 mg sodium
1,860 calories
86 g fat
(43 g saturated)

Your blood pressure rises just reading the menu: biscuits stuffed with fried chicken and topped with eggs, gravy, and cheese. Makes Chinese fare look like health food for the hypertensive.

Pancake Topping
TOTEM POLE

Sugar Free Pancake Syrup
25 calories
0 g sugars

Strawberry Compote
170 calories
39 g sugars

Blueberry Compote
190 calories
43 g sugars

Apricot Syrup
240 calories
54 g sugars

Pancake Syrup
290 calories
59 g sugars

PF Chang's

PF Chang's

D+

A plague of quadruple-digit entrées turns PF Chang's menu into a minefield. Noodle dishes and foods from the grill all come with dangerously high fat and calorie counts, while traditional stir-fries are sinking in a sea of excess sodium. Chang's does have a great variety of low-cal appetizers and an ordering flexibility that allows for easy substitutions and tweaks, like the great low-fat "wok velveted" option.

SURVIVAL STRATEGY

Order a lean appetizer like an order of dumplings or the Seared Ahi Tuna for the table, and resolve to split one of the more reasonable entrées between two people. Earn bonus points by tailoring your dish to be light on the oil and sauce.

146

Eat This

Cantonese Shrimp

430 calories

20 g fat
(4 g saturated)

1,900 mg sodium

Grabbing a booth at Chang's is an invitation for a full-throttle sodium shower no matter how you wok it. With that in mind, this is the best seafood dish on the menu, with a nice balance of protein, fat, and carbs.

Other Picks

Hong Kong Beef with Snow Peas

620 calories
28 g fat (6 g saturated)
1,852 mg sodium

Asian Grilled Norwegian Salmon

690 calories
12 g fat (4 g saturated)
1,430 mg sodium

Steamed Pork Dumplings with Potsticker Sauce

410 calories
14 g fat (6 g saturated)
1,360 mg sodium

840 calories

51 g fat
(9 g saturated)

3,249 mg sodium

Not That!

Kung Pao Shrimp

According to the nutritional information, this one dish contains three separate servings. In fact, most of the meals are broken up into multiple servings to help soften Chang's atrocious numbers. Why don't they just make healthier dishes instead?

Other Passes

1,011 calories
45 g fat (12 g saturated)
4,020 mg sodium

Mongolian Beef

1,020 calories
66 g fat (9 g saturated)
3,129 mg sodium

Hunan-Style Hot Fish

1,350 calories
104 g fat (17 g saturated)
1,080 mg sodium

Crispy Green Beans with Dipping Sauce

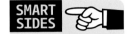

SMART SIDES

Shanghai Cucumbers
(small)
60 calories
3 g fat (0 g saturated)
1,115 mg sodium

Spinach Stir-Fried with Garlic
80 calories
4.5 g fat (2 g saturated)
450 mg sodium

Garlic Snap Peas
96 calories
3 g fat (0 g saturated)
161 mg sodium

Spicy Green Beans
165 calories
9 g fat (2 g saturated)
1,080 mg sodium

Sichuan-Style Asparagus
150 calories
9 g fat (2 g saturated)
1,095 mg sodium

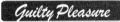

Mini Great Wall of Chocolate

160 calories
7 g fat
(2.5 g saturated)
150 mg sodium

Chang's modest lineup of mini desserts provides a perfect postmeal compromise. The Mini Great Wall is by far the best deal in the house, with the scaled-down version containing 1,280 fewer calories than the regular version.

147

Pizza Hut

C In an attempt to push the menu beyond the ill-reputed pizza, Pizza Hut expanded into pastas, salads, and something called a P'Zone. Sound like an improvement? Think again. Calzone-like P'Zones all pack more than 1,200 calories a piece. The salads aren't much better, and the pastas are actually worse. The thin crust pizzas and the Fit 'N Delicious offer redemption with sub-200-calorie slices. Eat a couple of those, and you'll do just fine.

SURVIVAL STRATEGY

Start with a few Baked Hot Wings, then turn to a ham or vegetable Thin 'N Crispy pie or anything on the Fit 'N Delicious menu for slices with as little as 150 calories.

148

Eat This

Pepperoni and Mushroom Hand-Tossed Style Pizza

(2 slices, 12" medium pie) and All American Traditional Wings (2)

500 calories
21 g fat
(8.5 g saturated)
1,370 mg sodium

If executed properly, the wing-pizza two-pronged attack can be an effective way to blunt hunger. Start with the wings and then by the time you finish the second slice, the protein from the chicken will have worked its satiety-rousing magic on your belly.

Other Picks

Chicken, Red Onion & Green Pepper Fit 'N Delicious Pizza
(2 slices, 12" pie)

360 calories
9 g fat (3 g saturated)
1,020 mg sodium

Veggie Lover's Personal Pan Pizza
(6" pie)

550 calories
20 g fat (8 g saturated)
1,190 mg sodium

Baked Hot Wings (2)

100 calories
6 g fat (2 g saturated)
430 mg sodium

740 calories

41 g fat
(13 g saturated)

1,830 mg sodium

Not That!

Cheese Hand-Tossed Style Pizza

(2 slices, 12" medium pie) and Crispy Bone-In Garlic Parmesan Wings (2)

We're not sure what Pizza Hut is doing to these wings (slow-poaching them in butter or injecting them with molten pig fat are two guesses), but each one packs an incredible 150 calories and 12.5 grams of fat—more than doubling the vital stats of the more subdued All American Traditional wings.

Other Passes

540 calories
26 g fat (9 g saturated)
1,120 mg sodium

Italian Sausage & Red Onion Pan Pizza
(2 slices, 12" medium pie)

1,010 calories
38 g fat (14 g saturated, 0.5 g trans)
2,240 mg sodium

Veggie Lover's Personal PANormous Pizza (9" pie)

210 calories
8 g fat (1.5 g saturated)
690 mg sodium

Spicy Asian Bone-Out Wings (2)

WEAPON OF MASS DESTRUCTION
Meaty P'Zone

1,420 calories
62 g fat
(30 g saturated,
2 g trans)
3,600 mg sodium

In July 2009, competitive eater Takero Kobayashi avenged a loss to Joey Chestnut by downing 5¾ P'Zones in 6 minutes. In those 360 seconds, Kobayahsi ingested 7,245 calories' worth of P'Zones. Put down just one of these massive meat pockets and you'll be taking in more calories than you'd find in 7 Krispy Kreme original glazed doughnuts.

ALL THIS

Ham & Pineapple Personal Pan Pizza and 7 All American Traditional Wings

OR

THAT

Supreme Stuffed Crust Pizza
(2 slices, large pie)
840 calories

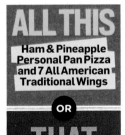

Popeyes

B-

Early in 2011, Popeyes introduced the Louisiana Leaux menu, featuring chicken tenders, a wrap, and a po' boy. All three entrées slide in with fewer than 350 calories. It's a commendable move, but unfortunately the menu is still marred by oversized side dishes, trans fatty flare ups, and the conspicuous lack of grilled chicken.

SURVIVAL STRATEGY

Skip the chicken-and-biscuit combo meals. Popeyes' chicken harbors more fat than the Original Recipe pieces at KFC, and the biscuit adds an extra 160 calories to your plate. Tenders and nuggets are relatively safe, but when it comes time for sides, settle for nothing less than non-fried foods. A large order of fries, for instance, delivers 3.5 grams of trans fatty acids.

Eat This

Loaded Chicken Wrap

400 calories
17 g fat
(6 g saturated)
1,100 mg sodium

This wrap is the best of both worlds: fried chicken and their signature Red Beans & Rice all rolled into one. Want more? It contains 19 grams of protein and 4 grams of fiber.

Other Picks

Spicy Chicken Leg and Wing
(with skin and breading)

240 calories
14 g fat (5.5 g saturated)
520 mg sodium

Chicken Biscuit

350 calories
20 g fat (9 g saturated)
930 mg sodium

Chicken Sausage Jambalaya

220 calories
11 g fat (3 g saturated)
760 mg sodium

630 calories

31 g fat
(8 g saturated,
1 g trans)

1,480 mg sodium

Not That!

Deluxe Mild Sandwich

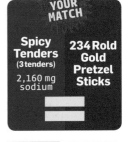

MEET YOUR MATCH

Spicy Tenders (3 tenders)
2,160 mg sodium

=

234 Rold Gold Pretzel Sticks

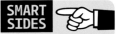

SMART SIDES

Green beans is the only side dish with fewer than 100 calories. They're full of antioxidants shown to improve cardiovascular health and contain a measly 1 gram of fat.

Know what you don't need on a piece of crispy fried chicken? Mayo. Trade it for a few shakes of hot sauce and you'll save 150 calories, inching this sandwich back toward the realms of respectability.

MENU MAGIC

You don't have a lot of flexibility in altering calorie counts at Popeye's, but the one option is a big help—choose chicken without skin or breading. The skin is packed with calories. The breading is just refined carbohydrates boiled in oil. Stripping away those two things will save you at least 50 calories for every leg and wing and a whopping 200 or more calories per thigh and breast.

Other Passes

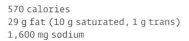

360 calories
22 g fat (8 g saturated, 0.5 g trans)
760 mg sodium

Spicy Chicken Breast
(with skin and breading)

570 calories
29 g fat (10 g saturated, 1 g trans)
1,600 mg sodium

Chicken Bowl

320 calories
19 g fat (6 g saturated)
710 mg sodium

Red Beans & Rice
(regular)

Quiznos

Submarine sandwiches can only be so bad, right? We thought so, too, until we saw some of the outrageous offerings on the Quiznos menu. The bigger subs can easily supply a full day's worth of saturated fat and close to 2 days' worth of sodium, and the oversize salads aren't much better. Sammies used to be the easy way out of trouble at Quiznos, but as their calorie counts continue to climb, options for healthy dining grow ever slimmer.

SURVIVAL STRATEGY

Avoid the salads, large subs, and soups that come in bread bowls. Stick with a small sub (at 310 calories, the Honey Bourbon Chicken is easily the best), or pair a Sammie with a cup of soup.

Eat This

Chicken Cordon Bleu Sub
(small)

440 calories

19.5 g fat
(4 g saturated)

980 mg sodium

While Quiznos can't compete with Subway when it comes to low-calorie fare, it does offer a few small subs capable of squashing your hunger for fewer than 500 calories. Along with the Cordon Bleu, the Turkey Cuban and the Traditional are solid standbys.

Other Picks

Beef, Bacon & Cheddar Toasty Bullet

445 calories
17.5 g fat (5.5 g saturated)
1,325 mg sodium

Turkey Ranch & Swiss Sub (small)

410 calories
17.5 g fat (3 g saturated)
1,210 mg sodium

Raspberry Vinaigrette Chicken Chopped Salad (small) **and Chili** (cup)

515 calories
16.5 g fat (4.5 g saturated)
1,530 mg sodium

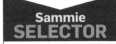

760 calories

46 g fat
(11 g saturated)

2,270 mg sodium

Not That!

Smoky Chipotle Turkey
Flatbread Sammies

(2)

We applauded Quiznos when it released its line of low-calorie Sammies 3 years ago, but the once-reliable lineup is rapidly deteriorating. Even a pair of Roadhouse Steak Sammies now clears 500 calories. Until Quiznos rights this wrong, stick with a single Sammie and pair it with soup.

Sammie SELECTOR

Roadhouse Steak
260 calories
6 g fat (1 g fat)

Cantina Chicken
275 calories
7 g fat (1.5 g saturated)

Veggie
340 calories
20 g fat (5 g saturated)

Smoky Chipotle Turkey
380 calories
23 g fat
(5.5 g saturated)

Italiano
390 calories
23 g fat (5 g saturated)

Bistro Steak Melt
395 calories
22.5 g fat
(5.5 g saturated)

CONDIMENT CATASTROPHE

Creamy Chipotle Salad Dressing
With 520 calories and 9 grams of saturated fat, this may be the worst salad dressing in America. Too bad the honey mustard, peppercorn Caesar, and ranch are also horrendous. Stick to the raspberry vinaigrette and nix the flatbread or tortilla strips to shave a few hundred calories off your salad.

Other Passes

640 calories
37 g fat (11 g saturated, 0.5 g trans)
1,395 mg sodium

Prime Rib on Garlic Bread Sub
(small)

560 calories
32.5 g fat (9 g saturated)
1,420 mg sodium

Ultimate Turkey Club Sub
(small)

840 calories
61 g fat (14 g saturated, 0.5 g trans)
1,555 mg sodium

Honey Mustard Chicken Chopped Salad (regular)

Red Lobster

Compared with the other major sit-down chains and their four-digit fare, Red Lobster looks like a paradigm of sound nutrition. The daily rotating fish specials are the centerpiece of a menu long on low-calorie, high-protein entrées and reasonable sides. That's why Red Lobster is one of America's healthiest chain restaurants. The only flaw you'll find is an overreliance on the deep fryer and the salt shaker.

SURVIVAL STRATEGY

Avoid calorie-heavy Cajun sauces, combo dishes, and anything labeled "crispy." And tell the waiter to keep those biscuits for himself. You'll never go wrong with simple broiled or grilled fish and a vegetable side.

Eat This

Seafood-Stuffed Flounder, Fresh Broccoli

and Garden Salad (with balsamic vinaigrette)

535 calories
20.5 g fat
(4.5 g saturated)
2,015 mg sodium

Although both of these entrées are based on baked fillets of flaky white fish, Red Lobster's lean crab-and-seafood stuffing is a smarter meal upgrade than the fatty layer of bread and cheese blanketing the tilapia.

Other Picks

Peach-Bourbon BBQ Shrimp and Scallops

540 calories
27 g fat (4.5 g saturated)
1,440 mg sodium

Pan-Seared Crab Cakes

280 calories
14 g fat (2.5 g saturated)
1,110 mg sodium

Manhattan Clam Chowder (cup)

80 calories
1 g fat (0 g saturated)
690 mg sodium

1,080 calories

62 g fat
(21.5 g saturated)

3,150 mg sodium

Not That!

Parmesan-Crusted Tilapia

(full portion) and Caesar Salad

Red Lobster might have some of the healthiest restaurant fare in the country (though this dish dampens our enthusiasm), but it still needs to lighten up on the salt. Always have broccoli for a big dose of sodium-balancing potassium.

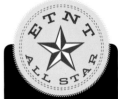

Fresh Fish Menu

Red Lobster may have built its name on crustaceans, but it's the daily selection of 25 fresh fish that represents why this is still the best sit-down chain in America. Try any of the fish (minus the cobia) blackened with a side of mango salsa for an amazing low-cal meal.

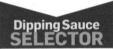

Dipping Sauce SELECTOR

Pico de Gallo
10 calories
0 g fat

Marinara
25 calories
1 g fat (0 g saturated)

Cocktail
40 calories
0 g fat

Piña Colada
80 calories
4 g fat (3 g saturated)

Honey Mustard
280 calories
26 g fat (4 g saturated)

100% Pure Melted Butter
350 calories
38 g fat (23 g saturated)

Other Passes

735 calories
25 g fat (4 g saturated)
3,780 mg sodium

Pecan-Crusted Jumbo Shrimp

650 calories
26 g fat (4.5 g saturated)
2,380 mg sodium

Wood-Grilled Shrimp Bruschetta

230 calories
17 g fat (10 g saturated)
680 mg sodium

New England Clam Chowder
(cup)

155

B-

Last year, we commended Macaroni Grill's efforts to revamp a pretty miserable menu by cutting calories and adding menu items such as rosemary spiedinis. This year, we challenge them to improve the menu even more. Far too many dishes still have at least 20 grams of saturated fat, and 21 entrées still carry more than 800 calories. You've come so far, Mac Grill, please don't stop now.

SURVIVAL STRATEGY

Besides a few outliers (pizza, pork chops, Mama's Trio, cheesecake), this menu is relatively safe. Choose a spiedini, grilled salmon or chicken, or a pasta sans sausage or cream sauce and you'll have enough wiggle room to end the meal with a bowl of vanilla gelato.

Eat This

Center-Cut Lamb Spiedini

490 calories
24 g fat
(5 g saturated)
750 mg sodium

Adding a variety of spiedini to a lineup of dishes in desperate need of fewer empty pasta carbohydrates was a genius move by Mac Grill. Extra credit for being one of the only chains in America to serve lamb, a meat both leaner and more delicious than its scarcity would suggest.

Other Picks

Snapper "Acqua Pazza"
400 calories
13 g fat (2.5 g saturated)
1,420 mg sodium

Pollo Caprese
550 calories
20 g fat (5 g saturated)
1,660 mg sodium

Scallops & Spinach Salad
340 calories
31 g fat (6 g saturated)
820 mg sodium

Not That!

Honey Balsamic Chicken

990 calories

47 g fat
(7 g saturated)

1,380 mg sodium

It looks like the picture of perfect health: grilled chicken with steamed broccoli. The reality, sadly, is just another restaurant dish with squandered potential.

Sauce SELECTOR
(Create Your Own Pasta Menu)

**Pomodoro
(Tomato Basil)**
160 calories
11 g fat (2 g saturated)
580 mg sodium

**Arrabbiata
(Spicy Red Sauce)**
180 calories
13 g fat (2 g saturated)
650 mg sodium

Roasted Garlic Cream
360 calories
29 g fat (13 g saturated)
1,160 mg sodium

**Bolognese
(Meat Sauce)**
430 calories
32 g fat (5 g saturated)
1,140 mg sodium

Alfredo
610 calories
59 g fat
(31 g saturated)
960 mg sodium

Other Passes

1,160 calories
73 g fat (25 g saturated)
1,240 mg sodium

King Salmon

980 calories
38 g fat (17 g saturated)
2,830 mg sodium

Penne Rustica

730 calories
49 g fat (11 g saturated)
1,840 mg sodium

Insalata Blu with Chicken

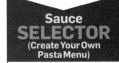

21

The number of entrées on Romano's menu that still carry 20 or more grams of saturated fat

157

Ruby Tuesday

Ru··y Tu ·d· y

C-

The chain earned its infamy off a hearty selection of hamburgers. The problem is, they average 91 grams of fat—about 150 percent of your recommended daily limit. And now that Ruby Tuesday has finally released full sodium counts, it's apparent it's been harboring one of the saltiest menus in America. But with the addition of the Fit & Trim and Petite menus this year, Ruby's earns a bump up on its report card.

SURVIVAL STRATEGY

Solace lies in the 3 S's: sirloin, salmon, and shrimp all make for relatively innocuous eating, especially when paired with one of Ruby Tuesday's half-dozen healthy sides, such as mashed cauliflower and sautéed portabellas.

158

Eat This

Jumbo Lump Crab Cake

with White Cheddar Mashed Potatoes and Fresh Steamed Broccoli

441 calories
34 g fat
(N/A g saturated)
925 mg sodium

It's hard not to love this dish: a rich crab cake, cheesy mashed potatoes, and a pile of fresh broccoli. Normally comfort food like this comes with an uncomfortable caloric load, but every once in a while Ruby Tuesday does its best to surprise us.

Other Picks

Top Sirloin with Creamy Mashed Cauliflower and Sautéed Baby Portabella Mushrooms

524 calories
24 g fat (N/A g saturated)
1,487 mg sodium

Salmon Florentine (without sides)

392 calories
21 g fat (N/A g saturated)
1,135 mg sodium

Red Velvet Cupcake

285 calories
11 g fat (N/A g saturated)
45 g carbohydrates

692 calories

38 g fat
(N/A g saturated)

2,036 mg sodium

Not That!

Petite Parmesan Shrimp Pasta

We love the fact that Ruby Tuesday's has done what few restaurants in this country have been willing to entertain: They've shrunk their food. Unfortunately, the results aren't always as impressive as we'd hoped. Worst of all is this "petite" pasta, which still packs more calories than you should consume in a single meal.

Other Passes

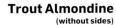

1,023 calories
52 g fat (N/A g saturated)
1,668 mg sodium

Chef's Cut 12-Ounce Sirloin
with Plain Baked Potato

684 calories
49 g fat (N/A g saturated)
560 mg sodium

Trout Almondine
(without sides)

630 calories
27 g fat (N/A g saturated)
88 g carbohydrates

Blondie for One

STEALTH HEALTH

Spaghetti Squash Marinara

406 calories
21 g fat
(N/A g saturated)
989 mg sodium

Replacing empty carbohydrates with vegetables is always key, and spaghetti squash provides more flavor and texture than a heap of bland noodles. Try making this simple dish at home for even fewer calories—and at a fraction of the cost.

Smoothie King

Smoothie King, the older and smaller of the two smoothie titans, suffers from portion problems. The smallest adult option is 20 ounces, which makes it that much harder to keep the calories from sugar remotely reasonable. Added sugars and honey don't make things any better. (Isn't fruit sweet enough?) Still, the menu boasts some great all-fruit smoothies, light options, and an excellent portfolio of smoothie enhancers.

SURVIVAL STRATEGY

Favor the Stay Healthy and Trim Down portions of the menu, and be sure to stick to 20-ounce smoothies made from nothing but real fruit. No matter what you do, avoid anything listed under the Indulge section—it's pure trouble.

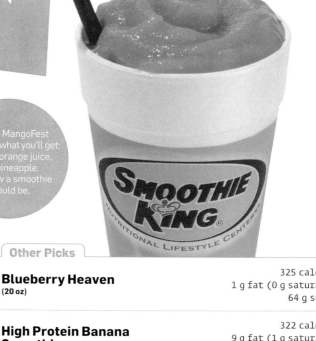

Eat This

MangoFest Smoothie
(20 fl oz)

285 calories

0 g fat

69 g sugars

Order a MangoFest and this is what you'll get: mango, orange juice, and pineapple. Just how a smoothie should be.

SMOOTHIE KING.
NUTRITIONAL LIFESTYLE CENTERS

Other Picks

Blueberry Heaven
(20 oz)

325 calories
1 g fat (0 g saturated)
64 g sugars

High Protein Banana Smoothie (20 fl oz)

322 calories
9 g fat (1 g saturated)
23 g sugars

Island Impact Smoothie
(20 fl oz)

311 calories
0 g fat
65 g sugars

465 calories

0 g fat

108 g sugars

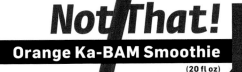

Not That!

Orange Ka-BAM Smoothie

(20 fl oz)

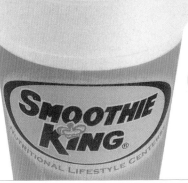

This might be labeled a "Stay Healthy" smoothie, but there's nothing healthy about an extra 100 calories from 23 grams of added sugars. Avoid the unnecessary sweetness by always asking for your drink "skinny."

Other Passes

554 calories
1 g fat (0 g saturated)
96 g sugars

Cranberry Supreme
(20 oz)

749 calories
22 g fat (4 g saturated)
107 g sugars

Peanut Power Plus Grape Smoothie **(20 fl oz)**

498 calories
1 g fat (0 g saturated)
96 g sugars

Kiwi Island Treat Smoothie **(20 fl oz)**

WEAPON OF MASS DESTRUCTION
The Hulk Strawberry Smoothie
(40 fl oz)

2,070 calories
64 g fat
(26 g saturated)
250 g sugars

We understand that Jamba's Hulk line is intended for those trying to bulk up, but this superhuman smoothie is completely unnecessary. There are ways to fuel up that don't include more sugar than three 20-ounce bottles of Mountain Dew.

STEALTH HEALTH

Green Tea Tango Smoothie

282 calories
3 g fat
(2 g saturated)
40 g sugars

The base of this beverage is matcha green tea, which is a high-quality green tea that comes loaded with antioxidants called catechins, which have been shown in studies to boost metabolism. Of course, it takes two to tango, which means this smoothie also gets stocked with a vitamin-rich fruit of your choice.

Sonic

C+

In many respects, the fried-and-fatty pitfalls are more dramatic at Sonic than they are at other chains. You have an oversized selection of deep-fried sides, a tempting lineup of frozen sodas, and an expansive catalogue of shakes, malts, and Sonic Blasts. That said, the chain offers most of its indulgences in small portions, making possible a Jr. Burger with Small Tots and Small Slush for 630 calories—a relative bargain considering what you'd suffer elsewhere.

SURVIVAL STRATEGY

Sounds crazy, but corn dogs, 6-inch hot dogs, and Jr. Burgers are your safest options. Just avoid the shakes. Even a 14-ounce cup can stick you with 600 calories.

Eat This

Corn Dogs
(2)

420 calories
22 g fat
(7 g saturated)
1,060 mg sodium

Corn dogs are pretty far from nutritious, but compared with Sonic's bloated lineup of burgers and sandwiches, these are pure gold.

Other Picks

Jr. Deluxe Burger with Green Chilis and Tots
(medium)

555 calories
33 g fat (8.5 g saturated, 0.5 g trans)
885 mg sodium

Ham, Egg & Cheese Breakfast Toaster

488 calories
27 g fat (8 g saturated)
1,720 mg sodium

Junior Banana Split

200 calories
6 g fat (4.5 g saturated)
22 g sugars

770 calories

43 g fat
(17 g saturated,
2 g trans)

1,100 mg sodium

Not That!

Sonic Cheeseburger
(with mustard)

Sonic's three single-patty Jr. burgers are the only burgers on the menu that have fewer than 500 calories, 10 grams of saturated fat, and 1.5 grams of trans fats. You've been warned.

Other Passes

1,180 calories
76 g fat (32 g saturated, 3.5 g trans)
1,600 mg sodium

SuperSonic Cheeseburger with Jalapeño

690 calories
44 g fat (18 g saturated, 1 g trans)
1,770 mg sodium

Sausage Biscuit Dippers with Gravy (3)

500 calories
22 g fat (16 g saturated)
41 g sugars

Chocolate Sundae

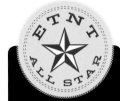

ETNT ALL STAR

Tots (small)

130 calories
8 g fat
(1.5 g saturated)
270 mg sodium

In the world of fried potatoes, the humble tot reigns supreme. A small order has a whole 100 calories fewer than a small McDonald's fries. Just keep the chili and the cheese off of them, okay?

Frozen Treat
TOTEM POLE
(regular, 14 fl oz)

Floats
Ice Cream + Soda
260 to 340 calories

CreamSlush Treats
Ice Cream + Ice + Flavor
350 to 370 calories

Shakes
Ice Cream + Milk
460 to 660 calories

Limeade Chillers
Ice Cream + Limeade
620 to 680 calories

Sonic Blasts
Ice Cream + Candy
680 to 750 calories

Starbucks

B+

The Starbucks logo might have gotten a makeover, but the menu still looks pretty much the same. And that's not a bad thing. A solid line of breakfast and lunch sandwiches buttressed by oatmeal, parfaits, and snack plates make this coffee shop a reliable place to tame a growling stomach on the go. Just ignore the carb-fueled confections. As for the drinks? The simpler the better.

SURVIVAL STRATEGY

There's no beating a regular cup of joe or unsweetened tea, but if you need a specialty fix, stick with fat-free milk, sugar-free syrup, and no whipped cream. As for food, go with the Perfect Oatmeal or an Egg White, Spinach, and Feta Wrap.

Eat This

Mocha Light Frappucino

(grande) and Chicken on Flatbread with Hummus Artisan Snack Plate

390 calories
10 g fat
(0 g saturated)
710 mg sodium
32 g sugars

Lose the whipped cream, switch to nonfat milk, and suddenly a notoriously indulgent beverage becomes a modest treat. And with 17 grams of protein for only 250 calories, the Chicken on Flatbread is Starbucks' best snack.

Other Picks

Greek Yogurt Honey Parfait

300 calories
12 g fat (6 g saturated)
32 g sugars

Tazo Shaken Iced Passion Tea (grande)

80 calories
0 g fat
20 g sugars

Red Velvet Whoopie Pie (Petite menu)

190 calories
11 g fat (5 g saturated)
19 g sugars

650 calories

30.5 g fat
(12 g saturated,
0.5 g trans)

640 mg sodium

52 g sugars

Not That!

Iced Nonfat
Caramel Macchiato

**(grande) and Fruit,
Nut & Cheese Artisan
Snack Plate**

Don't be fooled by the "nonfat" label. The macchiato's vanilla-flavored syrup and caramel drizzle are the culprits behind this sugar rush. As for the snack plate, we love everything on it, but a snack shouldn't have as many calories as a burger.

Other Passes

Raspberry Scone

500 calories
26 g fat (15 g saturated)
18 g sugars

Tazo Awake Tea Latte
(grande, 2% milk)

200 calories
5 g fat (3 g saturated)
31 g sugars

Red Velvet Cupcake

430 calories
26 g fat (14 g saturated)
34 g sugars

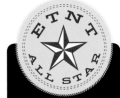

Iced Caffè
Americano
(grande)

15 calories
0 g fat
0 g sugars

Whether taken hot or cold, an Americano (a mixture of espresso and water) should be the base for all Starbucks orders. Add a pump of flavored syrup and you still have a low-calorie beverage on your hands.

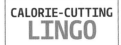

CALORIE-CUTTING
LINGO

HOLD THE WHIP
Cuts the cream and saves you anywhere from 50 to 110 calories

NONFAT
Uses fat-free milk instead of whole or 2%

SUGAR-FREE SYRUP
Use instead of regular syrup and save up to 150 calories a drink

SKINNY
Your drink will be made with sugar-free syrup and fat-free milk

Steak 'n Shake

Steak 'n Shake

B-

For a chain named after two of the most precarious foods on the planet, Steak 'n Shake could be far more dangerous. A single Steakburger with Cheese delivers a modest 330 calories, and not a single salad exceeds 500. Too bad we can't make a similar claim about the shakes. Even the smalls commonly eclipse 600 calories, and at least one—the large M&M shake—has more sugar than 7 Klondike Bars.

SURVIVAL STRATEGY

Go ahead and order a burger, but keep it simple. If you're feeling extra hungry, add a second steak patty for 110 calories. What you want to avoid are the tricked-out chili dishes. Anything entrée-size will saddle you with 830 to 1,220 calories.

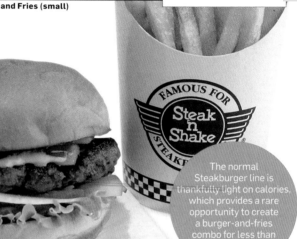

Eat This

Single Steakburger

and Fries (small)

520 calories
22 g fat
(6.5 g saturated)
390 mg sodium

The normal Steakburger line is thankfully light on calories, which provides a rare opportunity to create a burger-and-fries combo for less than 600 calories.

Other Picks

Turkey Club

420 calories
16 g fat (3.5 g saturated)
1,270 mg sodium

Frisco Steakburger Shooters with Cheese (2)

380 calories
22 g fat (8 g saturated)
820 mg sodium

Bacon Shooters (2) and Yogurt Parfait

550 calories
22 g fat (9.5 g saturated)
935 mg sodium

770 calories

56 g fat
(16 g saturated,
1.5 g trans)

920 mg sodium

Not That!

Grilled Portobello 'n Swiss Steakburger

The flagship Steakburger line doesn't have the blowout calories we expected, but seven greasy gut bombs still top 600 calories and trans fats run rampant.

HIDDEN DANGER

The Chili Menu

We usually rave about chili. Its beef, beans, and tomatoes are a reliable source of lean protein, fiber, and antioxidants. But six of the eight offerings on Steak 'n Shake's menu of chilis are 830 calories or more, and not one has less than a third of your day's fat.

Chili Deluxe
(bowl)

1,220 calories
74 g fat
(39 g saturated,
1.5 g trans)
2,560 mg sodium

Other Passes

580 calories
31 g fat (6 g saturated)
1,440 mg sodium

Guacamole Grilled Chicken Sandwich

750 calories
53 g fat (17 g saturated, 1.5 g trans)
1,160 mg sodium

Frisco Melt

890 calories
70 g fat (20 g saturated, 0.5 g trans)
1,030 mg sodium

Cheddar Scrambler and Hash Browns

Subway

A

This year, Subway became the first major fast-food chain to carry avocado, and all the heart-healthy fats found within, in every one of its 24,200 US stores. That's huge, but not nearly as huge as the chain's other initiative. This year, Subway cut sodium by 15 percent in its regular sandwiches and 28 percent in its Fresh Fit sandwiches. If the chain weren't already America's healthiest chain, it certainly is now.

SURVIVAL STRATEGY

Trouble lurks in three areas at Subway: 1) hot subs, 2) foot-longs, 3) chips and soda. Stick to 6-inch cold subs made with ham, turkey, roast beef, or chicken. Load up on veggies, and be extra careful about your condiment choices.

Eat This

Buffalo Chicken Toasted Sandwich

(6") and Berry Lishus Fruizle Express (small)

530 calories
15 g fat
(3 g saturated)
1,220 mg sodium

The new line of Refresher Fruizle Expresses all have fewer calories and sugars than a 12-ounce Coke and deliver between 120 and 210 percent of your daily vitamin C requirement.

Other Picks

Subway Club Sub (6")

310 calories
4.5 g fat (1.5 g saturated)
880 mg sodium

Black Forest Ham, Egg and Cheese Muffin Melts (2)

340 calories
8 g fat (3 g saturated)
1,220 mg sodium

Steak and Cheese Sub (6")

380 calories
10 g fat (4.5 g saturated)
1,060 mg sodium

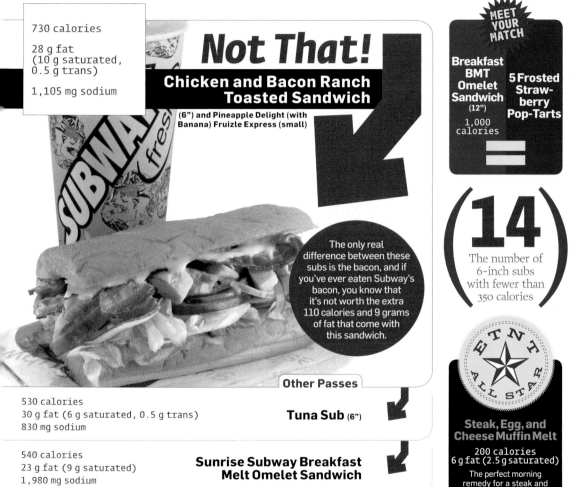

730 calories

28 g fat
(10 g saturated,
0.5 g trans)

1,105 mg sodium

Not That!

Chicken and Bacon Ranch Toasted Sandwich

(6") and Pineapple Delight (with Banana) Fruizle Express (small)

The only real difference between these subs is the bacon, and if you've ever eaten Subway's bacon, you know that it's not worth the extra 110 calories and 9 grams of fat that come with this sandwich.

MEET YOUR MATCH

Breakfast BMT Omelet Sandwich (12")

1,000 calories

=

5 Frosted Strawberry Pop-Tarts

(14)

The number of 6-inch subs with fewer than 350 calories

ETNT ALL STAR

Steak, Egg, and Cheese Muffin Melt

200 calories
6 g fat (2.5 g saturated)

The perfect morning remedy for a steak and eggs craving. Each Melt carries between 12 and 18 grams of protein, and a stellar 6 grams of fiber.

Other Passes

530 calories
30 g fat (6 g saturated, 0.5 g trans)
830 mg sodium

Tuna Sub (6")

540 calories
23 g fat (9 g saturated)
1,980 mg sodium

Sunrise Subway Breakfast Melt Omelet Sandwich

520 calories
18 g fat (9 g saturated, 1 g trans)
1,370 mg sodium

The Big Philly Cheesesteak (6")

TGI Friday's

We salute Friday's for its smaller-portions menu; the option to order reduced-size servings ought to be the new model, dethroning the bigger-is-better principle that dominates chain restaurants. But Friday's still refuses to provide nutrition info, and our research shows why: The menu is awash in atrocious appetizers, frightening salads, and entrées with embarrassingly high calorie counts.

SURVIVAL STRATEGY

Danger is waiting in every crack and corner of Friday's menu. Your best bets? The 400-calorie Shrimp Key West, the 480-calorie Dragonfire Chicken, or finding another restaurant entirely.

Eat This

Jack Daniel's Chicken

with Coleslaw and Fresh Broccoli

640 calories

This is one of only four entrées with fewer than 700 calories, and that's only because these are the two best sides on the menu. Get mashed potatoes and the fresh vegetable medley and you're looking at a punishing 1,030 calories.

Other Picks

Bruschetta Chicken Pasta

640 calories

Dragonfire Chicken

420 calories

Grilled Chicken Cobb Salad
with Low-Fat Balsamic Vinaigrette

590 calories

1,590 calories

Not That!

Jack Daniel's Chicken Sandwich

with Fries

Sweet potatoes are almost always a better option than white potatoes. Opting for the sweet version will administer a dose of the supernutrient beta-carotene, which has been shown to bolster eye health and cognitive performance. Most importantly at Friday's, choosing the sweet potato fries over regular fries for the table will cut the calories in half —from 800 to 400.

Friday's menu is saturated with excess fats. Take this grilled chicken sandwich. It's basted in Jack Daniel's glaze; topped with bacon, a blanket of cheese, and Cajun onion straws; and slathered with Jack Daniel's mayo. A model of American excess if we've ever seen one.

Other Passes

1,240 calories	**Sizzling Chicken & Shrimp**
1,220 calories	**Captain Morgan Caribbean Chicken Sandwich** with Fries
1,360 calories	**Pecan-Crusted Chicken Salad**

ALL THIS

Southwest Chicken Quesadillas, Cheeseburger Sliders, and Shrimp Cocktail

OR

THAT

Loaded Potato Skins

2,070 calories

Taco Bell

The Bell made a bold play in 2010 when they began to play up their menu as a potentially healthy dieting option. A bit far-fetched, but can you blame them? Taco Bell combines two things with bad nutritional reputations—Mexican food and fast food—but provides dozens of ways for you to keep your meal under 500 calories. Stick to the Fresco Menu, where no single item exceeds 350 calories. Not a diet, but close.

SURVIVAL STRATEGY

Stay away from Grilled Stuft Burritos, food served in a bowl, and anything prepared with multiple "layers"—they're all trouble. Instead, order any two of the following: crunchy tacos, bean burritos, or anything on the Fresco menu.

Eat This

Nacho Cheese Chicken Gordita

and Fresco Grilled Steak Soft Taco

430 calories
14.5 g fat
(3 g saturated)
1,090 mg sodium

Despite the name ("little fat one"), they have fewer calories than Taco Bell's burritos and chalupas but still pack in the protein, making them the perfect item to build a meal around. Tack on a Fresco taco or Pintos 'n Cheese for a near-perfect meal.

Other Picks

Taco Supremes
(crunchy, 2)

400 calories
24 g fat (10 g saturated)
700 mg sodium

Steak Burrito Supreme

390 calories
13 g fat (5 g saturated)
1,100 mg sodium

Fresco Chicken Soft Tacos
(2) and Pintos 'n Cheese

470 calories
13 g fat (5 g saturated)
1,540 mg sodium

530 calories

28 g fat
(12 g saturated,
0.5 g trans)

1,210 mg sodium

Not That!

Chicken Quesadilla

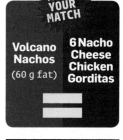

CONDIMENT CATASTROPHE

Zesty Dressing

200 calories
20 g fat
(3.5 g saturated)
250 mg sodium

Taco Bell offers an array of low-calorie sauces, but this isn't one of them. As if being filled with chemist-concocted ingredients such as carboxymethylcellulose isn't bad enough, one serving eats up a third of your day's fat allowance.

How much cheese goes into one of these? Well, just one chicken quesadilla has as much saturated fat as eight small orders of McDonald's french fries.

Other Passes

700 calories
30 g fat (10 g saturated)
1,520 mg sodium

Cheesy Double Decker Tacos (2)

540 calories
21 g fat (8 g saturated)
1,320 mg sodium

Beefy 5-Layer Burrito

650 calories
24 g fat (7 g saturated)
1,580 mg sodium

Chicken Grilled Stuft Burrito

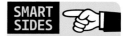

SMART SIDES

Cinnamon Twists

170 calories
7 g fat (0 g saturated)
200 mg sodium

The essential oils in cinnamon act as an antimicrobial agent in your body and cinnamon has also been shown to help control your postmeal blood sugar level, delaying hunger for longer.

173

Tim Hortons

B+

When it comes to sandwiches, Tim Horton's trumps the competition. Not a single lunch sandwich tops 500 calories, and its worst breakfast item is a 550-calorie sausage, egg, and cheese bagel. Supplement a lighter sandwich with Tim's oatmeal, yogurt, or soup, and you're golden. The menu still houses a variety of confections and empty carbohydrates, though, so don't let your guard down.

SURVIVAL STRATEGY

More than ever, it's about the quality of your calories instead of quantity. Your best bet at breakfast is the fruit-topped yogurt or brown sugar oatmeal. For lunch, choose either two wraps or one sandwich and a zero-calorie beverage, and you'll be on solid ground.

Eat This

English Muffin
with Hickory Smoked Ham, Egg, and Cheese and Iced Coffee (16 fl oz, with cream and sugar)

380 calories
16 g fat
(7 g saturated)
990 mg sodium
12 g sugars

Canada's answer to the Egg McMuffin, Horton's ham-laced handheld breakfast sandwich, jump-starts your day with 18 grams of protein. Pair it with an 80-calorie iced coffee and you'll be firing on all cylinders by the time the workday beckons.

Other Picks

Chicken Salad Sandwich
340 calories
9 g fat (1.5 g saturated)
970 mg sodium

Honey Dip Donut
210 calories
8 g fat (3.5 g saturated)
11 g sugars

Strawberry Filled Donut
230 calories
8 g fat (3.5 g saturated)
12 g sugars

Not That!

Bagel BELT
and Iced Cappuccino (12 fl oz)

770 calories

32 g fat
(16 g saturated)

1,060 mg sodium

47 g sugars

This is a decent-enough sandwich, but it only provides an extra 3 grams of protein for 160 extra calories over the English muffin sandwich. You can blame most of that on the big, doughy bagel.

Other Passes

420 calories
18 g fat (5 g saturated)
830 mg sodium

BLT

320 calories
19 g fat (9 g saturated)
23 g sugars

Honey Cruller

400 calories
15 g fat (4 g saturated)
29 g sugars

Whole Grain Raspberry Muffin

MENU MAGIC

Want the deliciousness of the French Vanilla Cappuccino but not its 240 calories? Hortons offers no-calorie syrups to spice up any drink. Order a medium coffee with one sugar and one cream and ask for a shot of no-calorie vanilla flavor. It'll save you 165 calories.

Uno Chicago Grill

Uno stikes a curious (if not altogether healthy) balance between oversize sandwiches and burgers, lean grilled steaks and fish entrées, and one of the world's most calorie-dense foods, deep dish pizza, which Uno's invented. It may pride itself on its nutrition transparency, but the only thing that's truly transparent is that there are far too many dishes here that pack 1,000 calories or more.

SURVIVAL STRATEGY

Stick with flatbread instead of deep-dish pizzas—this one move could save you more than 1,000 calories at a sitting. Beyond that, turn to the Smoke, Sizzle & Splash section of the menu for nutrition salvation.

Eat This

Chicken Tikka Masala

560 calories

24 g fat
(5 g saturated)

1,600 mg sodium

It's nice to see an American chain finally embracing the world-class cuisine of the Indian subcontinent. The potent flavor profile behind tikka masala comes from antioxidant-rich spices like cardamom, turmeric, and cayenne pepper. This is healthy eating at its most delicious.

Other Picks

Grilled Chicken Sandwich

450 calories
16.5 g fat (1.5 g saturated)
1,305 mg sodium

Chopped Power Salad

540 calories
14 g fat (3 g saturated)
1,220 mg sodium

BBQ Chicken on Five-Grain Crust Pizza (⅓ pie)

340 calories
12 g fat (5 g saturated)
500 mg sodium

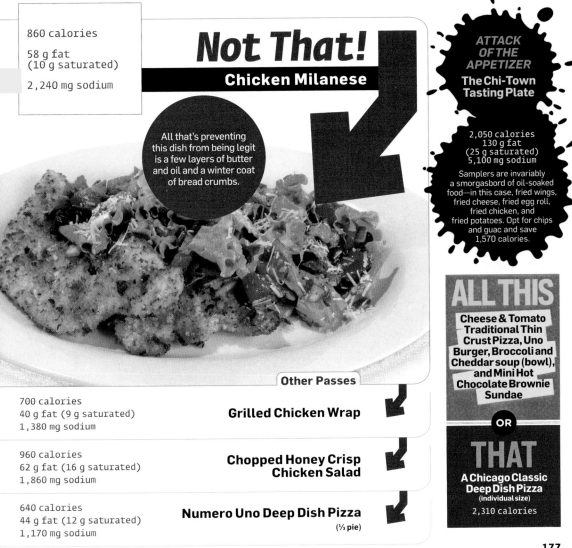

860 calories

58 g fat
(10 g saturated)

2,240 mg sodium

Not That!

Chicken Milanese

All that's preventing this dish from being legit is a few layers of butter and oil and a winter coat of bread crumbs.

ATTACK OF THE APPETIZER

The Chi-Town Tasting Plate

2,050 calories
130 g fat
(25 g saturated)
5,100 mg sodium

Samplers are invariably a smorgasbord of oil-soaked food—in this case, fried wings, fried cheese, fried egg roll, fried chicken, and fried potatoes. Opt for chips and guac and save 1,570 calories.

ALL THIS

Cheese & Tomato Traditional Thin Crust Pizza, Uno Burger, Broccoli and Cheddar soup (bowl), and Mini Hot Chocolate Brownie Sundae

OR

THAT

A Chicago Classic Deep Dish Pizza
(individual size)

2,310 calories

Other Passes

700 calories
40 g fat (9 g saturated)
1,380 mg sodium

Grilled Chicken Wrap

960 calories
62 g fat (16 g saturated)
1,860 mg sodium

Chopped Honey Crisp Chicken Salad

640 calories
44 g fat (12 g saturated)
1,170 mg sodium

Numero Uno Deep Dish Pizza
(⅓ pie)

177

Wendy's

B+

Scoring a decent meal at Wendy's is just about as easy as scoring a bad one, and that's a big compliment to pay a burger joint. Options such as chili and mandarin oranges offer the side-order variety that's missing from less-evolved fast-food chains like Dairy Queen and Burger King. Plus, Wendy's offers a handful of Jr. Burgers that don't stray far above 300 calories. Where Wendy's errs is in the expanded line of desserts and the roster of double- and triple-patty burgers.

SURVIVAL STRATEGY

Choose a grilled chicken sandwich or a wrap—they don't exceed 320 calories. Or opt for a small burger and pair it with chili or a side salad.

Eat This

Jr. Hamburger and Broccoli and Cheese Potato

560 calories
10 g fat
(4 g saturated,
0.5 g trans)

950 mg sodium

Wendy's Broccoli and Cheese Potato should get more love. It has 90 fewer calories than a medium order of fries, but it delivers 6 more grams of protein. Oh, and it has 8 grams of fiber and 110 percent of your daily vitamin C intake.

BURG

Other Picks

Chicken Nuggets
(10) with Sweet & Sour Nuggets Sauce

500 calories
29 g fat (6 g saturated)
970 mg sodium

Crispy Chicken Sandwich

350 calories
15 g fat (3 g saturated)
830 mg sodium

Ultimate Chicken Grill

370 calories
7 g fat (1.5 g saturated)
1,150 mg sodium

740 calories

47 g fat
(17 g saturated,
1.5 g trans)

1,990 mg sodium

Not That!

Baja Salad

(full size)

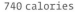

A salad with trans fats is a serious problem. Then again, all of Wendy's Garden Sensations are problems. The best one contains a barely acceptable 580 calories and comes saddled with 9 grams of saturated fat.

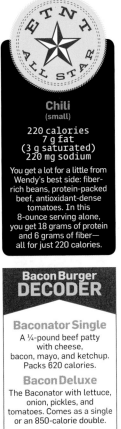

ETNT
ALL STAR

Chili
(small)

220 calories
7 g fat
(3 g saturated)
220 mg sodium

You get a lot for a little from Wendy's best side: fiber-rich beans, protein-packed beef, antioxidant-dense tomatoes. In this 8-ounce serving alone, you get 18 grams of protein and 6 grams of fiber— all for just 220 calories.

Bacon Burger DECODER

Baconator Single
A ¼-pound beef patty with cheese, bacon, mayo, and ketchup. Packs 620 calories.

Bacon Deluxe
The Baconator with lettuce, onion, pickles, and tomatoes. Comes as a single or an 850-calorie double.

Junior Bacon Cheeseburger
A smaller beef patty on a smaller bun with produce—at a full 290 fewer calories than the Single Bacon Deluxe, it's far and away your best option.

Other Passes

660 calories
33 g fat (10 g saturated)
1,660 mg sodium

Asiago Ranch Chicken Club
with Spicy Chicken Fillet

500 calories
24 g fat (4 g saturated)
1,010 mg sodium

Premium Fish Fillet Sandwich

580 calories
27 g fat (9 g saturated)
1,590 mg sodium

Apple Pecan Chicken Salad

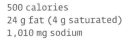

179

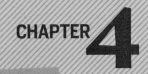

At the Supermarket

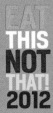

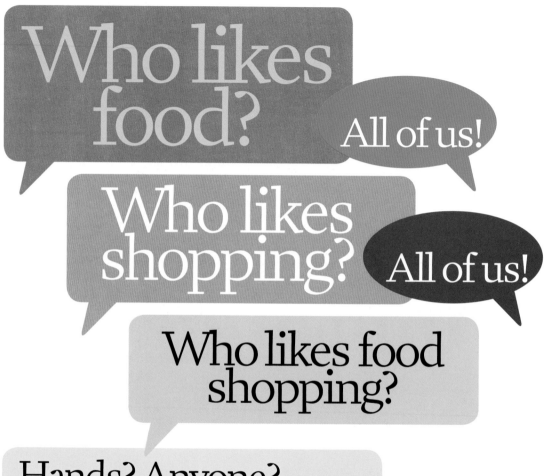

The answer is, almost nobody likes food shopping. A trip to the grocery store means spending an hour or so parsing specious nutritional claims and confusing price schemes and annoying, cloying packaging tricks, and then doling out more money than you ever imagined you'd have to under soul-sucking florescent lighting that could make Brooklyn Decker look like the Crypt Keeper.

All those mendacious marketing techniques in the supermarket are designed to populate your cart with foodlike substances that trick your taste buds while doing maximum damage to your waistline. It doesn't matter how thorough your command of the English language is; Eminem couldn't pronounce half of what's on an ingredients list, and only Don Draper could make sense of marketing gobbledygook like "Part of a Well-Balanced Diet" and "Loaded with Nine Essential Nutrients." There are about 40,000 products in your average supermarket, and unless you're swooping through the aisles with a math whiz (to calculate what the *real* calorie counts are), a dietician (to explain what all

those crazy words on the ingredients lists mean), and a marketing expert (to decode phrases like "all natural" and "heart healthy"), chances are you're going to make a few mistakes.

Make the same mistake over and over, and you could be shelling out extra money and gaining extra pounds. What you need is a cheat sheet that will lead you away from the worst offenders and toward the nutritionally safe options. Fortunately, you've got one in your hands.

For sure, shopping smart is harder than ever, in part because food is more expensive than ever. This past February, for example, wholesale food prices shot up by 3.9 percent on a year-over-year basis, the largest 1-month price increase since 1974. And a recent survey by the International Food Information Council Foundation found that 79 percent of consumers say that price impacts their decisions about what foods and drinks to buy, up from 64 percent back in 2006. Only 66 percent consider "healthfulness" an important aspect.

But in reality, over the long haul, healthy food is cheaper—because the less nutrition you get from the food you eat, the more you have to eat to satisfy your body. That means you're spending more money on junk—and gaining more fat. Fortunately, there's an answer: The foods in this chapter are the very best in class—the ultimate tickets to a leaner belly, a fatter wallet, and a happier image looking back at you from the mirror. But before you fire up your food cart, lock and load your coupons, and head down to the grocery store, remember these essential tips on how to buy more nutrition for less money.

Demand to see a birth certificate!

That whole wacky controversy over the presidency may be over (it's over, okay?), but that doesn't mean there aren't plenty of imposters still lurking out there. And they're not in the White House—they're in your house! I'm talking about food imposters—things that are sold like food, but are only partially food. The supermarket is filled with mini Manchurian candidates,

products that started out as innocents but were corrupted along the way. Consider that container of applesauce, for example: When apples are turned into applesauce, manufacturers can double their caloric load by adding high-fructose corn syrup (HFCS) while also stripping off the peel, which is where much of the fiber and other nutrients are found. So which will help your health more: an apple, or a mash of apple, water, and HFCS? Bottom line: The closer to the food's original form you can get, the better.

Buy nutrition, not calories.

Which is the better yogurt buy: 5.3 ounces of Fage Total 2% with Peach for $2.08, or 6 ounces of Yoplait Original 99% Fat Free Harvest Peach for exactly half that amount—$1.04? No-brainer, right? But think again: By paying half the price for the Yoplait, you're getting less than half the protein (5 grams versus 12), one-third more sugar, and 30 additional calories. Since protein is the stuff that makes you feel full, and sugar is the stuff that leads to up-and-down food cravings, that sounds like a bad investment: Over time, you're likely to wind up buying, and eating, and smuggling along your waistline more of the sugary Yoplait than you should. Or consider the choice of Kashi TLC Honey Toasted 7 Grain Crunchy granola bars ($4.19 for a box of 12) versus Nature Valley Crunchy Oats 'n Honey granola bars ($3.59 for a box of 12). Pretty equal in size, and they both sound pretty healthy. Another no-brainer, right? But shell out the additional 60 cents for the Kashi—that's about 17 percent more money—and you're buying double the fiber, 50 percent more protein, and one-third less sugar.

Don't plan a quickie.

Planning a shopping trip is a chore, what with the list and the unpacking all the bags and the kids hanging out of the cart trying to snag a box of anything decorated with Dora, Diego, SpongeBob, Jillian Michaels, or other characters. It's tempting to make a bunch of short, quick trips instead. But a recent study found that shoppers who stopped by for quickies ended up spending an average of 54 percent more on groceries than they had planned. You're not sneaking into Pakistan to pop Bin Laden, after all; you're implementing your family's long-term health and nutrition strategy. A quick exit isn't your primary goal. A well-stocked fridge is. (Hint: Few people know this, but supermarket shopping is the reason God invented MP3 players. The aisles are a lot less intimidating when Lady Gaga is singing "Born This Way" into your ears.)

Focus on the top dog.

By law, ingredients have to be listed by weight, so whatever's at the top of the list is what's most prevalent in the food. The top two or three ingredients are all you really need to focus on; they'll tell you all you need to know about the relative healthfulness of a product. A package of Oreos, for example, has 20 ingredients on its side. The very first ingredient? Sugar.

Sweet Cereals

Eat This

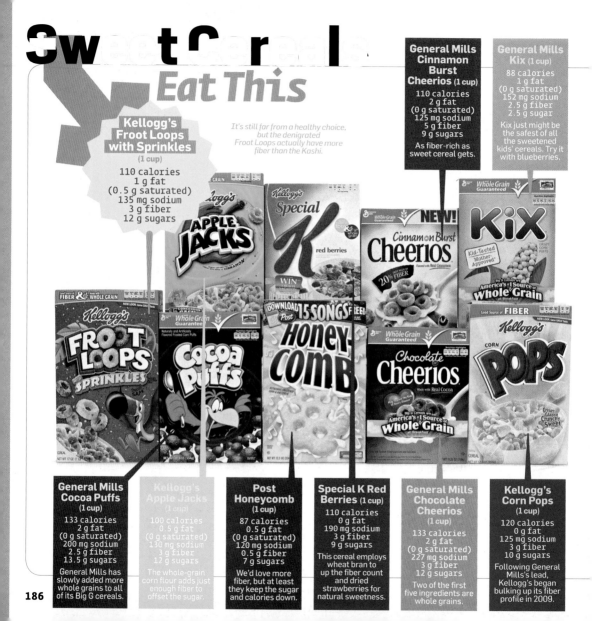

Kellogg's Froot Loops with Sprinkles
(1 cup)
110 calories
1 g fat
(0.5 g saturated)
135 mg sodium
3 g fiber
12 g sugars

It's still far from a healthy choice, but the denigrated Froot Loops actually have more fiber than the Kashi.

General Mills Cinnamon Burst Cheerios (1 cup)
110 calories
2 g fat
(0 g saturated)
125 mg sodium
5 g fiber
9 g sugars

As fiber-rich as sweet cereal gets.

General Mills Kix (1 cup)
88 calories
1 g fat
(0 g saturated)
152 mg sodium
2.5 g fiber
2.5 g sugar

Kix just might be the safest of all the sweetened kids' cereals. Try it with blueberries.

General Mills Cocoa Puffs
(1 cup)
133 calories
2 g fat
(0 g saturated)
200 mg sodium
2.5 g fiber
13.5 g sugars

General Mills has slowly added more whole grains to all of its Big G cereals.

Kellogg's Apple Jacks
(1 cup)
100 calories
0.5 g fat
(0 g saturated)
130 mg sodium
3 g fiber
12 g sugars

The whole-grain corn flour adds just enough fiber to offset the sugar.

Post Honeycomb
(1 cup)
87 calories
0.5 g fat
(0 g saturated)
120 mg sodium
0.5 g fiber
7 g sugars

We'd love more fiber, but at least they keep the sugar and calories down.

Special K Red Berries (1 cup)
110 calories
0 g fat
190 mg sodium
3 g fiber
9 g sugars

This cereal employs wheat bran to up the fiber count and dried strawberries for natural sweetness.

General Mills Chocolate Cheerios
(1 cup)
133 calories
2 g fat
(0 g saturated)
227 mg sodium
3 g fiber
12 g sugars

Two of the first five ingredients are whole grains.

Kellogg's Corn Pops
(1 cup)
120 calories
0 g fat
125 mg sodium
3 g fiber
10 g sugars

Following General Mills's lead, Kellogg's began bulking up its fiber profile in 2009.

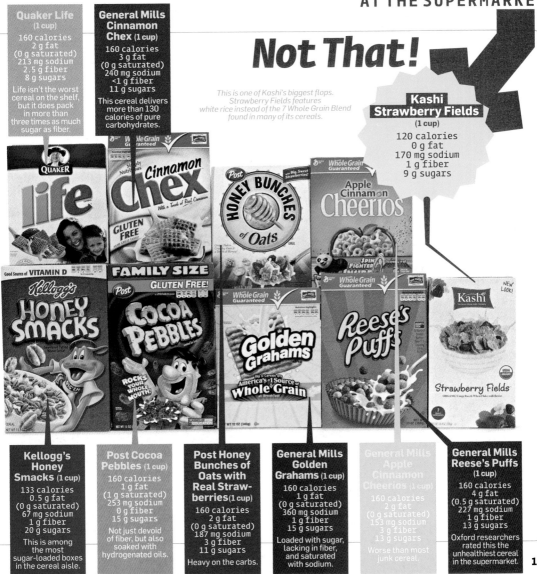

Not That!

Quaker Life
(1 cup)

160 calories
2 g fat
(0 g saturated)
213 mg sodium
2.5 g fiber
8 g sugars

Life isn't the worst cereal on the shelf, but it does pack in more than three times as much sugar as fiber.

General Mills Cinnamon Chex (1 cup)

160 calories
3 g fat
(0 g saturated)
240 mg sodium
<1 g fiber
11 g sugars

This cereal delivers more than 130 calories of pure carbohydrates.

This is one of Kashi's biggest flops. Strawberry Fields features white rice instead of the 7 Whole Grain Blend found in many of its cereals.

Kashi Strawberry Fields
(1 cup)

120 calories
0 g fat
170 mg sodium
1 g fiber
9 g sugars

Kellogg's Honey Smacks (1 cup)

133 calories
0.5 g fat
(0 g saturated)
67 mg sodium
1 g fiber
20 g sugars

This is among the most sugar-loaded boxes in the cereal aisle.

Post Cocoa Pebbles (1 cup)

160 calories
1 g fat
(1 g saturated)
253 mg sodium
0 g fiber
15 g sugars

Not just devoid of fiber, but also soaked with hydrogenated oils.

Post Honey Bunches of Oats with Real Strawberries (1 cup)

160 calories
2 g fat
(0 g saturated)
187 mg sodium
3 g fiber
11 g sugars

Heavy on the carbs.

General Mills Golden Grahams (1 cup)

160 calories
1 g fat
(0 g saturated)
360 mg sodium
1 g fiber
15 g sugars

Loaded with sugar, lacking in fiber, and saturated with sodium.

General Mills Apple Cinnamon Cheerios (1 cup)

160 calories
2 g fat
(0 g saturated)
153 mg sodium
3 g fiber
13 g sugars

Worse than most junk cereal.

General Mills Reese's Puffs
(1 cup)

160 calories
4 g fat
(0.5 g saturated)
227 mg sodium
1 g fiber
13 g sugars

Oxford researchers rated this the unhealthiest cereal in the supermarket.

Wholesome Cereals

Eat This

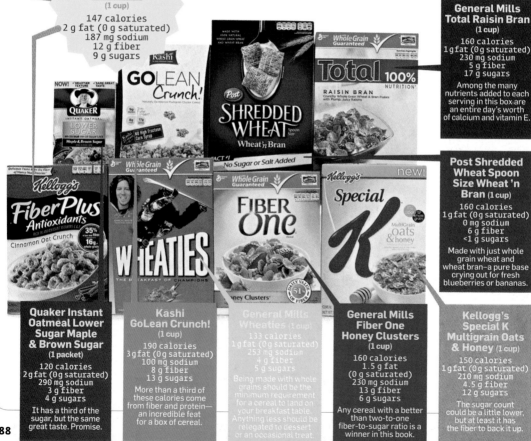

Kellogg's FiberPlus Cinnamon Oat Crunch
(1 cup)

147 calories
2 g fat (0 g saturated)
187 mg sodium
12 g fiber
9 g sugars

Cinnamon is a worthwhile addition to any cereal. Studies show that it helps your body manage blood sugar.

General Mills Total Raisin Bran
(1 cup)

160 calories
1 g fat (0 g saturated)
230 mg sodium
5 g fiber
17 g sugars

Among the many nutrients added to each serving in this box are an entire day's worth of calcium and vitamin E.

Post Shredded Wheat Spoon Size Wheat 'n Bran (1 cup)

160 calories
1 g fat (0 g saturated)
0 mg sodium
6 g fiber
<1 g sugars

Made with just whole grain wheat and wheat bran–a pure base crying out for fresh blueberries or bananas.

Quaker Instant Oatmeal Lower Sugar Maple & Brown Sugar
(1 packet)

120 calories
2 g fat (0 g saturated)
290 mg sodium
3 g fiber
4 g sugars

It has a third of the sugar, but the same great taste. Promise.

Kashi GoLean Crunch!
(1 cup)

190 calories
3 g fat (0 g saturated)
100 mg sodium
8 g fiber
13 g sugars

More than a third of these calories come from fiber and protein— an incredible feat for a box of cereal.

General Mills Wheaties (1 cup)

133 calories
1 g fat (0 g saturated)
253 mg sodium
4 g fiber
5 g sugars

Being made with whole grains should be the minimum requirement for a cereal to land on your breakfast table. Anything less should be relegated to dessert or an occasional treat.

General Mills Fiber One Honey Clusters
(1 cup)

160 calories
1.5 g fat
(0 g saturated)
230 mg sodium
13 g fiber
6 g sugars

Any cereal with a better than two-to-one fiber-to-sugar ratio is a winner in this book.

Kellogg's Special K Multigrain Oats & Honey (1 cup)

150 calories
1 g fat (0 g saturated)
210 mg sodium
4.5 g fiber
12 g sugars

The sugar count could be a little lower, but at least it has the fiber to back it up.

Not That!

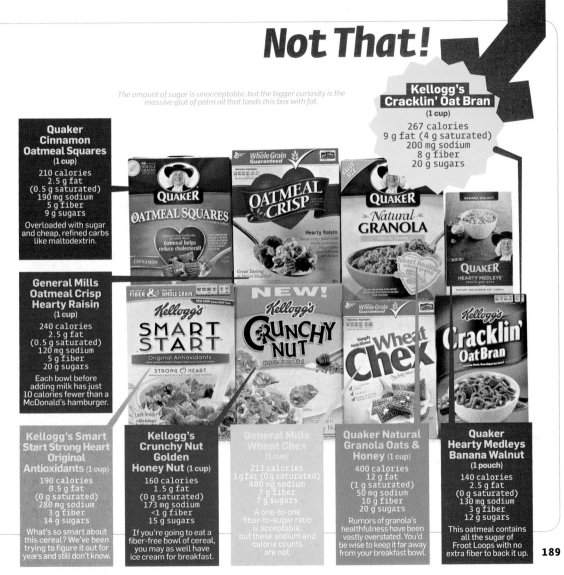

The amount of sugar is unacceptable, but the bigger curiosity is the massive glut of palm oil that loads this box with fat.

Kellogg's Cracklin' Oat Bran
(1 cup)

267 calories
9 g fat (4 g saturated)
200 mg sodium
8 g fiber
20 g sugars

Quaker Cinnamon Oatmeal Squares
(1 cup)

210 calories
2.5 g fat
(0.5 g saturated)
190 mg sodium
5 g fiber
9 g sugars

Overloaded with sugar and cheap, refined carbs like maltodextrin.

General Mills Oatmeal Crisp Hearty Raisin
(1 cup)

240 calories
2.5 g fat
(0.5 g saturated)
120 mg sodium
5 g fiber
20 g sugars

Each bowl before adding milk has just 10 calories fewer than a McDonald's hamburger.

Kellogg's Smart Start Strong Heart Original Antioxidants (1 cup)

190 calories
0.5 g fat
(0 g saturated)
280 mg sodium
3 g fiber
14 g sugars

What's so smart about this cereal? We've been trying to figure it out for years and still don't know.

Kellogg's Crunchy Nut Golden Honey Nut (1 cup)

160 calories
1.5 g fat
(0 g saturated)
173 mg sodium
<1 g fiber
15 g sugars

If you're going to eat a fiber-free bowl of cereal, you may as well have ice cream for breakfast.

General Mills Wheat Chex
(1 cup)

213 calories
1 g fat (0 g saturated)
400 mg sodium
7 g fiber
7 g sugars

A one-to-one fiber-to-sugar ratio is acceptable, but these sodium and calorie counts are not.

Quaker Natural Granola Oats & Honey (1 cup)

400 calories
12 g fat
(1 g saturated)
50 mg sodium
10 g fiber
20 g sugars

Rumors of granola's healthfulness have been vastly overstated. You'd be wise to keep it far away from your breakfast bowl.

Quaker Hearty Medleys Banana Walnut
(1 pouch)

140 calories
2.5 g fat
(0 g saturated)
130 mg sodium
3 g fiber
12 g sugars

This oatmeal contains all the sugar of Froot Loops with no extra fiber to back it up.

189

Breakfast Breads

Eat This

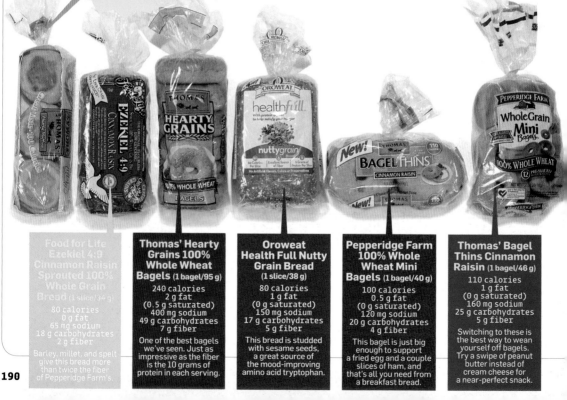

Thomas' Light Multi-Grain English Muffins
(1 muffin/57 g)

100 calories
1 g fat (0 g saturated)
180 mg sodium
26 g carbohydrates
8 g fiber

Outside of green vegetables, you'll find very few foods that manage to pack 8 grams of fiber into 100 calories. That makes this an unbeatable foundation for breakfast sandwiches.

Food for Life Ezekiel 4:9 Cinnamon Raisin Sprouted 100% Whole Grain Bread (1 slice/34 g)

80 calories
0 g fat
65 mg sodium
18 g carbohydrates
2 g fiber

Barley, millet, and spelt give this bread more than twice the fiber of Pepperidge Farm's.

Thomas' Hearty Grains 100% Whole Wheat Bagels (1 bagel/95 g)

240 calories
2 g fat
(0.5 g saturated)
400 mg sodium
49 g carbohydrates
7 g fiber

One of the best bagels we've seen. Just as impressive as the fiber is the 10 grams of protein in each serving.

Oroweat Health Full Nutty Grain Bread (1 slice/38 g)

80 calories
1 g fat
(0 g saturated)
150 mg sodium
17 g carbohydrates
5 g fiber

This bread is studded with sesame seeds, a great source of the mood-improving amino acid tryptophan.

Pepperidge Farm 100% Whole Wheat Mini Bagels (1 bagel/40 g)

100 calories
0.5 g fat
(0 g saturated)
120 mg sodium
20 g carbohydrates
4 g fiber

This bagel is just big enough to support a fried egg and a couple slices of ham, and that's all you need from a breakfast bread.

Thomas' Bagel Thins Cinnamon Raisin (1 bagel/46 g)

110 calories
1 g fat
(0 g saturated)
160 mg sodium
25 g carbohydrates
5 g fiber

Switching to these is the best way to wean yourself off bagels. Try a swipe of peanut butter instead of cream cheese for a near-perfect snack.

Not That!

The more fiber you work into your breakfast, the more likely you'll be to make it to lunch without experiencing hunger pangs. That means this muffin is a recipe for midmorning cravings.

Sara Lee Original English Muffins
(1 muffin/66 g)

140 calories
1 g fat (0 g saturated)
210 mg sodium
27 g carbohydrates
2 g fiber

Thomas' Plain Mini Bagels
(1 bagel/43 g)

120 calories
1 g fat
(0 g saturated)
240 mg sodium
24 g carbohydrates
<1 g fiber

Once your palate is accustomed to whole grains, flavorless, nutritionless breads like this will taste boring.

Otis Spunkmeyer Harvest Bran Muffins
(1 muffin/57 g)

200 calories
9 g fat
(1.5 g saturated)
210 mg sodium
29 g carbohydrates
2 g fiber

Most muffins are just cupcakes in disguise. The 16 grams of sugars in this Spunkmeyer dud just prove the point.

Nature's Pride 100% Natural Nutty Oat Bread
(1 slice/43 g)

120 calories
2 g fat
(0 g saturated)
150 mg sodium
20 g carbohydrates
3 g fiber

You should demand far more fiber than this from a 120-calorie slice of bread.

Sara Lee Deluxe Bagels Plain
(1 bagel/95 g)

260 calories
1 g fat
(0 g saturated)
400 mg sodium
50 g carbohydrates
2 g fiber

This is a wedge of refined carbohydrates, and as such, it will induce a blood sugar roller coaster that will wreak havoc on your energy reserves.

Pepperidge Farm Brown Sugar Cinnamon Swirl Bread
(1 slice/38 g)

110 calories
2 g fat
(0 g saturated)
140 mg sodium
21 g carbohydrates
<1 g fiber

This bread contains five different forms of sugar.

Yogurts

It takes Fage more than a pound of raw milk to make one container of this yogurt, which is why it's so thick and loaded with protein. Equally as commendable is the fact that Fage eschews preservatives and artificial thickeners.

Fage Total 2% with Peach
(1 container/5.3 oz)

130 calories
2.5 g fat
(1.5 g saturated)
0 g fiber
17 g sugars
10 g protein

Stonyfield Oikos Organic Greek Yogurt Honey
(1 container/5.3 oz)

120 calories
0 g fat
0 g fiber
17 g sugars
13 g protein

Oikos uses honey to turn this into a lightly sweetened treat, not a sugar-saturated breakfast blunder.

Yoplait Fiber One Nonfat Strawberry
(1 container/4 oz)

50 calories
0 g fat
5 g fiber
4 g sugars
3 g protein

Fiber One has fewer than half the calories and nearly double the fiber of its competitor.

Dannon Light & Fit Cherry
(1 container/6 oz)

80 calories
0 g fat
0 g fiber
11 g sugars
5 g protein

We prefer a yogurt with more protein, but it's tough to argue against a yogurt with just 80 calories per serving.

So Delicious Cultured Soy Milk Vanilla
(1 container/6 oz)

130 calories
2.5 g fat
(0 g saturated)
5 g fiber
19 g sugars
3 g protein

It's not the soy that makes this yogurt great, it's the organic agave sweetener and 5 grams of chicory root fiber.

Breyer's YoCrunch 100 Calorie Vanilla
with Chocolate Cookie Pieces
(1 container/106 g)

100 calories
1.5 g fat
(0.5 g saturated)
0 g fiber
13 g sugars
3 g protein

Impressively low-cal for a cookie-strewn treat.

Not That!

Yoplait commits the cardinal sin of fruit-flavored yogurts by candying these peaches with more sugar than you'd find in a two-pack of Reese's Peanut Butter Cups. The only yogurts worth eating are those that are unflavored or that can claim to have more fruit than sugar.

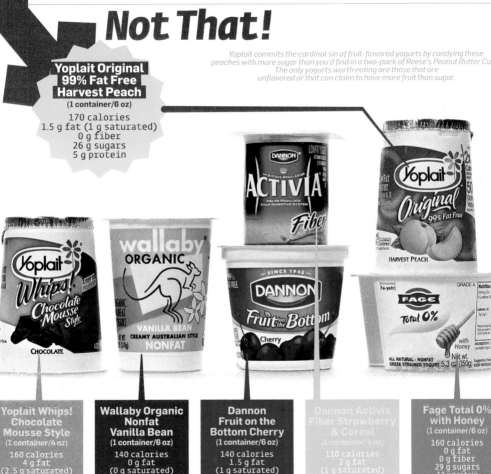

Yoplait Original 99% Fat Free Harvest Peach
(1 container/6 oz)

170 calories
1.5 g fat (1 g saturated)
0 g fiber
26 g sugars
5 g protein

Yoplait Whips! Chocolate Mousse Style
(1 container/4 oz)

160 calories
4 g fat (2.5 g saturated)
0 g fiber
22 g sugars
5 g protein

You'd be better off eating a small scoop of Breyers All Natural ice cream.

Wallaby Organic Nonfat Vanilla Bean
(1 container/6 oz)

140 calories
0 g fat (0 g saturated)
0 g fiber
22 g sugars
6 g protein

Organic dairy is worth celebrating, but you shouldn't bend your nutritional standards to get it.

Dannon Fruit on the Bottom Cherry
(1 container/6 oz)

140 calories
1.5 g fat (1 g saturated)
0 g fiber
24 g sugars
6 g protein

"Fruit on the bottom" means a few cherries muddled with sugar, fructose, and high-fructose corn syrup.

Dannon Activia Fiber Strawberry & Cereal
(1 container/4 oz)

110 calories
2 g fat (1 g saturated)
3 g fiber
16 g sugars
3 g protein

With a sugar level more than five times that of the level of fiber, this cup fails as a healthy snack.

Fage Total 0% with Honey
(1 container/6 oz)

160 calories
0 g fat
0 g fiber
29 g sugars
11 g protein

We are unabashed Fage junkies, but this is a serious buzzkill. Honey may be better than sugar, but it's not so good that you should eat it by the cupful.

193

Ch**ee**se

Eat This

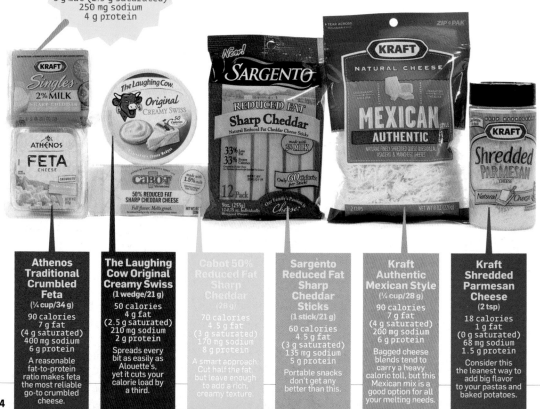

Cheese adds a creamy texture to your foods and flab-fighting calcium to your diet. But to keep the calories in check, use it smartly—which is to say, sparingly.

Kraft Singles 2% Milk Sharp Cheddar
(1 slice/19 g)

45 calories
3 g fat (1.5 g saturated)
250 mg sodium
4 g protein

Athenos Traditional Crumbled Feta
(¼ cup/34 g)

90 calories
7 g fat
(4 g saturated)
400 mg sodium
6 g protein

A reasonable fat-to-protein ratio makes feta the most reliable go-to crumbled cheese.

The Laughing Cow Original Creamy Swiss
(1 wedge/21 g)

50 calories
4 g fat
(2.5 g saturated)
210 mg sodium
2 g protein

Spreads every bit as easily as Alouette's, yet it cuts your calorie load by a third.

Cabot 50% Reduced Fat Sharp Cheddar
(28 g)

70 calories
4.5 g fat
(3 g saturated)
170 mg sodium
8 g protein

A smart approach: Cut half the fat, but leave enough to add a rich, creamy texture.

Sargento Reduced Fat Sharp Cheddar Sticks
(1 stick/21 g)

60 calories
4.5 g fat
(3 g saturated)
135 mg sodium
5 g protein

Portable snacks don't get any better than this.

Kraft Authentic Mexican Style
(¼ cup/28 g)

90 calories
7 g fat
(4 g saturated)
200 mg sodium
6 g protein

Bagged cheese blends tend to carry a heavy caloric toll, but this Mexican mix is a good option for all your melting needs.

Kraft Shredded Parmesan Cheese
(2 tsp)

18 calories
1 g fat
(0 g saturated)
68 mg sodium
1.5 g protein

Consider this the leanest way to add big flavor to your pastas and baked potatoes.

Not That!

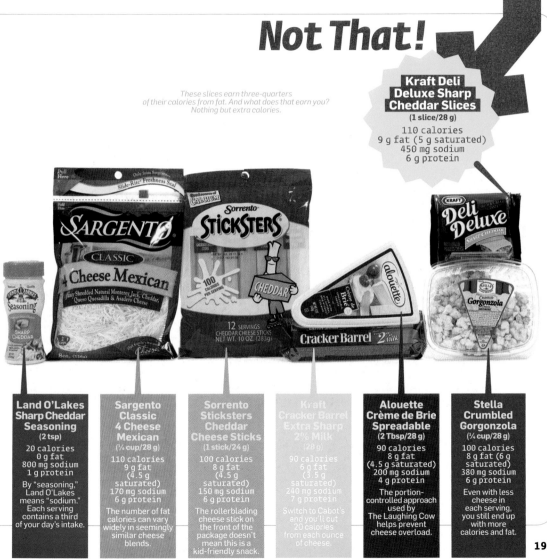

These slices earn three-quarters of their calories from fat. And what does that earn you? Nothing but extra calories.

Kraft Deli Deluxe Sharp Cheddar Slices
(1 slice/28 g)

110 calories
9 g fat (5 g saturated)
450 mg sodium
6 g protein

Land O'Lakes Sharp Cheddar Seasoning
(2 tsp)

20 calories
0 g fat
800 mg sodium
1 g protein

By "seasoning," Land O'Lakes means "sodium." Each serving contains a third of your day's intake.

Sargento Classic 4 Cheese Mexican
(¼ cup/28 g)

110 calories
9 g fat
(4.5 g saturated)
170 mg sodium
6 g protein

The number of fat calories can vary widely in seemingly similar cheese blends.

Sorrento Sticksters Cheddar Cheese Sticks
(1 stick/24 g)

100 calories
8 g fat
(4.5 g saturated)
150 mg sodium
6 g protein

The rollerblading cheese stick on the front of the package doesn't mean this is a kid-friendly snack.

Kraft Cracker Barrel Extra Sharp 2% Milk
(28 g)

90 calories
6 g fat
(3.5 g saturated)
240 mg sodium
7 g protein

Switch to Cabot's and you'll cut 20 calories from each ounce of cheese.

Alouette Crème de Brie Spreadable
(2 Tbsp/28 g)

90 calories
8 g fat
(4.5 g saturated)
200 mg sodium
4 g protein

The portion-controlled approach used by The Laughing Cow helps prevent cheese overload.

Stella Crumbled Gorgonzola
(¼ cup/28 g)

100 calories
8 g fat (6 g saturated)
380 mg sodium
6 g protein

Even with less cheese in each serving, you still end up with more calories and fat.

Deli Meats

Eat This

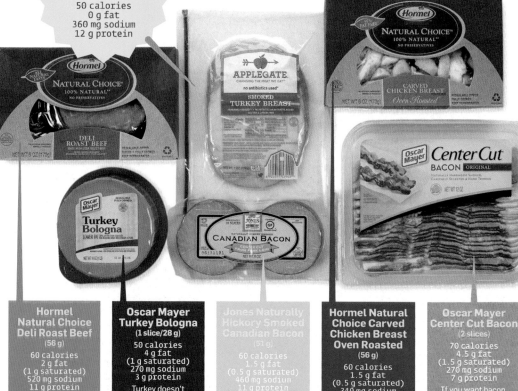

Applegate Smoked Turkey Breast
(56 g)

50 calories
0 g fat
360 mg sodium
12 g protein

Applegate Farms eschews antibiotics, producing some of the most pristine, natural meats in the supermarket.

Hormel Natural Choice Deli Roast Beef
(56 g)

60 calories
2 g fat
(1 g saturated)
520 mg sodium
11 g protein

One of the few deli brands to forgo all nitrites, nitrates, and other preservatives.

Oscar Mayer Turkey Bologna
(1 slice/28 g)

50 calories
4 g fat
(1 g saturated)
270 mg sodium
3 g protein

Turkey doesn't always mean healthier. This time it does.

Jones Naturally Hickory Smoked Canadian Bacon
(51 g)

60 calories
1.5 g fat
(0.5 g saturated)
460 mg sodium
11 g protein

The easiest swap in the supermarket; you get twice as much food for half the calories.

Hormel Natural Choice Carved Chicken Breast Oven Roasted
(56 g)

60 calories
1.5 g fat
(0.5 g saturated)
340 mg sodium
12 g protein

This chicken is almost pure protein.

Oscar Mayer Center Cut Bacon
(2 slices)

70 calories
4.5 g fat
(1.5 g saturated)
270 mg sodium
7 g protein

If you want bacon, eat bacon. You won't take in any extra calories or fat grams and you'll actually cut sodium.

Not That!

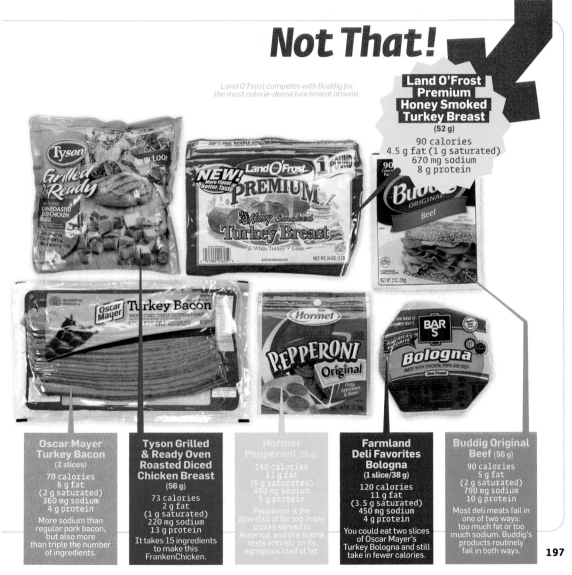

Land O'Frost competes with Buddig for the most calorie-dense lunchmeat around.

Land O'Frost Premium Honey Smoked Turkey Breast
(52 g)

90 calories
4.5 g fat (1 g saturated)
670 mg sodium
8 g protein

Oscar Mayer Turkey Bacon
(2 slices)

70 calories
6 g fat
(2 g saturated)
360 mg sodium
4 g protein

More sodium than regular pork bacon, but also more than triple the number of ingredients.

Tyson Grilled & Ready Oven Roasted Diced Chicken Breast
(56 g)

73 calories
2 g fat
(1 g saturated)
220 mg sodium
13 g protein

It takes 15 ingredients to make this FrankenChicken.

Hormel Pepperoni (28 g)

140 calories
13 g fat
(6 g saturated)
490 mg sodium
5 g protein

Pepperoni is the downfall of far too many pizzas served in America, and the blame rests entirely on its egregious load of fat.

Farmland Deli Favorites Bologna
(1 slice/38 g)

120 calories
11 g fat
(3.5 g saturated)
450 mg sodium
4 g protein

You could eat two slices of Oscar Mayer's Turkey Bologna and still take in fewer calories.

Buddig Original Beef (56 g)

90 calories
5 g fat
(2 g saturated)
790 mg sodium
10 g protein

Most deli meats fail in one of two ways: too much fat or too much sodium. Buddig's products routinely fail in both ways.

197

Hot Dogs and Sausages

Eat This

There's no reason to fear hot dogs.
A recent study from Kansas State University found that
microwave-cooked hot dogs have fewer cancer-causing compounds
than even rotisserie chicken. Stick with low-calorie brands
and you're never far from a quick, healthy, and protein-packed meal.

Hebrew National 97% Fat Free Beef Franks
(1 frank/45 g)

40 calories
1 g fat (0 g saturated)
520 mg sodium
6 g protein

Johnsonville Chicken Sausage Chipotle Monterey Jack Cheese (1 link/85 g)

170 calories
12 g fat
(4 g saturated)
770 mg sodium
13 g protein

We're glad to see the sausage behemoth get on board with the chicken variety.

Applegate Farms The Great Organic Hot Dogs
(1 frank/56 g)

110 calories
8 g fat
(3 g saturated)
330 mg sodium
7 g protein

Applegate Farms has re-created the famous frank of New York, but it's done so without resorting to dubious waste cuts or antibiotic-heavy meat.

Aidells Cajun Style Andouille
(1 link/85 g)

160 calories
11 g fat
(4 g saturated)
600 mg sodium
15 g protein

Remember Aidells. It's one of the most reliable purveyors in the deli fridge.

Al Fresco Chipotle Chorizo Chicken Sausage
(1 link/85 g)

140 calories
7 g fat
(2 g saturated)
420 mg sodium
15 g protein

Our love for Al Fresco runs deep. No company offers a wider variety of bold-flavored, low-calorie sausages.

Jennie-O Turkey Breakfast Sausage Links Lean (2 links/56 g)

90 calories
5 g fat
(1.5 g saturated)
370 mg sodium
10 g protein

Cutting fat doesn't just drop the calorie count, it also makes more space for protein.

Not That!

Hot dogs vary widely in terms of fat content,
so it's important to flip the package and scan the ingredients list.
Case in point: You could eat half a dozen of
the Hebrew National dogs on the opposite page and still not reach
the fat load of these "light" franks.

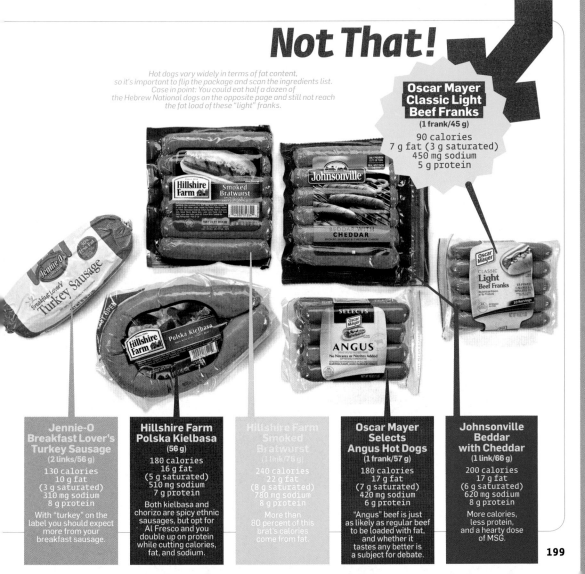

Oscar Mayer Classic Light Beef Franks
(1 frank/45 g)

90 calories
7 g fat (3 g saturated)
450 mg sodium
5 g protein

Jennie-O Breakfast Lover's Turkey Sausage
(2 links/56 g)

130 calories
10 g fat
(3 g saturated)
310 mg sodium
8 g protein

With "turkey" on the label you should expect more from your breakfast sausage.

Hillshire Farm Polska Kielbasa
(56 g)

180 calories
16 g fat
(5 g saturated)
510 mg sodium
7 g protein

Both kielbasa and chorizo are spicy ethnic sausages, but opt for Al Fresco and you double up on protein while cutting calories, fat, and sodium.

Hillshire Farm Smoked Bratwurst
(1 link/76 g)

240 calories
22 g fat
(8 g saturated)
780 mg sodium
8 g protein

More than 80 percent of this brat's calories come from fat.

Oscar Mayer Selects Angus Hot Dogs
(1 frank/57 g)

180 calories
17 g fat
(7 g saturated)
420 mg sodium
6 g protein

"Angus" beef is just as likely as regular beef to be loaded with fat, and whether it tastes any better is a subject for debate.

Johnsonville Beddar with Cheddar
(1 link/66 g)

200 calories
17 g fat
(6 g saturated)
620 mg sodium
8 g protein

More calories, less protein, and a hearty dose of MSG.

199

Condiments

Eat This

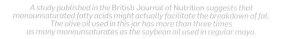

A study published in the British Journal of Nutrition suggests that monounsaturated fatty acids might actually facilitate the breakdown of fat. The olive oil used in this jar has more than three times as many monounsaturates as the soybean oil used in regular mayo.

Kraft Mayo with Olive Oil
(1 Tbsp/15 g)

45 calories
4 g fat (0 g saturated)
95 mg sodium
<1 g sugars

The Rib House Medium BBQ Sauce
(2 Tbsp/31 g)

25 calories
0 g fat
240 mg sodium
6 g sugars

The Rib House's sauce earns a touch of sweetness from brown sugar, but its primary ingredients are tomato paste and vinegar. This is as good as barbecue sauce gets.

Annie's Naturals Organic Horseradish Mustard
(2 tsp/10 g)

10 calories
0 g fat
120 mg sodium
0 g sugars

This bottle contains no ingredients that you wouldn't have in your kitchen.

Annie's Naturals Organic Ketchup
(1 Tbsp/17 g)

15 calories
0 g fat
170 mg sodium
4 g sugars

Go ahead and spring for organic. Research shows that organically raised tomatoes produce nearly twice as much cancer-fighting lycopene.

Grey Poupon Savory Honey Mustard
(1 Tbsp/15 g)

30 calories
0 g fat
15 mg sodium
3 g sugars

Made mostly from mustard seeds, which are loaded with omega-3 fatty acids.

Ocean Spray Whole Berry Cranberry Sauce
(2 Tbsp/35 g)

55 calories
0 g fat
5 g carbohydrates
5 mg sodium
11 g sugars

Not just for Thanksgiving anymore. Turn to cranberry sauce for a low-calorie, high-antioxidant sandwich companion.

McCormick Fat Free Tartar Sauce
(2 Tbsp/32 g)

30 calories
0 g fat
250 mg sodium
5 g sugars

Although by no means a nutritious condiment, this light take on tartar does eliminate more than 100 calories per serving.

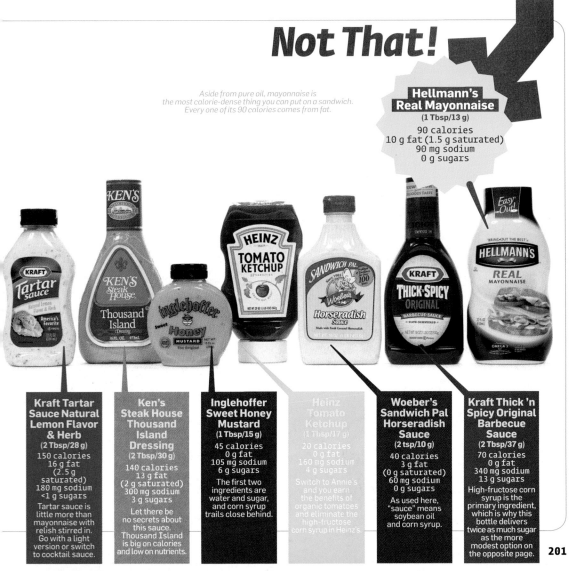

Not That!

*Aside from pure oil, mayonnaise is
the most calorie-dense thing you can put on a sandwich.
Every one of its 90 calories comes from fat.*

**Hellmann's
Real Mayonnaise**
(1 Tbsp/13 g)
90 calories
10 g fat (1.5 g saturated)
90 mg sodium
0 g sugars

**Kraft Tartar
Sauce Natural
Lemon Flavor
& Herb**
(2 Tbsp/28 g)
150 calories
16 g fat
(2.5 g
saturated)
180 mg sodium
<1 g sugars

Tartar sauce is
little more than
mayonnaise with
relish stirred in.
Go with a light
version or switch
to cocktail sauce.

**Ken's
Steak House
Thousand
Island
Dressing**
(2 Tbsp/30 g)
140 calories
13 g fat
(2 g saturated)
300 mg sodium
3 g sugars

Let there be
no secrets about
this sauce.
Thousand Island
is big on calories
and low on nutrients.

**Inglehoffer
Sweet Honey
Mustard**
(1 Tbsp/15 g)
45 calories
0 g fat
105 mg sodium
6 g sugars

The first two
ingredients are
water and sugar,
and corn syrup
trails close behind.

**Heinz
Tomato
Ketchup**
(1 Tbsp/17 g)
20 calories
0 g fat
160 mg sodium
4 g sugars

Switch to Annie's
and you earn
the benefits of
organic tomatoes
and eliminate the
high-fructose
corn syrup in Heinz's.

**Woeber's
Sandwich Pal
Horseradish
Sauce**
(2 tsp/10 g)
40 calories
3 g fat
(0 g saturated)
60 mg sodium
0 g sugars

As used here,
"sauce" means
soybean oil
and corn syrup.

**Kraft Thick 'n
Spicy Original
Barbecue
Sauce**
(2 Tbsp/37 g)
70 calories
0 g fat
340 mg sodium
13 g sugars

High-fructose corn
syrup is the
primary ingredient,
which is why this
bottle delivers
twice as much sugar
as the more
modest option on
the opposite page.

Breads

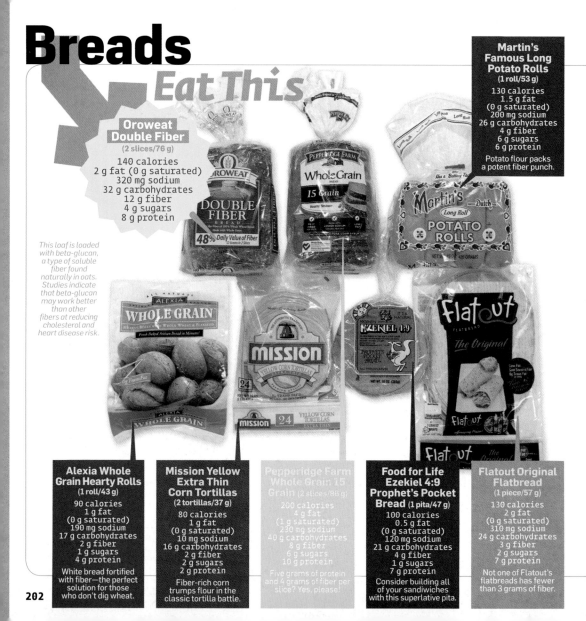

Eat This

Oroweat Double Fiber
(2 slices/76 g)

140 calories
2 g fat (0 g saturated)
320 mg sodium
32 g carbohydrates
12 g fiber
4 g sugars
8 g protein

This loaf is loaded with beta-glucan, a type of soluble fiber found naturally in oats. Studies indicate that beta-glucan may work better than other fibers at reducing cholesterol and heart disease risk.

Martin's Famous Long Potato Rolls
(1 roll/53 g)

130 calories
1.5 g fat
(0 g saturated)
200 mg sodium
26 g carbohydrates
4 g fiber
6 g sugars
6 g protein

Potato flour packs a potent fiber punch.

Alexia Whole Grain Hearty Rolls
(1 roll—43 g)

90 calories
1 g fat
(0 g saturated)
190 mg sodium
17 g carbohydrates
2 g fiber
1 g sugars
4 g protein

White bread fortified with fiber—the perfect solution for those who don't dig wheat.

Mission Yellow Extra Thin Corn Tortillas
(2 tortillas/37 g)

80 calories
1 g fat
(0 g saturated)
10 mg sodium
16 g carbohydrates
2 g fiber
2 g sugars
2 g protein

Fiber-rich corn trumps flour in the classic tortilla battle.

Pepperidge Farm Whole Grain 15 Grain (2 slices/86 g)

200 calories
4 g fat
(1 g saturated)
230 mg sodium
40 g carbohydrates
8 g fiber
6 g sugars
10 g protein

Five grams of protein and 4 grams of fiber per slice? Yes, please!

Food for Life Ezekiel 4:9 Prophet's Pocket Bread (1 pita/47 g)

100 calories
0.5 g fat
(0 g saturated)
120 mg sodium
21 g carbohydrates
4 g fiber
1 g sugars
7 g protein

Consider building all of your sandwiches with this superlative pita.

Flatout Original Flatbread
(1 piece/57 g)

130 calories
2 g fat
(0 g saturated)
310 mg sodium
24 g carbohydrates
3 g fiber
2 g sugars
7 g protein

Not one of Flatout's flatbreads has fewer than 3 grams of fiber.

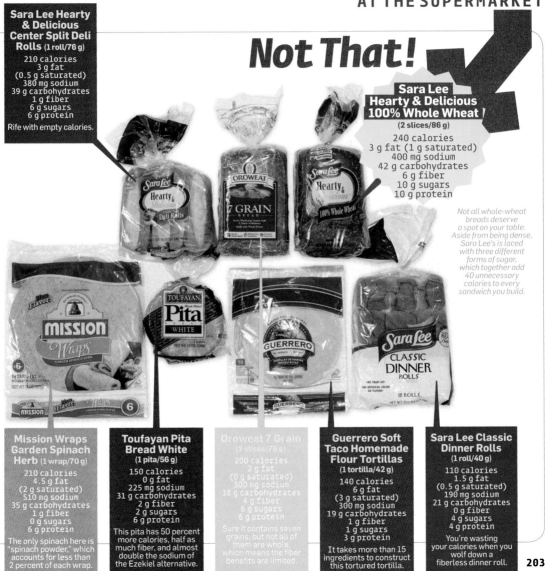

Not That!

Sara Lee Hearty & Delicious Center Split Deli Rolls (1 roll/76 g)

210 calories
3 g fat
(0.5 g saturated)
380 mg sodium
39 g carbohydrates
1 g fiber
6 g sugars
6 g protein

Rife with empty calories.

Sara Lee Hearty & Delicious 100% Whole Wheat (2 slices/86 g)

240 calories
3 g fat (1 g saturated)
400 mg sodium
42 g carbohydrates
6 g fiber
10 g sugars
10 g protein

Not all whole-wheat breads deserve a spot on your table. Aside from being dense, Sara Lee's is laced with three different forms of sugar, which together add 40 unnecessary calories to every sandwich you build.

Mission Wraps Garden Spinach Herb (1 wrap/70 g)

210 calories
4.5 g fat
(2 g saturated)
510 mg sodium
35 g carbohydrates
1 g fiber
0 g sugars
6 g protein

The only spinach here is "spinach powder," which accounts for less than 2 percent of each wrap.

Toufayan Pita Bread White (1 pita/56 g)

150 calories
0 g fat
225 mg sodium
31 g carbohydrates
2 g fiber
2 g sugars
6 g protein

This pita has 50 percent more calories, half as much fiber, and almost double the sodium of the Ezekiel alternative.

Oroweat 7 Grain (2 slices/76 g)

200 calories
2 g fat
(0 g saturated)
300 mg sodium
38 g carbohydrates
4 g fiber
6 g sugars
6 g protein

Sure it contains seven grains, but not all of them are whole, which means the fiber benefits are limited.

Guerrero Soft Taco Homemade Flour Tortillas (1 tortilla/42 g)

140 calories
6 g fat
(3 g saturated)
300 mg sodium
19 g carbohydrates
1 g fiber
1 g sugars
3 g protein

It takes more than 15 ingredients to construct this tortured tortilla.

Sara Lee Classic Dinner Rolls (1 roll/40 g)

110 calories
1.5 g fat
(0.5 g saturated)
190 mg sodium
21 g carbohydrates
0 g fiber
4 g sugars
4 g protein

You're wasting your calories when you wolf down a fiberless dinner roll.

203

Grains & Noodles
Eat This

Whole-grain pastas are loaded with fiber, and diets rich in fiber are shown to decrease your odds of developing either diabetes or heart disease. You want about 20 grams per day, and this spaghetti has 30 percent of that.

Near East Rice Pilaf Mix with Lentil (¼ cup/56 g dry)

180 calories
0.5 g fat
(0 g saturated)
650 mg sodium
36 g carbohydrates
8 g fiber

This box contains exactly seven ingredients, and you probably have every one of them in your pantry.

Ronzoni Healthy Harvest Whole Grain Spaghetti (56 g dry)

180 calories
1 g fat (0 g saturated)
41 g carbohydrates
6 g fiber

Ronzoni Smart Taste Penne Rigate (56 g dry)

170 calories
0.5 g fat
(0 g saturated)
40 g carbohydrates
5 g fiber

Whole-wheat pasta can be a gritty departure from normal noodles, but Smart Taste combines fiber with the taste of white pasta.

Minute Brown Rice (½ cup/43 g dry)

150 calories
1.5 g fat
(0 g saturated)
34 g carbohydrates
2 g fiber

Eating healthy doesn't take more time, just smart decisions in the supermarket.

House Foods Tofu Shirataki Angel Hair (113 g)

20 calories
0.5 g fat
(0 g saturated)
3 g carbohydrates
2 g fiber

These traditional Asian noodles are made from tofu and yam flour. Don't be afraid—they have a neutral flavor that's perfect for dressing up.

Eden Organic Red Quinoa (¼ cup/45 g dry)

170 calories
2 g fat
(0 g saturated)
32 g carbohydrates
5 g fiber

Quinoa contains every amino acid your body needs from food. That's a claim rice can't make.

Bob's Red Mill Pearl Barley (¼ cup/50 g dry)

180 calories
1 g fat
(0 g saturated)
39 g carbohydrates
8 g fiber

Perfect for adding nutritional heft to everyday soups. Try using it as a replacement for noodles in minestrone.

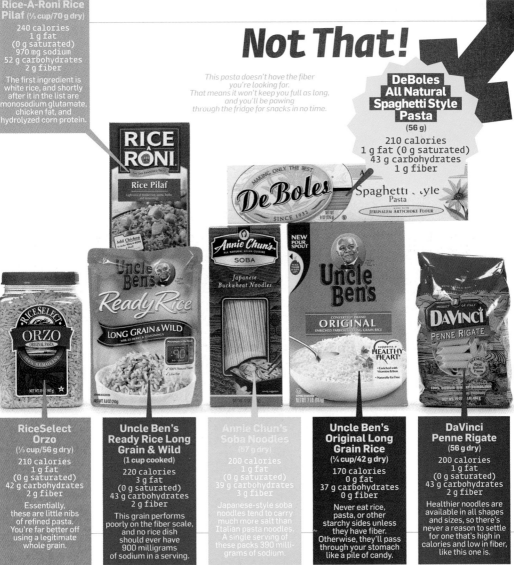

Not That!

Rice-A-Roni Rice Pilaf (⅓ cup/70 g dry)

240 calories
1 g fat
(0 g saturated)
970 mg sodium
52 g carbohydrates
2 g fiber

The first ingredient is white rice, and shortly after it in the list are monosodium glutamate, chicken fat, and hydrolyzed corn protein.

This pasta doesn't have the fiber you're looking for. That means it won't keep you full as long, and you'll be pawing through the fridge for snacks in no time.

DeBoles All Natural Spaghetti Style Pasta
(56 g)

210 calories
1 g fat (0 g saturated)
43 g carbohydrates
1 g fiber

RiceSelect Orzo
(⅓ cup/56 g dry)

210 calories
1 g fat
(0 g saturated)
42 g carbohydrates
2 g fiber

Essentially, these are little nibs of refined pasta. You're far better off using a legitimate whole grain.

Uncle Ben's Ready Rice Long Grain & Wild
(1 cup cooked)

220 calories
3 g fat
(0 g saturated)
43 g carbohydrates
2 g fiber

This grain performs poorly on the fiber scale, and no rice dish should ever have 900 milligrams of sodium in a serving.

Annie Chun's Soba Noodles
(57 g dry)

200 calories
1 g fat
(0 g saturated)
39 g carbohydrates
3 g fiber

Japanese-style soba noodles tend to carry much more salt than Italian pasta noodles. A single serving of these packs 390 milligrams of sodium.

Uncle Ben's Original Long Grain Rice
(¼ cup/42 g dry)

170 calories
0 g fat
37 g carbohydrates
0 g fiber

Never eat rice, pasta, or other starchy sides unless they have fiber. Otherwise, they'll pass through your stomach like a pile of candy.

DaVinci Penne Rigate
(56 g dry)

200 calories
1 g fat
(0 g saturated)
43 g carbohydrates
2 g fiber

Healthier noodles are available in all shapes and sizes, so there's never a reason to settle for one that's high in calories and low in fiber, like this one is.

Sauces

Eat This

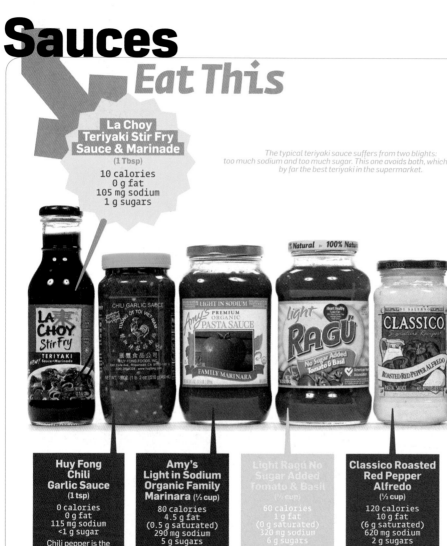

La Choy Teriyaki Stir Fry Sauce & Marinade

(1 Tbsp)

10 calories
0 g fat
105 mg sodium
1 g sugars

The typical teriyaki sauce suffers from two blights: too much sodium and too much sugar. This one avoids both, which makes it by far the best teriyaki in the supermarket.

Huy Fong Chili Garlic Sauce (1 tsp)

0 calories
0 g fat
115 mg sodium
<1 g sugar

Chili pepper is the primary ingredient, and it contains not a single gram of added sugar.

Amy's Light in Sodium Organic Family Marinara (½ cup)

80 calories
4.5 g fat
(0.5 g saturated)
290 mg sodium
5 g sugars

Stick with the low-sodium version. Amy's regular marinara has 290 mg more sodium.

Light Ragú No Sugar Added Tomato & Basil (½ cup)

60 calories
1 g fat
(0 g saturated)
320 mg sodium
6 g sugars

Think Italians add sugar to their marinara? Of course not—added sugars mask the naturally sweet flavor of cooked tomatoes.

Classico Roasted Red Pepper Alfredo (½ cup)

120 calories
10 g fat
(6 g saturated)
620 mg sodium
2 g sugars

Smart move: The roasted red peppers in this jar displace a heavy load of fatty cream and cheese calories.

Muir Glen Organic Cabernet Marinara (½ cup)

60 calories
1 g fat
(0 g saturated)
360 mg sodium
4 g sugars

Cabernet is king of the alcohol-imbued pasta sauces. It's rich and complex and doesn't require a glut of cream to impart its footprint on a bowl of spaghetti.

Not That!

If you end up with 2 tablespoons of this stuff on your plate, you'll be about to take in almost half your day's sodium and more sugar than you'd find in a scoop of Edy's Slow Churned Double Fudge Brownie Ice Cream.

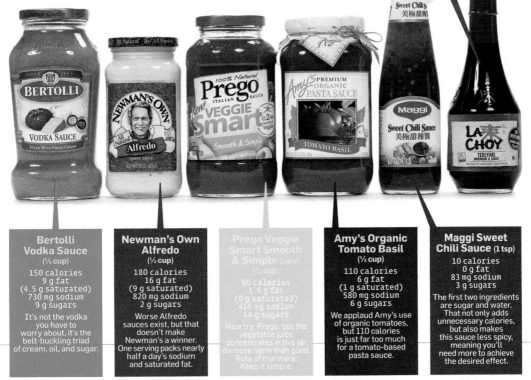

La Choy Teriyaki Marinade and Sauce
(1 Tbsp)
40 calories
0 g fat
570 mg sodium
8 g sugars

Bertolli Vodka Sauce
(½ cup)

150 calories
9 g fat
(4.5 g saturated)
730 mg sodium
9 g sugars

It's not the vodka you have to worry about, it's the belt-buckling triad of cream, oil, and sugar.

Newman's Own Alfredo
(½ cup)

180 calories
16 g fat
(9 g saturated)
820 mg sodium
2 g sugars

Worse Alfredo sauces exist, but that doesn't make Newman's a winner. One serving packs nearly half a day's sodium and saturated fat.

Prego Veggie Smart Smooth & Simple (new)
(½ cup)

90 calories
1.5 g fat
(0 g saturated)
410 mg sodium
14 g sugars

Nice try, Prego, but the vegetable juice concentrates in this jar do more harm than good. Rule of marinara: Keep it simple.

Amy's Organic Tomato Basil
(½ cup)

110 calories
6 g fat
(1 g saturated)
580 mg sodium
6 g sugars

We applaud Amy's use of organic tomatoes, but 110 calories is just far too much for a tomato-based pasta sauce.

Maggi Sweet Chili Sauce (1 tsp)

10 calories
0 g fat
83 mg sodium
3 g sugars

The first two ingredients are sugar and water. That not only adds unnecessary calories, but also makes this sauce less spicy, meaning you'll need more to achieve the desired effect.

Soups

Eat This

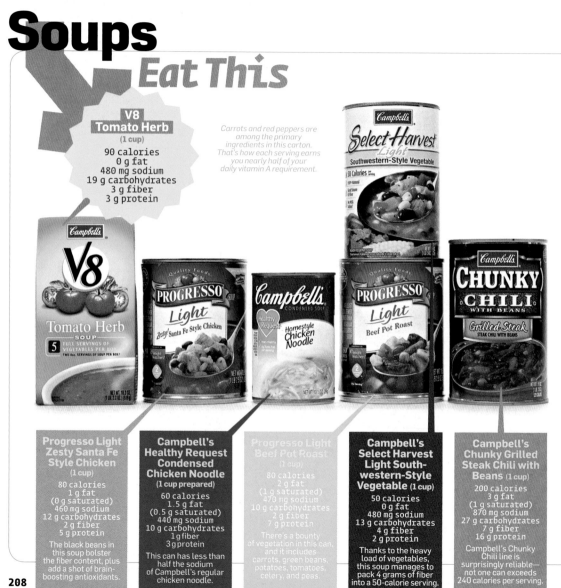

V8 Tomato Herb (1 cup)

90 calories
0 g fat
480 mg sodium
19 g carbohydrates
3 g fiber
3 g protein

Carrots and red peppers are among the primary ingredients in this carton. That's how each serving earns you nearly half of your daily vitamin A requirement.

Progresso Light Zesty Santa Fe Style Chicken (1 cup)

80 calories
1 g fat
(0 g saturated)
460 mg sodium
12 g carbohydrates
2 g fiber
5 g protein

The black beans in this soup bolster the fiber content, plus add a shot of brain-boosting antioxidants.

Campbell's Healthy Request Condensed Chicken Noodle (1 cup prepared)

60 calories
1.5 g fat
(0.5 g saturated)
440 mg sodium
10 g carbohydrates
1 g fiber
3 g protein

This can has less than half the sodium of Campbell's regular chicken noodle.

Progresso Light Beef Pot Roast (1 cup)

80 calories
2 g fat
(1 g saturated)
470 mg sodium
10 g carbohydrates
2 g fiber
7 g protein

There's a bounty of vegetation in this can, and it includes carrots, green beans, potatoes, tomatoes, celery, and peas.

Campbell's Select Harvest Light Southwestern-Style Vegetable (1 cup)

50 calories
0 g fat
480 mg sodium
13 g carbohydrates
4 g fiber
2 g protein

Thanks to the heavy load of vegetables, this soup manages to pack 4 grams of fiber into a 50-calorie serving.

Campbell's Chunky Grilled Steak Chili with Beans (1 cup)

200 calories
3 g fat
(1 g saturated)
870 mg sodium
27 g carbohydrates
7 g fiber
16 g protein

Campbell's Chunky Chili line is surprisingly reliable—not one can exceeds 240 calories per serving.

Not That!

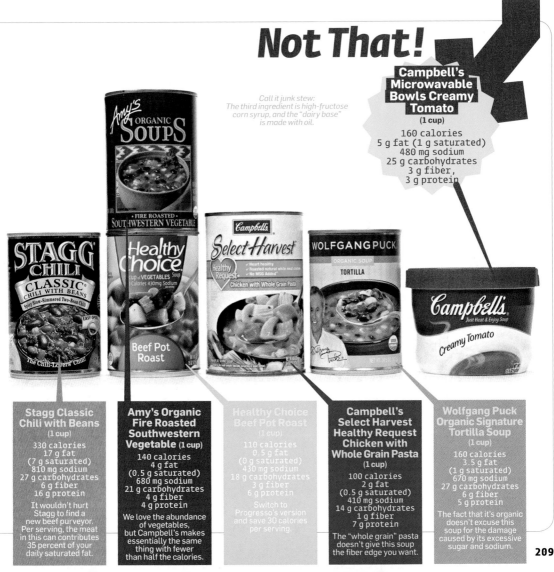

Call it junk stew:
The third ingredient is high-fructose
corn syrup, and the "dairy base"
is made with oil.

**Campbell's
Microwavable
Bowls Creamy
Tomato**
(1 cup)

160 calories
5 g fat (1 g saturated)
480 mg sodium
25 g carbohydrates
3 g fiber,
3 g protein

**Stagg Classic
Chili with Beans**
(1 cup)

330 calories
17 g fat
(7 g saturated)
810 mg sodium
27 g carbohydrates
6 g fiber
16 g protein

It wouldn't hurt
Stagg to find a
new beef purveyor.
Per serving, the meat
in this can contributes
35 percent of your
daily saturated fat.

**Amy's Organic
Fire Roasted
Southwestern
Vegetable** (1 cup)

140 calories
4 g fat
(0.5 g saturated)
680 mg sodium
21 g carbohydrates
4 g fiber
4 g protein

We love the abundance
of vegetables,
but Campbell's makes
essentially the same
thing with fewer
than half the calories.

**Healthy Choice
Beef Pot Roast**
(1 cup)

110 calories
0.5 g fat
(0 g saturated)
430 mg sodium
18 g carbohydrates
3 g fiber
6 g protein

Switch to
Progresso's version
and save 30 calories
per serving.

**Campbell's
Select Harvest
Healthy Request
Chicken with
Whole Grain Pasta**
(1 cup)

100 calories
2 g fat
(0.5 g saturated)
410 mg sodium
14 g carbohydrates
1 g fiber
7 g protein

The "whole grain" pasta
doesn't give this soup
the fiber edge you want.

**Wolfgang Puck
Organic Signature
Tortilla Soup**
(1 cup)

160 calories
3.5 g fat
(1 g saturated)
670 mg sodium
27 g carbohydrates
6 g fiber
5 g protein

The fact that it's organic
doesn't excuse this
soup for the damage
caused by its excessive
sugar and sodium.

209

Bars

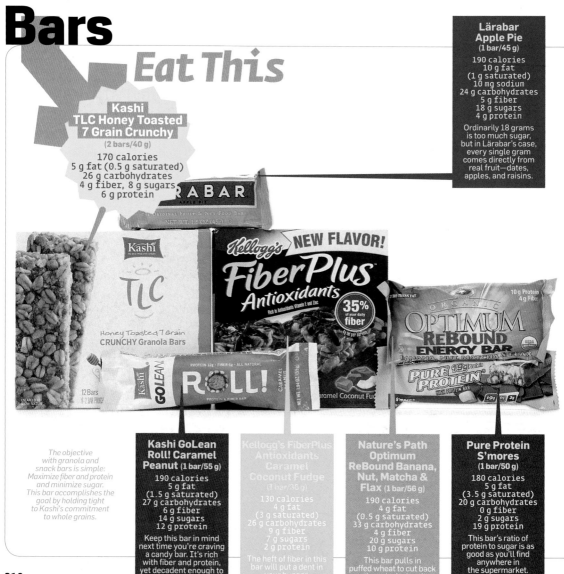

Eat This

Kashi TLC Honey Toasted 7 Grain Crunchy
(2 bars/40 g)

170 calories
5 g fat (0.5 g saturated)
26 g carbohydrates
4 g fiber, 8 g sugars
6 g protein

Lärabar Apple Pie
(1 bar/45 g)

190 calories
10 g fat
(1 g saturated)
10 mg sodium
24 g carbohydrates
5 g fiber
18 g sugars
4 g protein

Ordinarily 18 grams is too much sugar, but in Lärabar's case, every single gram comes directly from real fruit—dates, apples, and raisins.

The objective with granola and snack bars is simple: Maximize fiber and protein and minimize sugar. This bar accomplishes the goal by holding tight to Kashi's commitment to whole grains.

Kashi GoLean Roll! Caramel Peanut (1 bar/55 g)

190 calories
5 g fat
(1.5 g saturated)
27 g carbohydrates
6 g fiber
14 g sugars
12 g protein

Keep this bar in mind next time you're craving a candy bar. It's rich with fiber and protein, yet decadent enough to soothe a sweet tooth.

Kellogg's FiberPlus Antioxidants Caramel Coconut Fudge
(1 bar/30 g)

130 calories
4 g fat
(3 g saturated)
26 g carbohydrates
9 g fiber
7 g sugars
2 g protein

The heft of fiber in this bar will put a dent in your hunger.

Nature's Path Optimum ReBound Banana, Nut, Matcha & Flax (1 bar/56 g)

190 calories
4 g fat
(0.5 g saturated)
33 g carbohydrates
4 g fiber
20 g sugars
10 g protein

This bar pulls in puffed wheat to cut back on the caloric density.

Pure Protein S'mores
(1 bar/50 g)

180 calories
5 g fat
(3.5 g saturated)
20 g carbohydrates
0 g fiber
2 g sugars
19 g protein

This bar's ratio of protein to sugar is as good as you'll find anywhere in the supermarket.

Not That!

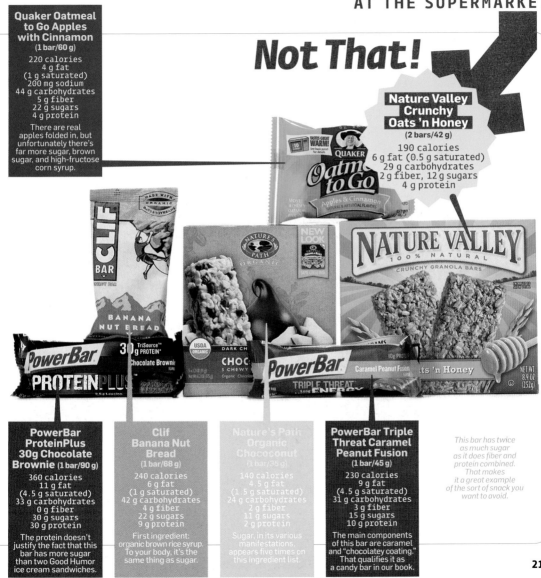

Quaker Oatmeal to Go Apples with Cinnamon
(1 bar/60 g)

220 calories
4 g fat
(1 g saturated)
200 mg sodium
44 g carbohydrates
5 g fiber
22 g sugars
4 g protein

There are real apples folded in, but unfortunately there's far more sugar, brown sugar, and high-fructose corn syrup.

Nature Valley Crunchy Oats 'n Honey
(2 bars/42 g)

190 calories
6 g fat (0.5 g saturated)
29 g carbohydrates
2 g fiber, 12 g sugars
4 g protein

PowerBar ProteinPlus 30g Chocolate Brownie (1 bar/90 g)

360 calories
11 g fat
(4.5 g saturated)
33 g carbohydrates
0 g fiber
30 g sugars
30 g protein

The protein doesn't justify the fact that this bar has more sugar than two Good Humor ice cream sandwiches.

Clif Banana Nut Bread (1 bar/68 g)

240 calories
6 g fat
(1 g saturated)
42 g carbohydrates
4 g fiber
22 g sugars
9 g protein

First ingredient: organic brown rice syrup. To your body, it's the same thing as sugar.

Nature's Path Organic Chococonut (1 bar/35 g)

140 calories
4.5 g fat
(1.5 g saturated)
24 g carbohydrates
2 g fiber
11 g sugars
2 g protein

Sugar, in its various manifestations, appears five times on this ingredient list.

PowerBar Triple Threat Caramel Peanut Fusion (1 bar/45 g)

230 calories
9 g fat
(4.5 g saturated)
31 g carbohydrates
3 g fiber
15 g sugars
10 g protein

The main components of this bar are caramel and "chocolaty coating." That qualifies it as a candy bar in our book.

This bar has twice as much sugar as it does fiber and protein combined. That makes it a great example of the sort of snack you want to avoid.

Crackers

Eat This

The primary ingredient here is whole-wheat fiber, which is precisely what you want. The extra fiber—a form of oat fiber that Nabisco adds to this Fiber Selects line—is just a bonus.

Wheat Thins Fiber Selects Garden Vegetable
(15 crackers/30 g)

120 calories
4 g fat (0.5 g saturated)
260 mg sodium
22 g carbohydrates
5 g fiber

Pepperidge Farm Baked Naturals Cheese Crisps
(20 pieces/30 g)

140 calories
6 g fat
(1 g saturated)
270 mg sodium
19 g carbohydrates
1 g fiber

A touch of fiber and the use of real cheese help keep Pepperidge Farm's new cracker just outside the junk category.

Special K Multi-Grain Crackers
(24 crackers/30 g)

120 calories
3 g fat
(0 g saturated)
250 mg sodium
23 g carbohydrates
3 g fiber

This is as few calories as you can reasonably expect in a serving of whole-grain crackers.

Nabisco Triscuit Thin Crisps Original
(15 crackers/30 g)

130 calories
5 g fat
(1 g saturated)
180 mg sodium
21 g carbohydrates
3 g fiber

You can't beat the purity of this recipe: whole wheat, oil, and salt. Period.

Kellogg's Special K Sea Salt Cracker Chips
(30 crackers/30 g)

110 calories
2.5 g fat
(0 g saturated)
230 mg sodium
23 g carbohydrates
3 g fiber

Potato starch is used to bolster this cracker chip's fiber content.

Nabisco Wheat Thins Crunch Stix Chipotle Pepper
(14 pieces/29 g)

130 calories
4 g fat
(0.5 g saturated)
170 mg sodium
22 g carbohydrates
2 g fiber

Whole-grain flour is the first ingredient, a rarity with flavored novelty crackers.

RyKrisp Seasoned Crackers
(4 crackers/28 g)

120 calories
2 g fat
(0 g saturated)
180 mg sodium
22 g carbohydrates
6 g fiber

Prevention of gallstones is among the many benefits of foods high in insoluble fiber.

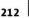

Not That!

As the name suggests, this cracker contains a handful of dehydrated vegetables. The problem is, the main ingredient is still refined flour, and it's bogged down with hydrogenated oils and high-fructose corn syrup.

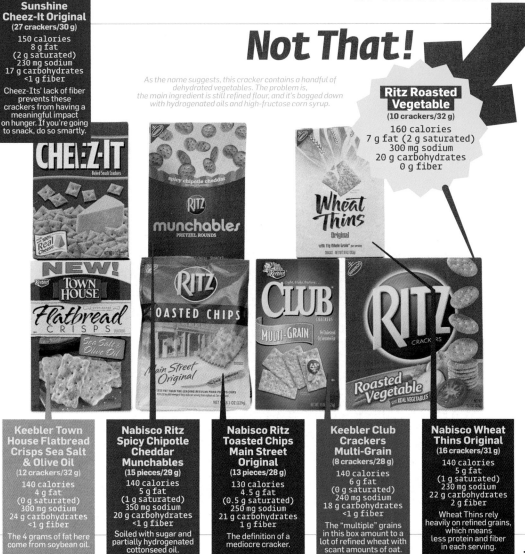

Sunshine Cheez-It Original
(27 crackers/30 g)

150 calories
8 g fat
(2 g saturated)
230 mg sodium
17 g carbohydrates
<1 g fiber

Cheez-Its' lack of fiber prevents these crackers from having a meaningful impact on hunger. If you're going to snack, do so smartly.

Ritz Roasted Vegetable
(10 crackers/32 g)

160 calories
7 g fat (2 g saturated)
300 mg sodium
20 g carbohydrates
0 g fiber

Keebler Town House Flatbread Crisps Sea Salt & Olive Oil
(12 crackers/32 g)

140 calories
4 g fat
(0 g saturated)
300 mg sodium
24 g carbohydrates
<1 g fiber

The 4 grams of fat here come from soybean oil.

Nabisco Ritz Spicy Chipotle Cheddar Munchables
(15 pieces/29 g)

140 calories
5 g fat
(1 g saturated)
350 mg sodium
20 g carbohydrates
<1 g fiber

Soiled with sugar and partially hydrogenated cottonseed oil.

Nabisco Ritz Toasted Chips Main Street Original
(13 pieces/28 g)

130 calories
4.5 g fat
(0.5 g saturated)
250 mg sodium
21 g carbohydrates
1 g fiber

The definition of a mediocre cracker.

Keebler Club Crackers Multi-Grain
(8 crackers/28 g)

140 calories
6 g fat
(0 g saturated)
240 mg sodium
18 g carbohydrates
<1 g fiber

The "multiple" grains in this box amount to a lot of refined wheat with scant amounts of oat.

Nabisco Wheat Thins Original
(16 crackers/31 g)

140 calories
5 g fat
(1 g saturated)
230 mg sodium
22 g carbohydrates
2 g fiber

Wheat Thins rely heavily on refined grains, which means less protein and fiber in each serving.

213

Chips

Eat This

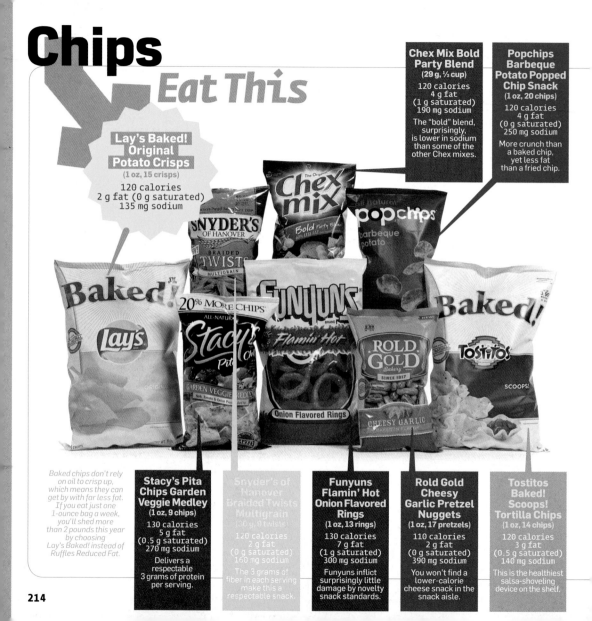

Chex Mix Bold Party Blend
(29 g, ⅓ cup)

120 calories
4 g fat
(1 g saturated)
190 mg sodium

The "bold" blend, surprisingly, is lower in sodium than some of the other Chex mixes.

Popchips Barbeque Potato Popped Chip Snack
(1 oz, 20 chips)

120 calories
4 g fat
(0 g saturated)
250 mg sodium

More crunch than a baked chip, yet less fat than a fried chip.

Lay's Baked! Original Potato Crisps

(1 oz, 15 crisps)

120 calories
2 g fat (0 g saturated)
135 mg sodium

Baked chips don't rely on oil to crisp up, which means they can get by with far less fat. If you eat just one 1-ounce bag a week, you'll shed more than 2 pounds this year by choosing Lay's Baked! instead of Ruffles Reduced Fat.

Stacy's Pita Chips Garden Veggie Medley
(1 oz, 9 chips)

130 calories
5 g fat
(0.5 g saturated)
270 mg sodium

Delivers a respectable 3 grams of protein per serving.

Snyder's of Hanover Braided Twists Multigrain
(30 g, 9 twists)

120 calories
2 g fat
(0 g saturated)
160 mg sodium

The 3 grams of fiber in each serving make this a respectable snack.

Funyuns Flamin' Hot Onion Flavored Rings
(1 oz, 13 rings)

130 calories
7 g fat
(1 g saturated)
300 mg sodium

Funyuns inflict surprisingly little damage by novelty snack standards.

Rold Gold Cheesy Garlic Pretzel Nuggets
(1 oz, 17 pretzels)

110 calories
2 g fat
(0 g saturated)
390 mg sodium

You won't find a lower-calorie cheese snack in the snack aisle.

Tostitos Baked! Scoops! Tortilla Chips
(1 oz, 14 chips)

120 calories
3 g fat
(0.5 g saturated)
140 mg sodium

This is the healthiest salsa-shoveling device on the shelf.

Not That!

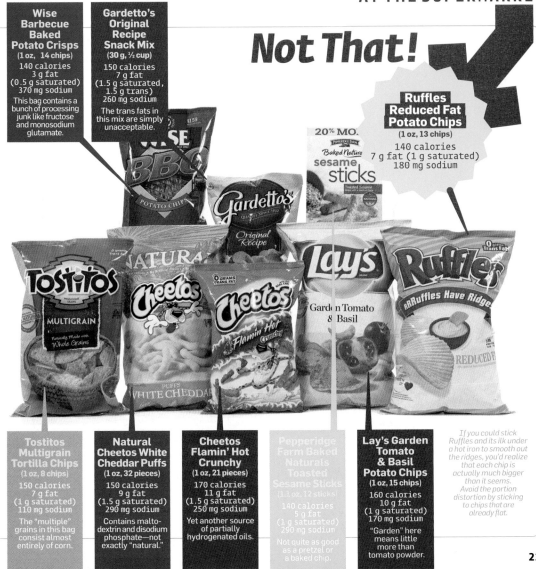

Wise Barbecue Baked Potato Crisps
(1 oz, 14 chips)
140 calories
3 g fat
(0.5 g saturated)
370 mg sodium

This bag contains a bunch of processing junk like fructose and monosodium glutamate.

Gardetto's Original Recipe Snack Mix
(30 g, ½ cup)
150 calories
7 g fat
(1.5 g saturated, 1.5 g trans)
260 mg sodium

The trans fats in this mix are simply unacceptable.

Ruffles Reduced Fat Potato Chips
(1 oz, 13 chips)
140 calories
7 g fat (1 g saturated)
180 mg sodium

Tostitos Multigrain Tortilla Chips
(1 oz, 8 chips)
150 calories
7 g fat
(1 g saturated)
110 mg sodium

The "multiple" grains in this bag consist almost entirely of corn.

Natural Cheetos White Cheddar Puffs
(1 oz, 32 pieces)
150 calories
9 g fat
(1.5 g saturated)
290 mg sodium

Contains maltodextrin and disodium phosphate—not exactly "natural."

Cheetos Flamin' Hot Crunchy
(1 oz, 21 pieces)
170 calories
11 g fat
(1.5 g saturated)
250 mg sodium

Yet another source of partially hydrogenated oils.

Pepperidge Farm Baked Naturals Toasted Sesame Sticks
(1.1 oz, 12 sticks)
140 calories
5 g fat
(1 g saturated)
290 mg sodium

Not quite as good as a pretzel or a baked chip.

Lay's Garden Tomato & Basil Potato Chips
(1 oz, 15 chips)
160 calories
10 g fat
(1 g saturated)
170 mg sodium

"Garden" here means little more than tomato powder.

If you could stick Ruffles and its ilk under a hot iron to smooth out the ridges, you'd realize that each chip is actually much bigger than it seems. Avoid the portion distortion by sticking to chips that are already flat.

Dips and Spreads

Eat This

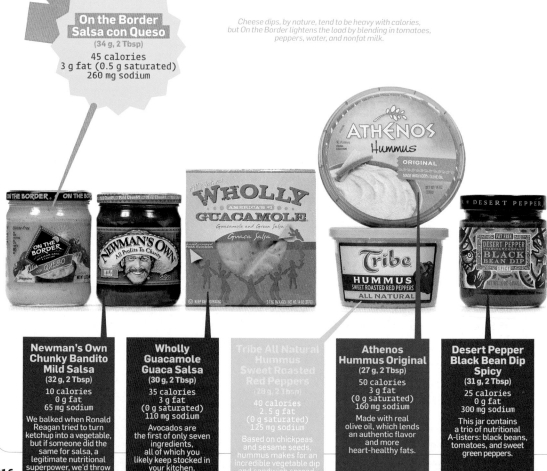

On the Border Salsa con Queso
(34 g, 2 Tbsp)

45 calories
3 g fat (0.5 g saturated)
260 mg sodium

Cheese dips, by nature, tend to be heavy with calories, but On the Border lightens the load by blending in tomatoes, peppers, water, and nonfat milk.

Newman's Own Chunky Bandito Mild Salsa
(32 g, 2 Tbsp)

10 calories
0 g fat
65 mg sodium

We balked when Ronald Reagan tried to turn ketchup into a vegetable, but if someone did the same for salsa, a legitimate nutritional superpower, we'd throw our support behind it.

Wholly Guacamole Guaca Salsa
(30 g, 2 Tbsp)

35 calories
3 g fat
(0 g saturated)
110 mg sodium

Avocados are the first of only seven ingredients, all of which you likely keep stocked in your kitchen.

Tribe All Natural Hummus Sweet Roasted Red Peppers
(28 g, 2 Tbsp)

40 calories
2.5 g fat
(0 g saturated)
125 mg sodium

Based on chickpeas and sesame seeds, hummus makes for an incredible vegetable dip and sandwich spread.

Athenos Hummus Original
(27 g, 2 Tbsp)

50 calories
3 g fat
(0 g saturated)
160 mg sodium

Made with real olive oil, which lends an authentic flavor and more heart-healthy fats.

Desert Pepper Black Bean Dip Spicy
(31 g, 2 Tbsp)

25 calories
0 g fat
300 mg sodium

This jar contains a trio of nutritional A-listers: black beans, tomatoes, and sweet green peppers.

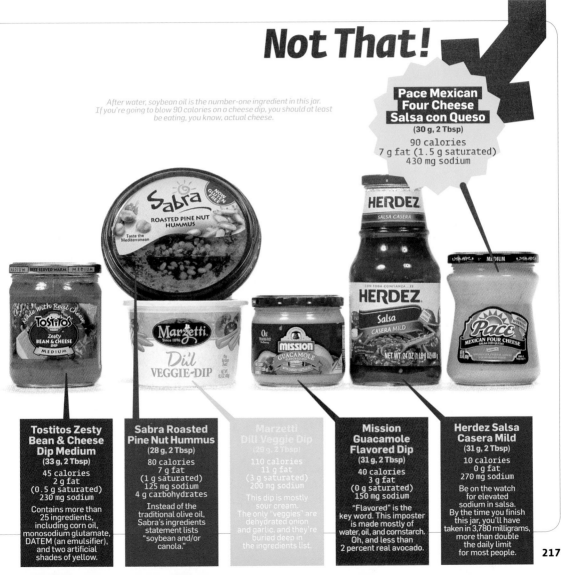

Not That!

After water, soybean oil is the number-one ingredient in this jar. If you're going to blow 90 calories on a cheese dip, you should at least be eating, you know, actual cheese.

Pace Mexican Four Cheese Salsa con Queso
(30 g, 2 Tbsp)

90 calories
7 g fat (1.5 g saturated)
430 mg sodium

Tostitos Zesty Bean & Cheese Dip Medium
(33 g, 2 Tbsp)

45 calories
2 g fat
(0.5 g saturated)
230 mg sodium

Contains more than 25 ingredients, including corn oil, monosodium glutamate, DATEM (an emulsifier), and two artificial shades of yellow.

Sabra Roasted Pine Nut Hummus
(28 g, 2 Tbsp)

80 calories
7 g fat
(1 g saturated)
125 mg sodium
4 g carbohydrates

Instead of the traditional olive oil, Sabra's ingredients statement lists "soybean and/or canola."

Marzetti Dill Veggie Dip
(29 g, 2 Tbsp)

110 calories
11 g fat
(3 g saturated)
200 mg sodium

This dip is mostly sour cream. The only "veggies" are dehydrated onion and garlic, and they're buried deep in the ingredients list.

Mission Guacamole Flavored Dip
(31 g, 2 Tbsp)

40 calories
3 g fat
(0 g saturated)
150 mg sodium

"Flavored" is the key word. This imposter is made mostly of water, oil, and cornstarch. Oh, and less than 2 percent real avocado.

Herdez Salsa Casera Mild
(31 g, 2 Tbsp)

10 calories
0 g fat
270 mg sodium

Be on the watch for elevated sodium in salsa. By the time you finish this jar, you'll have taken in 3,780 milligrams, more than double the daily limit for most people.

217

Dressings

Eat This

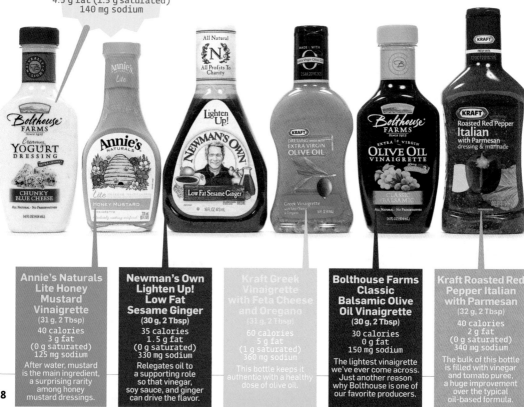

Bolthouse Farms Creamy Yogurt Dressing Chunky Blue Cheese
(30 g, 2 Tbsp)

50 calories
4.5 g fat (1.5 g saturated)
140 mg sodium

Bolthouse Farms casts yogurt as the star in classic flavors such as ranch, honey mustard, Thousand Island, and blue cheese, allowing you to swap out vegetable oil for worthwhile hits of calcium and probiotic bacteria.

Annie's Naturals Lite Honey Mustard Vinaigrette
(31 g, 2 Tbsp)

40 calories
3 g fat
(0 g saturated)
125 mg sodium

After water, mustard is the main ingredient, a surprising rarity among honey mustard dressings.

Newman's Own Lighten Up! Low Fat Sesame Ginger
(30 g, 2 Tbsp)

35 calories
1.5 g fat
(0 g saturated)
330 mg sodium

Relegates oil to a supporting role so that vinegar, soy sauce, and ginger can drive the flavor.

Kraft Greek Vinaigrette with Feta Cheese and Oregano
(31 g, 2 Tbsp)

60 calories
5 g fat
(1 g saturated)
360 mg sodium

This bottle keeps it authentic with a healthy dose of olive oil.

Bolthouse Farms Classic Balsamic Olive Oil Vinaigrette
(30 g, 2 Tbsp)

30 calories
0 g fat
150 mg sodium

The lightest vinaigrette we've ever come across. Just another reason why Bolthouse is one of our favorite producers.

Kraft Roasted Red Pepper Italian with Parmesan
(32 g, 2 Tbsp)

40 calories
2 g fat
(0 g saturated)
340 mg sodium

The bulk of this bottle is filled with vinegar and tomato puree, a huge improvement over the typical oil-based formula.

Not That!

Virtually every calorie in this bottle comes from soybean oil, which is a common theme in the dressing aisle. Consider them wasted calories; soybean oil doesn't have the same heart-healthy cachet as olive or canola oil.

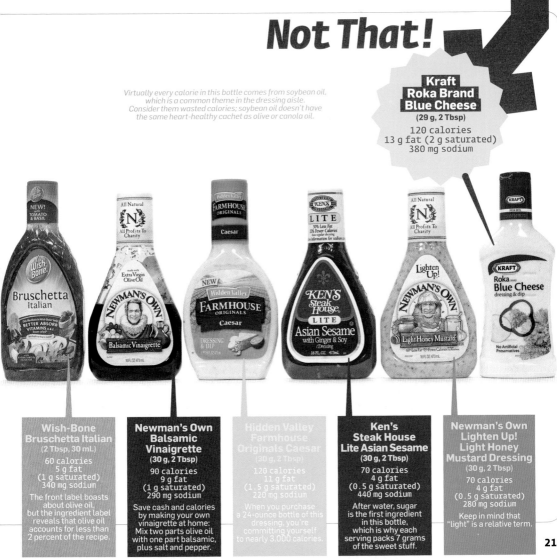

**Kraft
Roka Brand
Blue Cheese**
(29 g, 2 Tbsp)

120 calories
13 g fat (2 g saturated)
380 mg sodium

**Wish-Bone
Bruschetta Italian**
(2 Tbsp, 30 mL)

60 calories
5 g fat
(1 g saturated)
340 mg sodium

The front label boasts about olive oil, but the ingredient label reveals that olive oil accounts for less than 2 percent of the recipe.

**Newman's Own
Balsamic
Vinaigrette**
(30 g, 2 Tbsp)

90 calories
9 g fat
(1 g saturated)
290 mg sodium

Save cash and calories by making your own vinaigrette at home: Mix two parts olive oil with one part balsamic, plus salt and pepper.

**Hidden Valley
Farmhouse
Originals Caesar**
(30 g, 2 Tbsp)

120 calories
11 g fat
(1.5 g saturated)
220 mg sodium

When you purchase a 24-ounce bottle of this dressing, you're committing yourself to nearly 3,000 calories.

**Ken's
Steak House
Lite Asian Sesame**
(30 g, 2 Tbsp)

70 calories
4 g fat
(0.5 g saturated)
440 mg sodium

After water, sugar is the first ingredient in this bottle, which is why each serving packs 7 grams of the sweet stuff.

**Newman's Own
Lighten Up!
Light Honey
Mustard Dressing**
(30 g, 2 Tbsp)

70 calories
4 g fat
(0.5 g saturated)
280 mg sodium

Keep in mind that "light" is a relative term.

219

Cookies

Eat This

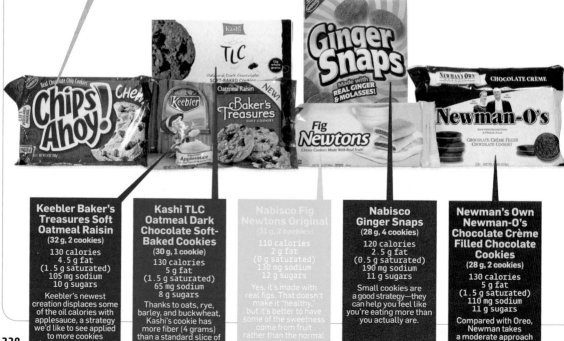

Chips Ahoy! Chewy
(27 g, 2 cookies)

120 calories
5 g fat (2.5 g saturated)
85 mg sodium
10 g sugars

This cookie isn't just the best of the Chips Ahoy! line, it's also one of the lowest-calorie cookies on the shelf.

Keebler Baker's Treasures Soft Oatmeal Raisin
(32 g, 2 cookies)

130 calories
4.5 g fat
(1.5 g saturated)
105 mg sodium
10 g sugars

Keebler's newest creation displaces some of the oil calories with applesauce, a strategy we'd like to see applied to more cookies in the elves' catalog.

Kashi TLC Oatmeal Dark Chocolate Soft-Baked Cookies
(30 g, 1 cookie)

130 calories
5 g fat
(1.5 g saturated)
65 mg sodium
8 g sugars

Thanks to oats, rye, barley, and buckwheat, Kashi's cookie has more fiber (4 grams) than a standard slice of whole-wheat bread.

Nabisco Fig Newtons Original
(31 g, 2 cookies)

110 calories
2 g fat
(0 g saturated)
130 mg sodium
12 g sugars

Yes, it's made with real figs. That doesn't make it "healthy," but it's better to have some of the sweetness come from fruit rather than the normal processed sugar rush.

Nabisco Ginger Snaps
(28 g, 4 cookies)

120 calories
2.5 g fat
(0.5 g saturated)
190 mg sodium
11 g sugars

Small cookies are a good strategy—they can help you feel like you're eating more than you actually are.

Newman's Own Newman-O's Chocolate Crème Filled Chocolate Cookies
(28 g, 2 cookies)

130 calories
5 g fat
(1.5 g saturated)
110 mg sodium
11 g sugars

Compared with Oreo, Newman takes a moderate approach to oil and sugar.

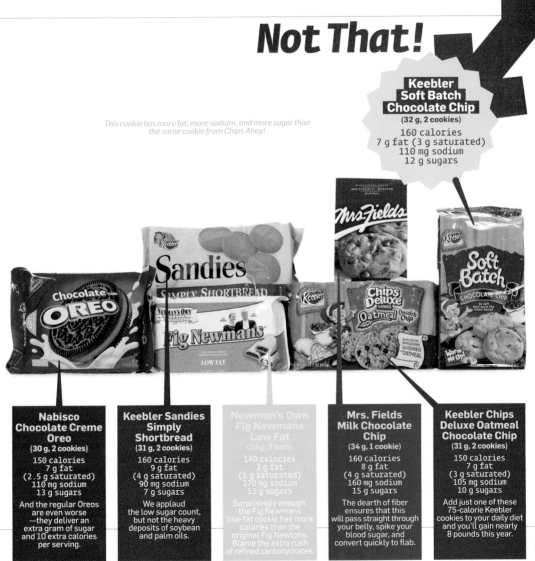

Not That!

This cookie has more fat, more sodium, and more sugar than the same cookie from Chips Ahoy!

Keebler Soft Batch Chocolate Chip
(32 g, 2 cookies)

160 calories
7 g fat (3 g saturated)
110 mg sodium
12 g sugars

Nabisco Chocolate Creme Oreo
(30 g, 2 cookies)

150 calories
7 g fat
(2.5 g saturated)
110 mg sodium
13 g sugars

And the regular Oreos are even worse —they deliver an extra gram of sugar and 10 extra calories per serving.

Keebler Sandies Simply Shortbread
(31 g, 2 cookies)

160 calories
9 g fat
(4 g saturated)
90 mg sodium
7 g sugars

We applaud the low sugar count, but not the heavy deposits of soybean and palm oils.

Newman's Own Fig Newmans Low Fat
(38 g, 2 bars)

140 calories
2 g fat
(1 g saturated)
170 mg sodium
13 g sugars

Surprisingly enough, the Fig Newmans low-fat cookie has more calories than the original Fig Newtons. Blame the extra rush of refined carbohydrates.

Mrs. Fields Milk Chocolate Chip
(34 g, 1 cookie)

160 calories
8 g fat
(4 g saturated)
160 mg sodium
15 g sugars

The dearth of fiber ensures that this will pass straight through your belly, spike your blood sugar, and convert quickly to flab.

Keebler Chips Deluxe Oatmeal Chocolate Chip
(31 g, 2 cookies)

150 calories
7 g fat
(3 g saturated)
105 mg sodium
10 g sugars

Add just one of these 75-calorie Keebler cookies to your daily diet and you'll gain nearly 8 pounds this year.

221

Candy Bars

Eat This

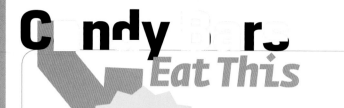

Pretzel M&M's
(32 g, 1 bag)
150 calories
5 g fat (3 g saturated)
16 g sugars

Hershey's Kit Kat
(43 g, 1 package)
210 calories
11 g fat
(7 g saturated)
21 g sugars

The wafer core is light and porous, which saves you calories over the denser bars.

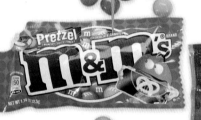

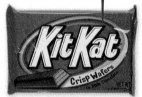

The latest spin on M&M's trounces everything else in the candy co.'s sugary arsenal. The original milk chocolate core has been replaced with pretzel, which is low in calories by confectionary standards. As a result, you trade in a boatload of sugar for a satisfying cookie-like crunch.

Life Savers Gummies
(40 g, 10 pieces)
130 calories
0 g fat
25 g sugars

The secret to the chew: gelatin. Starburst uses the same trick, but spoils it with a strange mix of oils.

York Peppermint Pattie
(39 g, 1 patty)
140 calories
2.5 g fat
(1.5 g saturated)
25 g sugars

For a smaller treat, go with York Miniatures. You can have three for about the same number of calories.

Nestlé 100 Grand
(43 g, 1 package)
190 calories
8 g fat
(5 g saturated)
30 g carbohydrates
22 g sugars

This is an *Eat This, Not That!* Hall of Famer, routinely beating out more common chocolate bars by 80 or more calories.

Hershey's Take 5
(42 g, 1 package)
200 calories
11 g fat
(5 g saturated)
18 g sugars

The pretzel core saves you a boatload of calories.

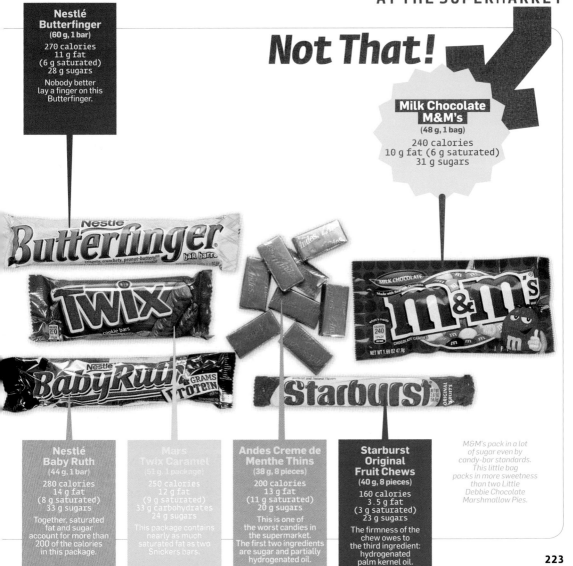

Not That!

Nestlé Butterfinger
(60 g, 1 bar)

270 calories
11 g fat
(6 g saturated)
28 g sugars

Nobody better lay a finger on this Butterfinger.

Milk Chocolate M&M's
(48 g, 1 bag)

240 calories
10 g fat (6 g saturated)
31 g sugars

Nestlé Baby Ruth
(44 g, 1 bar)

280 calories
14 g fat
(8 g saturated)
33 g sugars

Together, saturated fat and sugar account for more than 200 of the calories in this package.

Mars Twix Caramel
(51 g, 1 package)

250 calories
12 g fat
(9 g saturated)
33 g carbohydrates
24 g sugars

This package contains nearly as much saturated fat as two Snickers bars.

Andes Creme de Menthe Thins
(38 g, 8 pieces)

200 calories
13 g fat
(11 g saturated)
20 g sugars

This is one of the worst candies in the supermarket. The first two ingredients are sugar and partially hydrogenated oil.

Starburst Original Fruit Chews
(40 g, 8 pieces)

160 calories
3.5 g fat
(3 g saturated)
23 g sugars

The firmness of the chew owes to the third ingredient: hydrogenated palm kernel oil.

M&M's pack in a lot of sugar even by candy-bar standards. This little bag packs in more sweetness than two Little Debbie Chocolate Marshmallow Pies.

Frozen Breakfast Entrées

Eat This

An ideal breakfast includes a substantial load of protein, and this bowl has that nailed. Protein accounts for 40 percent of the calories, which increases your odds of making it to lunch without snacking.

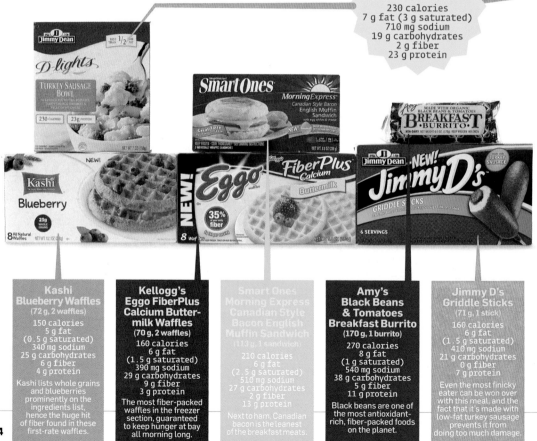

Jimmy Dean D-Lights Turkey Sausage Bowl
(198 g, 1 bowl)

230 calories
7 g fat (3 g saturated)
710 mg sodium
19 g carbohydrates
2 g fiber
23 g protein

Kashi Blueberry Waffles
(72 g, 2 waffles)

150 calories
5 g fat
(0.5 g saturated)
340 mg sodium
25 g carbohydrates
6 g fiber
4 g protein

Kashi lists whole grains and blueberries prominently on the ingredients list, hence the huge hit of fiber found in these first-rate waffles.

Kellogg's Eggo FiberPlus Calcium Buttermilk Waffles
(70 g, 2 waffles)

160 calories
6 g fat
(1.5 g saturated)
390 mg sodium
29 g carbohydrates
9 g fiber
3 g protein

The most fiber-packed waffles in the freezer section, guaranteed to keep hunger at bay all morning long.

Smart Ones Morning Express Canadian Style Bacon English Muffin Sandwich
(113 g, 1 sandwich)

210 calories
6 g fat
(2.5 g saturated)
510 mg sodium
27 g carbohydrates
2 g fiber
13 g protein

Next to ham, Canadian bacon is the leanest of the breakfast meats.

Amy's Black Beans & Tomatoes Breakfast Burrito
(170 g, 1 burrito)

270 calories
8 g fat
(1 g saturated)
540 mg sodium
38 g carbohydrates
5 g fiber
11 g protein

Black beans are one of the most antioxidant-rich, fiber-packed foods on the planet.

Jimmy D's Griddle Sticks
(71 g, 1 stick)

160 calories
6 g fat
(1.5 g saturated)
410 mg sodium
21 g carbohydrates
0 g fiber
7 g protein

Even the most finicky eater can be won over with this meal, and the fact that it's made with low-fat turkey sausage prevents it from doing too much damage.

Not That!

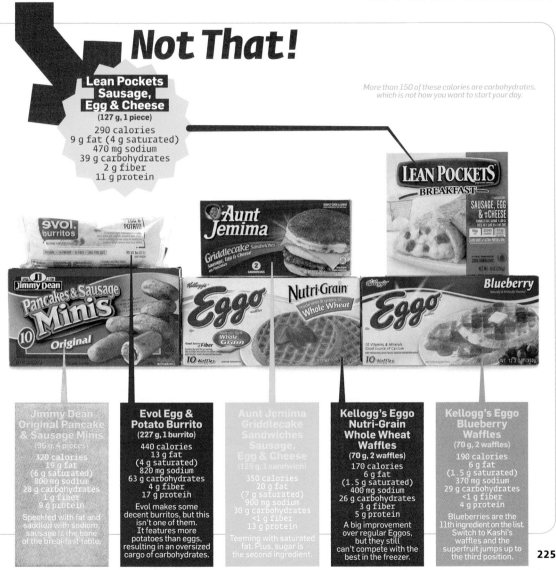

Lean Pockets Sausage, Egg & Cheese
(127 g, 1 piece)

290 calories
9 g fat (4 g saturated)
470 mg sodium
39 g carbohydrates
2 g fiber
11 g protein

More than 150 of these calories are carbohydrates, which is not how you want to start your day.

Jimmy Dean Original Pancake & Sausage Minis
(96 g, 4 pieces)

320 calories
19 g fat
(6 g saturated)
800 mg sodium
28 g carbohydrates
1 g fiber
9 g protein

Speckled with fat and saddled with sodium, sausage is the bane of the breakfast table.

Evol Egg & Potato Burrito
(227 g, 1 burrito)

440 calories
13 g fat
(4 g saturated)
820 mg sodium
63 g carbohydrates
4 g fiber
17 g protein

Evol makes some decent burritos, but this isn't one of them. It features more potatoes than eggs, resulting in an oversized cargo of carbohydrates.

Aunt Jemima Griddlecake Sandwiches Sausage, Egg & Cheese
(125 g, 1 sandwich)

350 calories
20 g fat
(7 g saturated)
900 mg sodium
30 g carbohydrates
<1 g fiber
13 g protein

Teeming with saturated fat. Plus, sugar is the second ingredient.

Kellogg's Eggo Nutri-Grain Whole Wheat Waffles
(70 g, 2 waffles)

170 calories
6 g fat
(1.5 g saturated)
400 mg sodium
26 g carbohydrates
3 g fiber
5 g protein

A big improvement over regular Eggos, but they still can't compete with the best in the freezer.

Kellogg's Eggo Blueberry Waffles
(70 g, 2 waffles)

190 calories
6 g fat
(1.5 g saturated)
370 mg sodium
29 g carbohydrates
<1 g fiber
4 g protein

Blueberries are the 11th ingredient on the list. Switch to Kashi's waffles and the superfruit jumps up to the third position.

Frozen Pizz

Eat This

Kashi Pesto Stone-Fired Thin Crust
(113 g, ⅓ pie)

240 calories
9 g fat (3.5 g saturated)
590 mg sodium
27 g carbohydrates
4 g fiber
14 g protein

This pie features more pesto than cheese, which means you end up with more monounsaturated fat from olive oil than saturated fat from dairy. That's a healthy swap.

Lean Cuisine French Bread Pepperoni Pizza
(148 g, 1 pie)

310 calories
7 g fat (2 g saturated)
690 mg sodium
48 g carbohydrates
4 g fiber
16 g protein

Cut the fat by more than half and double your fiber with this first-rate pizza package.

Amy's Cheese Pizza
(167 g, 1 pie)

420 calories
17 g fat (6 g saturated)
720 mg sodium
56 g carbohydrates
3 g fiber
18 g protein

For the rare times when you allow yourself the privilege of eating a whole pizza, this is where you should turn. Exactly what a personal serving size should be.

Newman's Own Uncured Pepperoni Thin & Crispy
(125 g, ⅓ pie)

320 calories
16 g fat (6 g saturated)
800 mg sodium
31 g carbohydrates
1 g fiber
15 g protein

Newman's eschews chemical nitrates and nitrites in favor of sea salt and celery juice for their uncured pepperoni.

Bagel Bites Cheese & Pepperoni
(88 g, 4 pieces)

190 calories
6 g fat
(2.5 g saturated)
380 mg sodium
29 g carbohydrates
2 g fiber
8 g protein

Each mini bagel contains fewer than 50 calories. As an occasional snack, you could do a lot worse.

Tofurky Vegan Cheese
(113 g, ⅓ pie)

240 calories
8 g fat (2.5 g saturated)
350 mg sodium
39 g carbohydrates
4 g fiber
6 g protein

Tofurky's "cheese" is made using a combination of protein, flour, and oils. It's a great alternative for those who are lactose intolerant.

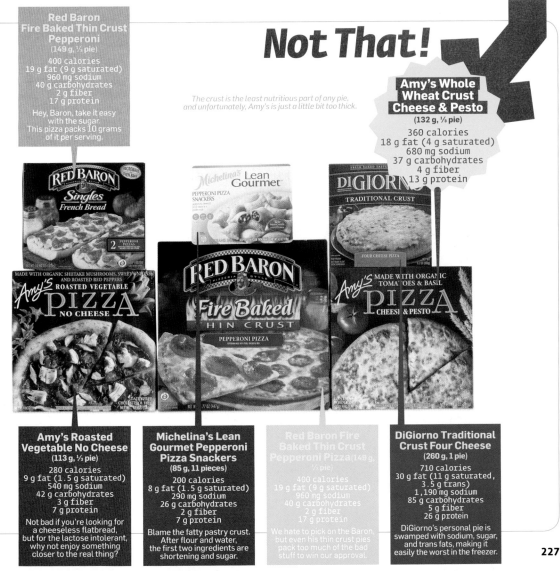

Red Baron Fire Baked Thin Crust Pepperoni
(149 g, ½ pie)

400 calories
19 g fat (9 g saturated)
960 mg sodium
40 g carbohydrates
2 g fiber
17 g protein

Hey, Baron, take it easy with the sugar. This pizza packs 10 grams of it per serving.

Not That!

The crust is the least nutritious part of any pie, and unfortunately, Amy's is just a little bit too thick.

Amy's Whole Wheat Crust Cheese & Pesto
(132 g, ⅓ pie)

360 calories
18 g fat (4 g saturated)
680 mg sodium
37 g carbohydrates
4 g fiber
13 g protein

Amy's Roasted Vegetable No Cheese
(113 g, ⅓ pie)

280 calories
9 g fat (1.5 g saturated)
540 mg sodium
42 g carbohydrates
3 g fiber
7 g protein

Not bad if you're looking for a cheeseless flatbread, but for the lactose intolerant, why not enjoy something closer to the real thing?

Michelina's Lean Gourmet Pepperoni Pizza Snackers
(85 g, 11 pieces)

200 calories
8 g fat (1.5 g saturated)
290 mg sodium
26 g carbohydrates
2 g fiber
7 g protein

Blame the fatty pastry crust. After flour and water, the first two ingredients are shortening and sugar.

Red Baron Fire Baked Thin Crust Pepperoni Pizza (149 g, ½ pie)

400 calories
19 g fat (9 g saturated)
960 mg sodium
40 g carbohydrates
2 g fiber
17 g protein

We hate to pick on the Baron, but even his thin crust pies pack too much of the bad stuff to win our approval.

DiGiorno Traditional Crust Four Cheese
(260 g, 1 pie)

710 calories
30 g fat (11 g saturated, 3.5 g trans)
1,190 mg sodium
85 g carbohydrates
5 g fiber
26 g protein

DiGiorno's personal pie is swamped with sodium, sugar, and trans fats, making it easily the worst in the freezer.

227

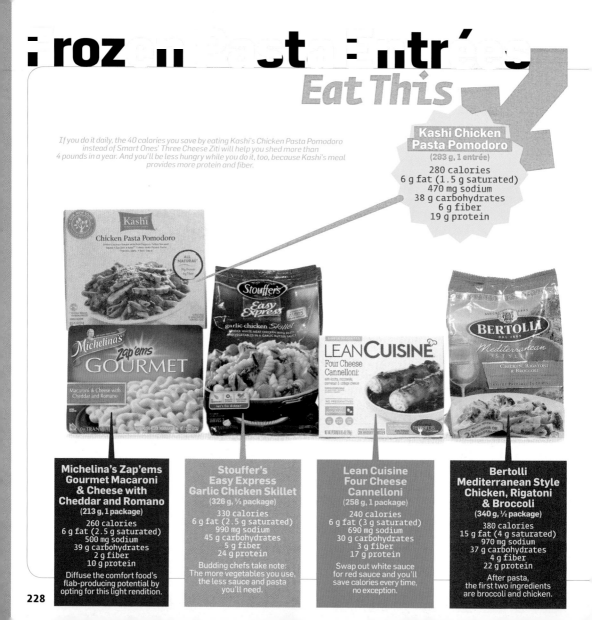

Frozen Pasta Entrées

Eat This

If you do it daily, the 40 calories you save by eating Kashi's Chicken Pasta Pomodoro instead of Smart Ones' Three Cheese Ziti will help you shed more than 4 pounds in a year. And you'll be less hungry while you do it, too, because Kashi's meal provides more protein and fiber.

Kashi Chicken Pasta Pomodoro
(293 g, 1 entrée)

280 calories
6 g fat (1.5 g saturated)
470 mg sodium
38 g carbohydrates
6 g fiber
19 g protein

Michelina's Zap'ems Gourmet Macaroni & Cheese with Cheddar and Romano
(213 g, 1 package)

260 calories
6 g fat (2.5 g saturated)
500 mg sodium
39 g carbohydrates
2 g fiber
10 g protein

Diffuse the comfort food's flab-producing potential by opting for this light rendition.

Stouffer's Easy Express Garlic Chicken Skillet
(326 g, ½ package)

330 calories
6 g fat (2.5 g saturated)
990 mg sodium
45 g carbohydrates
5 g fiber
24 g protein

Budding chefs take note: The more vegetables you use, the less sauce and pasta you'll need.

Lean Cuisine Four Cheese Cannelloni
(258 g, 1 package)

240 calories
6 g fat (3 g saturated)
690 mg sodium
30 g carbohydrates
3 g fiber
17 g protein

Swap out white sauce for red sauce and you'll save calories every time, no exception.

Bertolli Mediterranean Style Chicken, Rigatoni & Broccoli
(340 g, ½ package)

380 calories
15 g fat (4 g saturated)
970 mg sodium
37 g carbohydrates
4 g fiber
22 g protein

After pasta, the first two ingredients are broccoli and chicken.

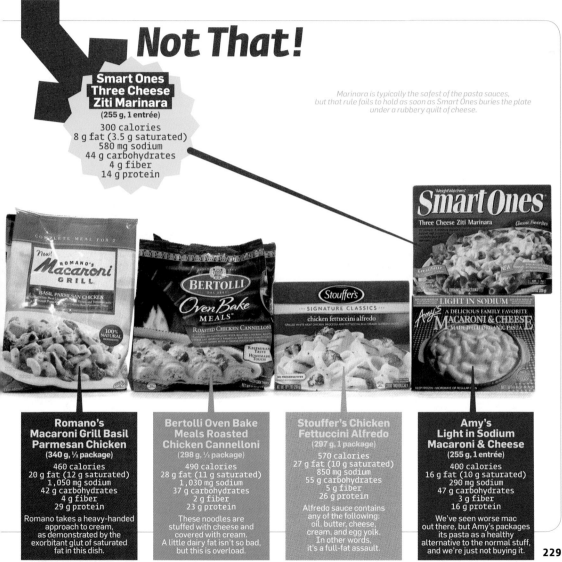

Not That!

Smart Ones Three Cheese Ziti Marinara
(255 g, 1 entrée)

300 calories
8 g fat (3.5 g saturated)
580 mg sodium
44 g carbohydrates
4 g fiber
14 g protein

Marinara is typically the safest of the pasta sauces, but that rule fails to hold as soon as Smart Ones buries the plate under a rubbery quilt of cheese.

Romano's Macaroni Grill Basil Parmesan Chicken
(340 g, ½ package)

460 calories
20 g fat (12 g saturated)
1,050 mg sodium
42 g carbohydrates
4 g fiber
29 g protein

Romano takes a heavy-handed approach to cream, as demonstrated by the exorbitant glut of saturated fat in this dish.

Bertolli Oven Bake Meals Roasted Chicken Cannelloni
(298 g, ½ package)

490 calories
28 g fat (11 g saturated)
1,030 mg sodium
37 g carbohydrates
2 g fiber
23 g protein

These noodles are stuffed with cheese and covered with cream. A little dairy fat isn't so bad, but this is overload.

Stouffer's Chicken Fettuccini Alfredo
(297 g, 1 package)

570 calories
27 g fat (10 g saturated)
850 mg sodium
55 g carbohydrates
5 g fiber
26 g protein

Alfredo sauce contains any of the following: oil, butter, cheese, cream, and egg yolk. In other words, it's a full-fat assault.

Amy's Light in Sodium Macaroni & Cheese
(255 g, 1 entrée)

400 calories
16 g fat (10 g saturated)
290 mg sodium
47 g carbohydrates
3 g fiber
16 g protein

We've seen worse mac out there, but Amy's packages its pasta as a healthy alternative to the normal stuff, and we're just not buying it.

229

Frozen Fish Entrées

Eat This

Gorton's Cajun Blackened Grilled Fillets
(108 g, 1 fillet)

90 calories
3 g fat (0.5 g saturated)
400 mg sodium
16 g protein

The smoky, spicy finesse of a blackening rub can imbue any fillet with massive flavor at no caloric cost. It's easily one of the healthiest ways to prepare meat and fish.

Cape Gourmet Cooked Shrimp
(3 oz)

50 calories
0.5 g fat
330 mg sodium
10 g protein

Unadulterated shrimp are one of the leanest sources of protein on the planet.

Northern King Bay Scallops
(4 oz)

150 calories
1 g fat
(0 g saturated)
155 mg sodium
29 g protein

Scallops are teeming with the amino acid tryptophan, which bolsters feelings of wellbeing and helps regulate sleep cycles.

Margaritaville Island Lime Shrimp
(4 oz, 6 shrimp)

240 calories
11 g fat
(3 g saturated)
330 mg sodium
12 g protein

These shrimp have also been tossed in butter. The difference is quantity; here it's a light bath, but in SeaPak's scampi it's a tidal wave.

SeaPak Salmon Burgers
(91 g, 1 burger)

110 calories
5 g fat
(1 g saturated)
340 mg sodium
16 g protein

Toss this on the grill, then sandwich it between a toasted bun with arugula, grilled onions, and Greek yogurt spiked with olive oil, garlic, and fresh dill.

Stouffer's Easy Express Shrimp Fried Rice Skillet
(354 g, ½ package)

290 calories
3 g fat
(0.5 g saturated)
980 mg sodium
14 g protein

American interpretations of Asian cuisine tend to be high in sodium, but 13 grams of fiber more than make up for it.

Not That!

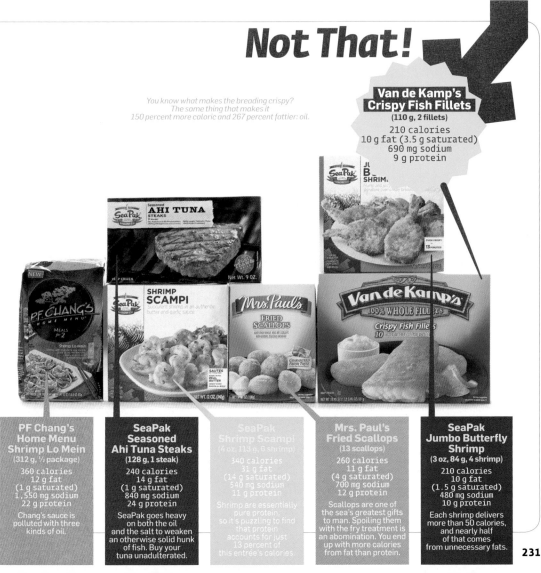

*You know what makes the breading crispy?
The same thing that makes it
150 percent more caloric and 267 percent fattier: oil.*

**Van de Kamp's
Crispy Fish Fillets**
(110 g, 2 fillets)
210 calories
10 g fat (3.5 g saturated)
690 mg sodium
9 g protein

**PF Chang's
Home Menu
Shrimp Lo Mein**
(312 g, ½ package)
360 calories
12 g fat
(1 g saturated)
1,550 mg sodium
22 g protein

Chang's sauce is
polluted with three
kinds of oil.

**SeaPak
Seasoned
Ahi Tuna Steaks**
(128 g, 1 steak)
240 calories
14 g fat
(1 g saturated)
840 mg sodium
24 g protein

SeaPak goes heavy
on both the oil
and the salt to weaken
an otherwise solid hunk
of fish. Buy your
tuna unadulterated.

**SeaPak
Shrimp Scampi**
(4 oz, 113 g, 6 shrimp)
340 calories
31 g fat
(14 g saturated)
540 mg sodium
11 g protein

Shrimp are essentially
pure protein,
so it's puzzling to find
that protein
accounts for just
13 percent of
this entrée's calories.

**Mrs. Paul's
Fried Scallops**
(13 scallops)
260 calories
11 g fat
(4 g saturated)
700 mg sodium
12 g protein

Scallops are one of
the sea's greatest gifts
to man. Spoiling them
with the fry treatment is
an abomination. You end
up with more calories
from fat than protein.

**SeaPak
Jumbo Butterfly
Shrimp**
(3 oz, 84 g, 4 shrimp)
210 calories
10 g fat
(1.5 g saturated)
480 mg sodium
10 g protein

Each shrimp delivers
more than 50 calories,
and nearly half
of that comes
from unnecessary fats.

231

Frozen Chicken Entrées

Eat This

Evol Bowls Teriyaki Chicken
(255 g, 1 bowl)

250 calories
6 g fat (1 g saturated)
490 mg sodium
34 g carbohydrates
4 g fiber
14 g protein

Evol's teriyaki bowl is made with brown rice, free-range chicken, and enough produce to meet 90 percent of your day's vitamin A needs.

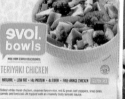

Banquet Chicken Fried Chicken Meal (286 g, 1 entrée)

350 calories
17 g fat
(4 g saturated)
930 mg sodium
35 g carbohydrates
5 g fiber
12 g protein

A thinner coating of breading and a heavier reliance on sides saves you 90 calories over Banquet's "premium" version of the same meal.

Ethnic Gourmet Chicken Tikka Masala (283 g, 1 package)

260 calories
6 g fat
(2 g saturated)
680 mg sodium
32 g carbohydrates
3 g fiber
19 g protein

The sauce is created with nonfat yogurt, which provides the thick heft of cream without all the calories.

Kashi Lemongrass Coconut Chicken (283 g, 1 entrée)

300 calories
8 g fat
(4 g saturated)
680 mg sodium
38 g carbohydrates
7 g fiber
18 g protein

Instead of the standard white noodles or rice, this meal rests on a whole-grain blend of oats, rye, red winter wheat, and quinoa.

Marie Callender's Fresh Flavor Steamer Chicken Teriyaki (283 g, 1 meal)

280 calories
3.5 g fat
(1 g saturated)
890 mg sodium
44 g carbohydrates
3 g fiber
17 g protein

Keeps the calories down by casting broccoli and carrots in leading roles.

Smart Ones Artisan Creations Grilled Flatbread Chicken Marinara with Mozzarella Cheese (170 g, 1 flatbread)

290 calories
6 g fat
(1.5 g saturated)
640 mg sodium
41 g carbohydrates
3 g fiber
18 g protein

Marinara adds big flavor but only a few calories.

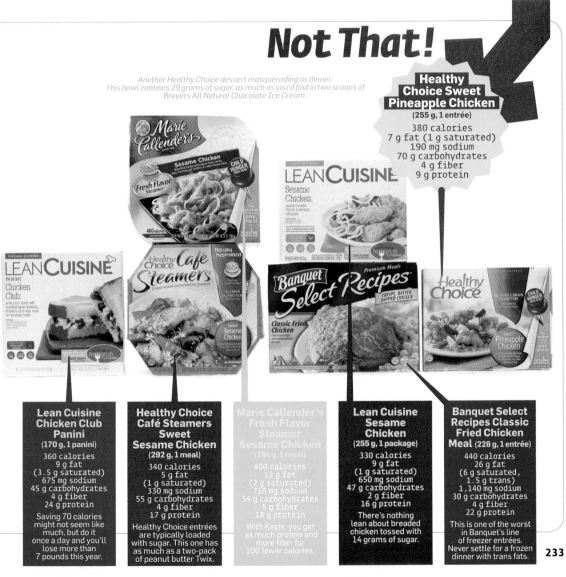

Not That!

*Another Healthy Choice dessert masquerading as dinner.
This bowl contains 29 grams of sugar, as much as you'd find in two scoops of Breyers All Natural Chocolate Ice Cream.*

Healthy Choice Sweet Pineapple Chicken
(255 g, 1 entrée)

380 calories
7 g fat (1 g saturated)
190 mg sodium
70 g carbohydrates
4 g fiber
9 g protein

Lean Cuisine Chicken Club Panini
(170 g, 1 panini)

360 calories
9 g fat
(3.5 g saturated)
675 mg sodium
45 g carbohydrates
4 g fiber
24 g protein

Saving 70 calories might not seem like much, but do it once a day and you'll lose more than 7 pounds this year.

Healthy Choice Café Steamers Sweet Sesame Chicken
(292 g, 1 meal)

340 calories
5 g fat
(1 g saturated)
330 mg sodium
55 g carbohydrates
4 g fiber
17 g protein

Healthy Choice entrées are typically loaded with sugar. This one has as much as a two-pack of peanut butter Twix.

Marie Callender's Fresh Flavor Steamer Sesame Chicken
(291 g, 1 meal)

400 calories
12 g fat
(2 g saturated)
710 mg sodium
54 g carbohydrates
5 g fiber
18 g protein

With Kashi, you get as much protein and more fiber for 100 fewer calories.

Lean Cuisine Sesame Chicken
(255 g, 1 package)

330 calories
9 g fat
(1 g saturated)
650 mg sodium
47 g carbohydrates
2 g fiber
16 g protein

There's nothing lean about breaded chicken tossed with 14 grams of sugar.

Banquet Select Recipes Classic Fried Chicken Meal (228 g, 1 entrée)

440 calories
26 g fat
(6 g saturated,
1.5 g trans)
1,140 mg sodium
30 g carbohydrates
4 g fiber
22 g protein

This is one of the worst in Banquet's line of freezer entrées. Never settle for a frozen dinner with trans fats.

233

Eat This

Stouffer's Homestyle Classics Beef Pot Roast
(251 g, 1 entrée)

230 calories
7 g fat (2 g saturated)
820 mg sodium
26 g carbohydrates
3 g fiber
16 g protein

If you'd rather eat a potpie, just pour this into a bowl and eat it with a piece of toasted whole-grain bread. There, all the potpie perks without the fat.

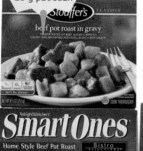

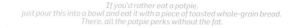

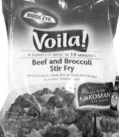

Smart Ones Homestyle Beef Roast
(255 g, 1 meal)

180 calories
4.5 g fat (2 g saturated)
670 mg sodium
18 g carbohydrates
4 g fiber
17 g protein

Most protein bars can't deliver this dose for so few calories. Tack on 4 g of fiber and you have an amazing 180-calorie package.

Hot Pockets Sideshots Cheeseburgers
(127 g, 2 buns)

290 calories
10 g fat (4 g saturated)
660 mg sodium
37 g carbohydrates
1 g fiber
12 g protein

A fairly innocuous snack to set in front of a group of hungry kids.

Banquet Meat Loaf Meal
(269 g, 1 meal)

280 calories
13 g fat (5 g saturated)
1,000 mg sodium
28 g carbohydrates
4 g fiber
12 g protein

When it comes to delivering comfort dishes for a reasonable number of calories, Banquet's regular line of entrées is among the best in the freezer.

Birds Eye Voila! Beef and Broccoli Stir Fry
(218 g, 1¼ cup)

210 calories
6 g fat (1.5 g saturated)
700 mg sodium
27 g carbohydrates
2 g fiber
10 g protein

The first ingredient in this bag is broccoli. In the cost-conscious world of processed foods, that's exceedingly rare.

Not That!

A potpie crust is essentially an oversized pastry, which is to say lots of carbohydrates glued together with saturated fat.

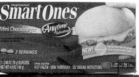

Banquet Beef Pot Pie
(198 g, 1 pie)

390 calories
22 g fat
(9 g saturated, 0.5 g trans)
1,010 mg sodium
36 g carbohydrates
3 g fiber
10 g protein

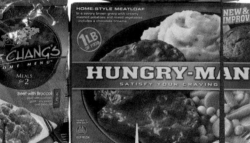

PF Chang's Home Menu Beef with Broccoli
(312 g, ½ package)

360 calories
18 g fat (3 g saturated)
1,330 mg sodium
26 g carbohydrates
4 g fiber
21 g protein

Chang's bagged meals suffer from the same malady as its restaurant fare, which is to say far too much sodium.

Hungry-Man Home-Style Meatloaf
(454 g, 1 package)

660 calories
35 g fat (12 g saturated)
1,660 mg sodium
61 g carbohydrates
5 g fiber
26 g protein

Word of advice to the calorie conscious: Purge Hungry-Man from your freezer for good. This is consistently the worst brand in the frozen-foods aisle.

Smart Ones Mini Cheeseburgers
(140 g, 2 mini-burgers)

400 calories
18 g fat (8 g saturated)
720 mg sodium
40 g carbohydrates
6 g fiber
20 g protein

Each burger has 20 percent of your day's saturated fat.

Healthy Choice Café Steamers Grilled Whiskey Steak
(269 g, 1 meal)

290 calories
4 g fat (1.5 g saturated)
480 mg sodium
47 g carbohydrates
5 g fiber
16 g protein

More than a quarter of the calories in this box come from added sugars.

235

Eat This

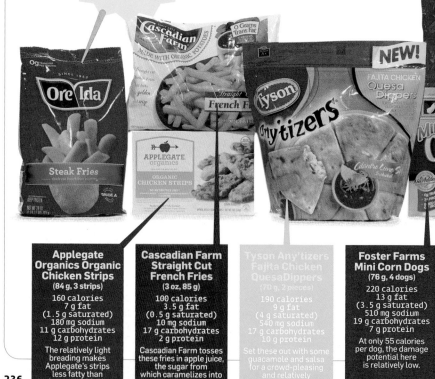

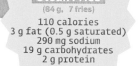

Ore-Ida Steak Fries
(84 g, 7 fries)

110 calories
3 g fat (0.5 g saturated)
290 mg sodium
19 g carbohydrates
2 g protein

A serving of these hulking spuds contains fewer than half the calories you'd find in the average medium order of fast-food fries.

Applegate Organics Organic Chicken Strips
(84 g, 3 strips)

160 calories
7 g fat
(1.5 g saturated)
180 mg sodium
11 g carbohydrates
12 g protein

The relatively light breading makes Applegate's strips less fatty than the competition's.

Cascadian Farm Straight Cut French Fries
(3 oz, 85 g)

100 calories
3.5 g fat
(0.5 g saturated)
10 mg sodium
17 g carbohydrates
2 g protein

Cascadian Farm tosses these fries in apple juice, the sugar from which caramelizes into a crisp golden crust.

Tyson Any'tizers Fajita Chicken QuesaDippers
(70 g, 2 pieces)

190 calories
9 g fat
(4 g saturated)
540 mg sodium
17 g carbohydrates
10 g protein

Set these out with some guacamole and salsa for a crowd-pleasing and relatively harmless hors d'oeuvre.

Foster Farms Mini Corn Dogs
(76 g, 4 dogs)

220 calories
13 g fat
(3.5 g saturated)
510 mg sodium
19 g carbohydrates
7 g protein

At only 55 calories per dog, the damage potential here is relatively low.

Hot Pockets Snackers Grilled Italian Style Bites (94 g, 4 pieces)

210 calories
6 g fat
(2.5 g saturated)
500 mg sodium
28 g carbohydrates
8 g protein

Each Snacker packs in 2 grams of protein. That doesn't make it healthy, but it's not a bad start.

Appetizers

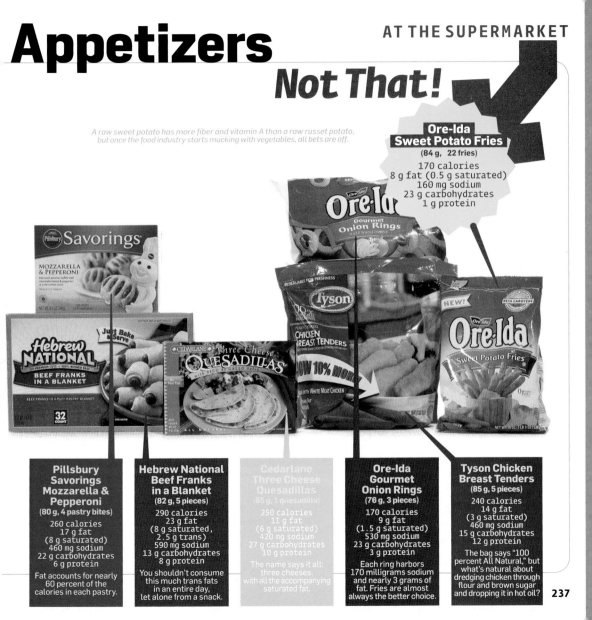

Not That!

A raw sweet potato has more fiber and vitamin A than a raw russet potato, but once the food industry starts mucking with vegetables, all bets are off.

Ore-Ida Sweet Potato Fries
(84 g, 22 fries)

170 calories
8 g fat (0.5 g saturated)
160 mg sodium
23 g carbohydrates
1 g protein

Pillsbury Savorings Mozzarella & Pepperoni
(80 g, 4 pastry bites)

260 calories
17 g fat
(8 g saturated)
460 mg sodium
22 g carbohydrates
6 g protein

Fat accounts for nearly 60 percent of the calories in each pastry.

Hebrew National Beef Franks in a Blanket
(82 g, 5 pieces)

290 calories
23 g fat
(8 g saturated,
2.5 g trans)
590 mg sodium
13 g carbohydrates
8 g protein

You shouldn't consume this much trans fats in an entire day, let alone from a snack.

Cedarlane Three Cheese Quesadillas
(85 g, 1 quesadilla)

250 calories
11 g fat
(6 g saturated)
420 mg sodium
27 g carbohydrates
10 g protein

The name says it all: three cheeses, with all the accompanying saturated fat.

Ore-Ida Gourmet Onion Rings
(76 g, 3 pieces)

170 calories
9 g fat
(1.5 g saturated)
530 mg sodium
23 g carbohydrates
3 g protein

Each ring harbors 170 milligrams sodium and nearly 3 grams of fat. Fries are almost always the better choice.

Tyson Chicken Breast Tenders
(85 g, 5 pieces)

240 calories
14 g fat
(3 g saturated)
460 mg sodium
15 g carbohydrates
12 g protein

The bag says "100 percent All Natural," but what's natural about dredging chicken through flour and brown sugar and dropping it in hot oil?

Ice Creams
Eat This

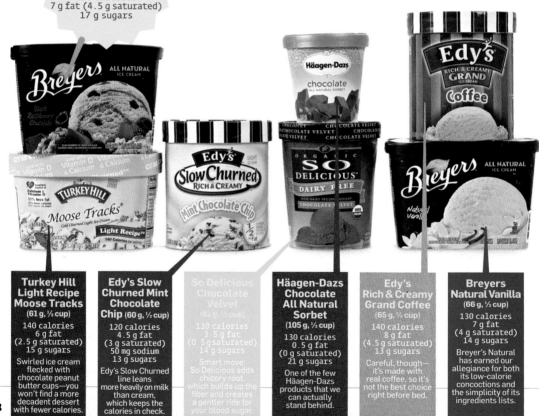

Breyers Black Raspberry Chocolate
(67 g, ½ cup)

150 calories
7 g fat (4.5 g saturated)
17 g sugars

The secret to a low-calorie ice cream is simple: lead off with something lighter than cream. This one uses regular milk first and cream second. Perfect.

Turkey Hill Light Recipe Moose Tracks
(61 g, ½ cup)

140 calories
6 g fat
(2.5 g saturated)
15 g sugars

Swirled ice cream flecked with chocolate peanut butter cups—you won't find a more decadent dessert with fewer calories.

Edy's Slow Churned Mint Chocolate Chip (60 g, ½ cup)

120 calories
4.5 g fat
(3 g saturated)
50 mg sodium
13 g sugars

Edy's Slow Churned line leans more heavily on milk than cream, which keeps the calories in check.

So Delicious Chocolate Velvet
(81 g, ½ cup)

130 calories
3.5 g fat
(0.5 g saturated)
14 g sugars

Smart move: So Delicious adds chicory root, which builds up the fiber and creates a gentler ride for your blood sugar.

Häagen-Dazs Chocolate All Natural Sorbet
(105 g, ½ cup)

130 calories
0.5 g fat
(0 g saturated)
21 g sugars

One of the few Häagen-Dazs products that we can actually stand behind.

Edy's Rich & Creamy Grand Coffee
(65 g, ½ cup)

140 calories
8 g fat
(4.5 g saturated)
13 g sugars

Careful, though—it's made with real coffee, so it's not the best choice right before bed.

Breyers Natural Vanilla
(66 g, ½ cup)

130 calories
7 g fat
(4 g saturated)
14 g sugars

Breyer's Natural has earned our allegiance for both its low-calorie concoctions and the simplicity of its ingredients lists.

Not That!

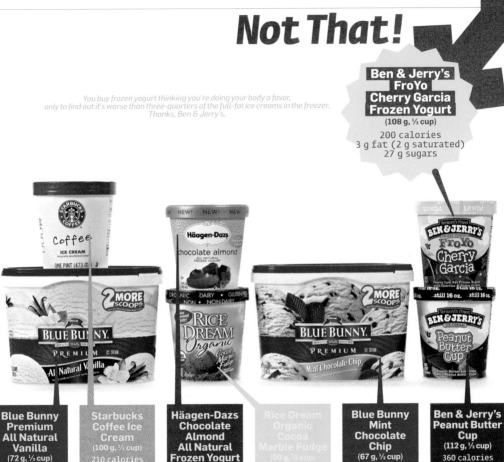

*You buy frozen yogurt thinking you're doing your body a favor,
only to find out it's worse than three-quarters of the full-fat ice creams in the freezer.
Thanks, Ben & Jerry's.*

Ben & Jerry's FroYo Cherry Garcia Frozen Yogurt
(108 g, ½ cup)

200 calories
3 g fat (2 g saturated)
27 g sugars

Blue Bunny Premium All Natural Vanilla
(72 g, ½ cup)

160 calories
9 g fat
(6 g saturated)
16 g sugars

The All Natural line is the worst among the many Blue Bunny vanilla ice creams.

Starbucks Coffee Ice Cream
(100 g, ½ cup)

210 calories
13 g fat
(8 g saturated)
19 g sugars

Starbuck's ice cream line follows the precedent of the Frappuccino: lots of fat, lots of sugar.

Häagen-Dazs Chocolate Almond All Natural Frozen Yogurt
(102 g, ½ cup)

190 calories
5 g fat
(1 g saturated)
19 g sugars

Leave it to Häagen-Dazs to find a way to mess up frozen yogurt.

Rice Dream Organic Cocoa Marble Fudge
(80 g, ¾ cup)

170 calories
6 g fat
(0.5 g saturated)
17 g sugars

Rice Dream adds vegetable oils to create a high-cal approximation of ice cream.

Blue Bunny Mint Chocolate Chip
(67 g, ½ cup)

160 calories
9 g fat
(6 g saturated)
16 g sugars

Not terrible, but just north of the calorie and fat counts you want out of your ice cream.

Ben & Jerry's Peanut Butter Cup
(112 g, ½ cup)

360 calories
26 g fat
(14 g saturated)
24 g sugars

Eat two scoops of this and you'll take in more calories than a McDonald's McDouble with a small side of french fries.

239

Frozen Treats
Eat This

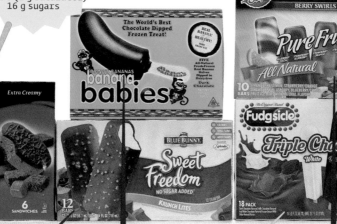

Breyers Smooth & Dreamy Chocolate Caramel Brownie Sandwich
(62 g, 1 sandwich)

160 calories
4 g fat (2 g saturated)
16 g sugars

This is a massive sandwich for only 160 calories. The secret, as with all low-cal ice cream treats, is in keeping cream off the top of the ingredients list. Bonus: It packs 3 grams of fiber.

Blue Bunny Sweet Freedom Krunch Lites
(40 g, 1 bar)

100 calories
7 g fat
(6 g saturated)
2 g sugars

No added sugar and made with low-fat ice cream.

Diana's Bananas Banana Babies Dark Chocolate
(60 g, 1 piece)

130 calories
6 g fat
(3.5 g saturated)
14 g sugars

Banana, chocolate, and peanut oil. You don't find a frozen treat with a simpler recipe.

Fudgsicle Triple Chocolate variety pack, Milk Chocolate
(43 g, 1 pop)

60 calories
1.5 g fat
(0 g saturated)
9 g sugars

The classic freezer treat is surprisingly easy on the waistline.

Breyers Pure Fruit Berry Swirls
(51 g, 1 bar)

40 calories
0 g fat
9 g sugars

Much of this sugar comes from the real fruit purees packed into these bars.

So Delicious Minis Vanilla
(37 g, 1 sandwich)

100 calories
3.5 g fat
(2.5 g saturated)
7 g sugars

This is a good treat to keep in mind, even if you're not lactose intolerant. It's low in sugar and laced with 2 grams of slow-digesting fiber.

Not That!

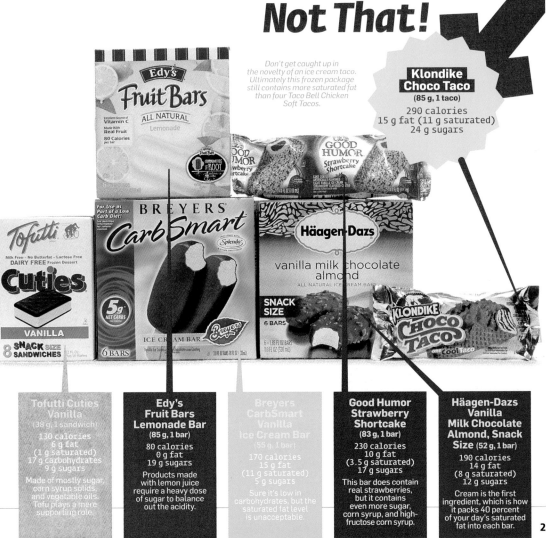

Don't get caught up in the novelty of an ice cream taco. Ultimately this frozen package still contains more saturated fat than four Taco Bell Chicken Soft Tacos.

Klondike Choco Taco
(85 g, 1 taco)
290 calories
15 g fat (11 g saturated)
24 g sugars

Tofutti Cuties Vanilla
(38 g, 1 sandwich)
130 calories
6 g fat
(1 g saturated)
17 g carbohydrates
9 g sugars

Made of mostly sugar, corn syrup solids, and vegetable oils. Tofu plays a mere supporting role.

Edy's Fruit Bars Lemonade Bar
(85 g, 1 bar)
80 calories
0 g fat
19 g sugars

Products made with lemon juice require a heavy dose of sugar to balance out the acidity.

Breyers CarbSmart Vanilla Ice Cream Bar
(55 g, 1 bar)
170 calories
15 g fat
(11 g saturated)
5 g sugars

Sure it's low in carbohydrates, but the saturated fat level is unacceptable.

Good Humor Strawberry Shortcake
(83 g, 1 bar)
230 calories
10 g fat
(3.5 g saturated)
17 g sugars

This bar does contain real strawberries, but it contains even more sugar, corn syrup, and high-fructose corn syrup.

Häagen-Dazs Vanilla Milk Chocolate Almond, Snack Size (52 g, 1 bar)
190 calories
14 g fat
(8 g saturated)
12 g sugars

Cream is the first ingredient, which is how it packs 40 percent of your day's saturated fat into each bar.

241

Juices

Drink This

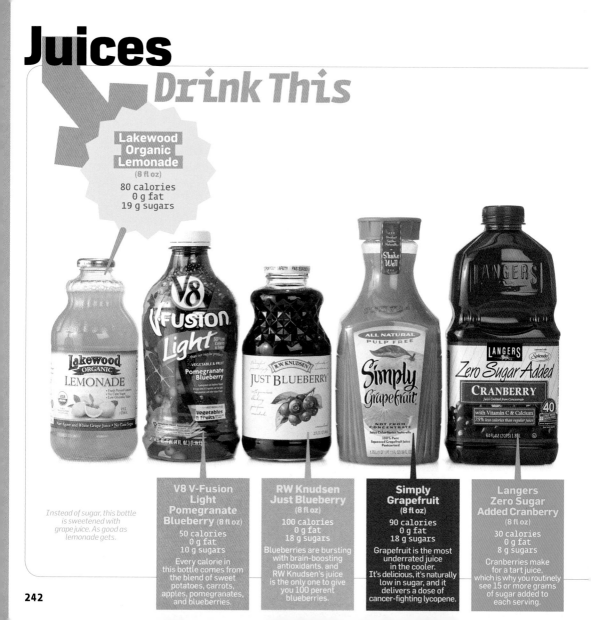

Lakewood Organic Lemonade
(8 fl oz)

80 calories
0 g fat
19 g sugars

Instead of sugar, this bottle is sweetened with grape juice. As good as lemonade gets.

V8 V-Fusion Light Pomegranate Blueberry (8 fl oz)

50 calories
0 g fat
10 g sugars

Every calorie in this bottle comes from the blend of sweet potatoes, carrots, apples, pomegranates, and blueberries.

RW Knudsen Just Blueberry (8 fl oz)

100 calories
0 g fat
18 g sugars

Blueberries are bursting with brain-boosting antioxidants, and RW Knudsen's juice is the only one to give you 100 perent blueberries.

Simply Grapefruit (8 fl oz)

90 calories
0 g fat
18 g sugars

Grapefruit is the most underrated juice in the cooler. It's delicious, it's naturally low in sugar, and it delivers a dose of cancer-fighting lycopene.

Langers Zero Sugar Added Cranberry (8 fl oz)

30 calories
0 g fat
8 g sugars

Cranberries make for a tart juice, which is why you routinely see 15 or more grams of sugar added to each serving.

Not That!

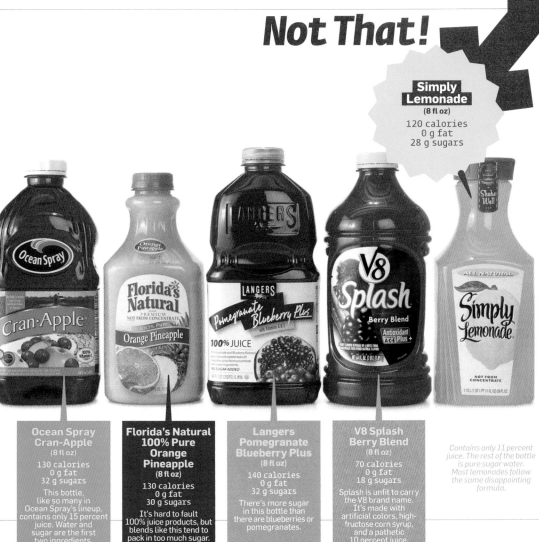

Simply Lemonade
(8 fl oz)

120 calories
0 g fat
28 g sugars

Ocean Spray Cran-Apple
(8 fl oz)

130 calories
0 g fat
32 g sugars

This bottle, like so many in Ocean Spray's lineup, contains only 15 percent juice. Water and sugar are the first two ingredients.

Florida's Natural 100% Pure Orange Pineapple
(8 fl oz)

130 calories
0 g fat
30 g sugars

It's hard to fault 100% juice products, but blends like this tend to pack in too much sugar.

Langers Pomegranate Blueberry Plus
(8 fl oz)

140 calories
0 g fat
32 g sugars

There's more sugar in this bottle than there are blueberries or pomegranates.

V8 Splash Berry Blend
(8 fl oz)

70 calories
0 g fat
18 g sugars

Splash is unfit to carry the V8 brand name. It's made with artificial colors, high-fructose corn syrup, and a pathetic 10 percent juice.

Contains only 11 percent juice. The rest of the bottle is pure sugar water. Most lemonades follow the same disappointing formula.

243

Teas

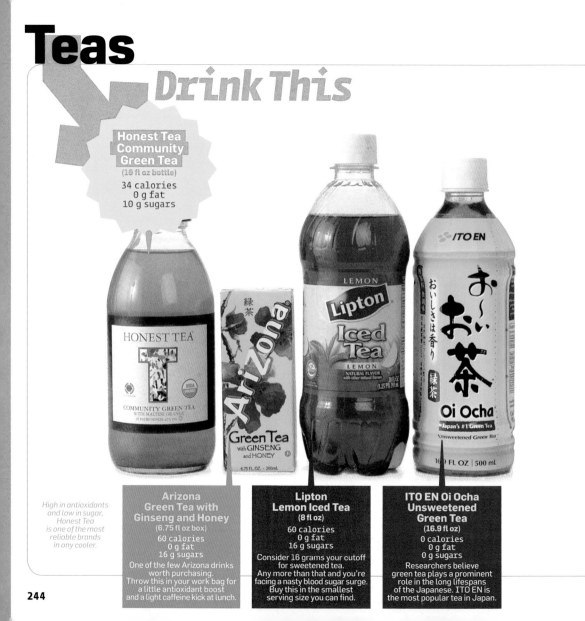

Drink This

Honest Tea Community Green Tea
(16 fl oz bottle)
34 calories
0 g fat
10 g sugars

High in antioxidants and low in sugar, Honest Tea is one of the most reliable brands in any cooler.

Arizona Green Tea with Ginseng and Honey
(6.75 fl oz box)
60 calories
0 g fat
16 g sugars
One of the few Arizona drinks worth purchasing. Throw this in your work bag for a little antioxidant boost and a light caffeine kick at lunch.

Lipton Lemon Iced Tea
(8 fl oz)
60 calories
0 g fat
16 g sugars
Consider 16 grams your cutoff for sweetened tea. Any more than that and you're facing a nasty blood sugar surge. Buy this in the smallest serving size you can find.

ITO EN Oi Ocha Unsweetened Green Tea
(16.9 fl oz)
0 calories
0 g fat
0 g sugars
Researchers believe green tea plays a prominent role in the long lifespans of the Japanese. ITO EN is the most popular tea in Japan.

Not That!

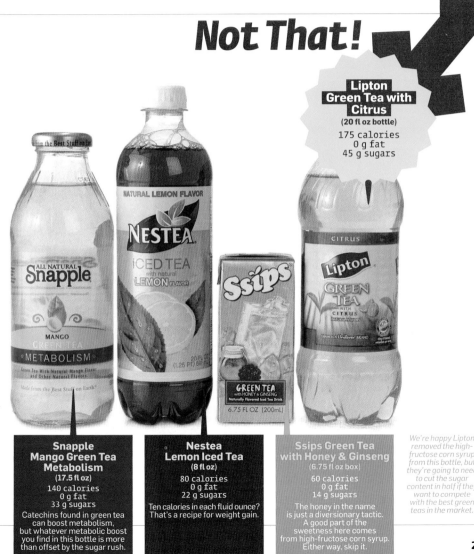

Lipton Green Tea with Citrus
(20 fl oz bottle)

175 calories
0 g fat
45 g sugars

Snapple Mango Green Tea Metabolism
(17.5 fl oz)

140 calories
0 g fat
33 g sugars

Catechins found in green tea can boost metabolism, but whatever metabolic boost you find in this bottle is more than offset by the sugar rush.

Nestea Lemon Iced Tea
(8 fl oz)

80 calories
0 g fat
22 g sugars

Ten calories in each fluid ounce? That's a recipe for weight gain.

Ssips Green Tea with Honey & Ginseng
(6.75 fl oz box)

60 calories
0 g fat
14 g sugars

The honey in the name is just a diversionary tactic. A good part of the sweetness here comes from high-fructose corn syrup. Either way, skip it.

We're happy Lipton removed the high-fructose corn syrup from this bottle, but they're going to need to cut the sugar content in half if they want to compete with the best green teas in the market.

245

Mixers

Drink This

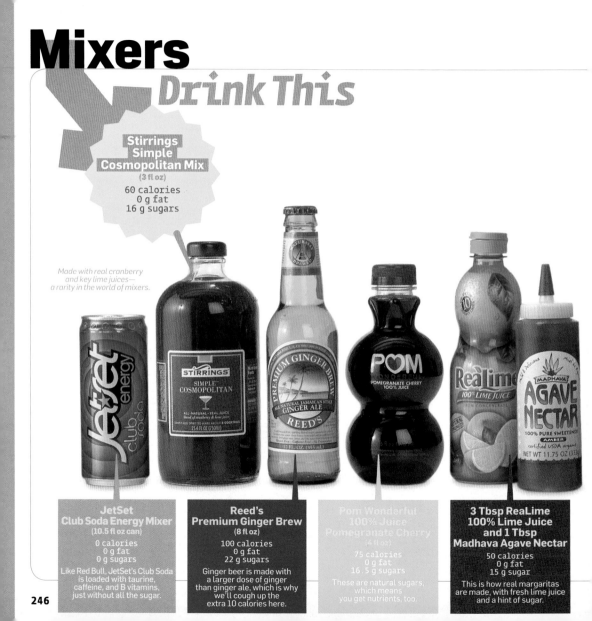

**Stirrings
Simple
Cosmopolitan Mix**
(3 fl oz)

60 calories
0 g fat
16 g sugars

*Made with real cranberry
and key lime juices—
a rarity in the world of mixers.*

**JetSet
Club Soda Energy Mixer**
(10.5 fl oz can)

0 calories
0 g fat
0 g sugars

Like Red Bull, JetSet's Club Soda
is loaded with taurine,
caffeine, and B vitamins,
just without all the sugar.

**Reed's
Premium Ginger Brew**
(8 fl oz)

100 calories
0 g fat
22 g sugars

Ginger beer is made with
a larger dose of ginger
than ginger ale, which is why
we'll cough up the
extra 10 calories here.

**Pom Wonderful
100% Juice
Pomegranate Cherry**
(4 fl oz)

75 calories
0 g fat
16.5 g sugars

These are natural sugars,
which means
you get nutrients, too.

**3 Tbsp ReaLime
100% Lime Juice
and 1 Tbsp
Madhava Agave Nectar**

50 calories
0 g fat
15 g sugar

This is how real margaritas
are made, with fresh lime juice
and a hint of sugar.

Not That!

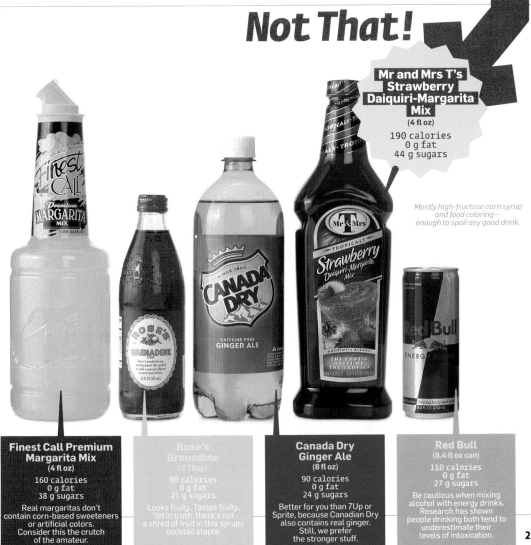

Mr and Mrs T's Strawberry Daiquiri-Margarita Mix
(4 fl oz)

190 calories
0 g fat
44 g sugars

Mostly high-fructose corn syrup and food coloring—enough to spoil any good drink.

Finest Call Premium Margarita Mix
(4 fl oz)

160 calories
0 g fat
38 g sugars

Real margaritas don't contain corn-based sweeteners or artificial colors. Consider this the crutch of the amateur.

Rose's Grenadine
(2 Tbsp)

90 calories
0 g fat
21 g sugars

Looks fruity. Tastes fruity. Yet in truth, there's not a shred of fruit in this syrupy cocktail staple.

Canada Dry Ginger Ale
(8 fl oz)

90 calories
0 g fat
24 g sugars

Better for you than 7Up or Sprite, because Canada Dry also contains real ginger. Still, we prefer the stronger stuff.

Red Bull
(8.4 fl oz can)

110 calories
0 g fat
27 g sugars

Be cautious when mixing alcohol with energy drinks. Research has shown people drinking both tend to underestimate their levels of intoxication.

Beers

Drink This

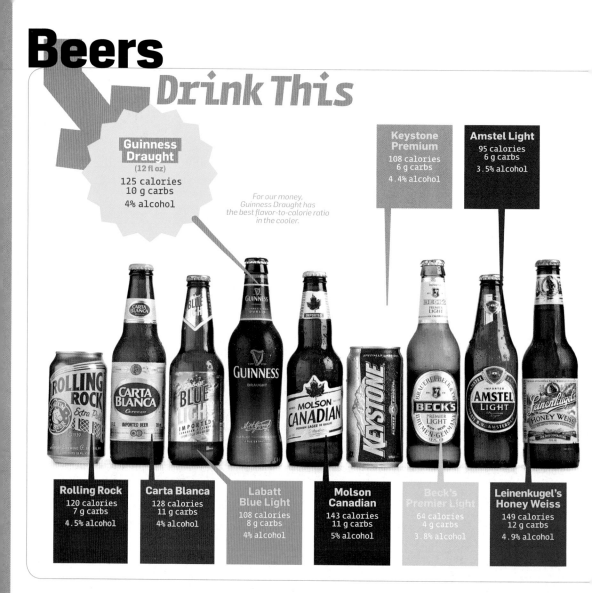

Guinness Draught
(12 fl oz)
125 calories
10 g carbs
4% alcohol

For our money, Guinness Draught has the best flavor-to-calorie ratio in the cooler.

Keystone Premium
108 calories
6 g carbs
4.4% alcohol

Amstel Light
95 calories
6 g carbs
3.5% alcohol

Rolling Rock
120 calories
7 g carbs
4.5% alcohol

Carta Blanca
128 calories
11 g carbs
4% alcohol

Labatt Blue Light
108 calories
8 g carbs
4% alcohol

Molson Canadian
143 calories
11 g carbs
5% alcohol

Beck's Premier Light
64 calories
4 g carbs
3.8% alcohol

Leinenkugel's Honey Weiss
149 calories
12 g carbs
4.9% alcohol

Not That!

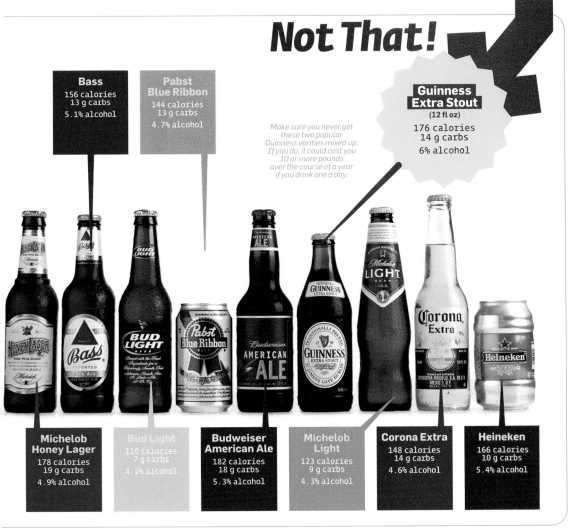

Bass
156 calories
13 g carbs
5.1% alcohol

Pabst Blue Ribbon
144 calories
13 g carbs
4.7% alcohol

Guinness Extra Stout
(12 fl oz)
176 calories
14 g carbs
6% alcohol

Make sure you never get these two popular Guinness varities mixed up. If you do, it could cost you 10 or more pounds over the course of a year if you drink one a day.

Michelob Honey Lager
178 calories
19 g carbs
4.9% alcohol

Bud Light
110 calories
7 g carbs
4.2% alcohol

Budweiser American Ale
182 calories
18 g carbs
5.3% alcohol

Michelob Light
123 calories
9 g carbs
4.3% alcohol

Corona Extra
148 calories
14 g carbs
4.6% alcohol

Heineken
166 calories
10 g carbs
5.4% alcohol

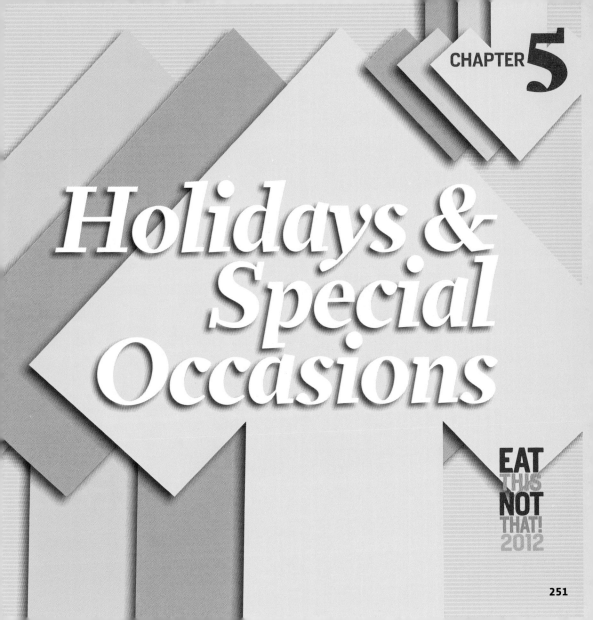

CHAPTER 5

Holidays &
Special
Occasions

EAT
THIS
NOT
THAT!
2012

Planning a traditional Thanksgiving dinner this year?

OF COURSE YOU ARE! What would this November's family gathering be without a heaping table laden with the very larder that fed the Pilgrims through their long first winter? Yummy! So go ahead—pass the platters of corn, the plates filled with root vegetables, the delightful desserts. And in the middle of it all, a big tray of hot, delicious roasted eels.

Eels? Eww!

Sorry, traditionalists, but if you really want to make like the Pilgrims, you'd better rethink your harvest. Wild turkeys—the kind that roamed the Americas in giant flocks when the first Old Worlders arrived in America—are almost impossible to hunt down with a bow and arrow or a musket. Fast, wily, and ugly as sin, turkeys were a very rare and special meal indeed, but if you lived or died by turkey, well, you died. Not the kind of food you'd try to make a feast out of. Indeed, the naturalist James Prosek claims that eels—abundant, high in fat and protein, and lethargic enough to catch with a spear in cold months—were almost certainly part of the main course at the first Thanksgiving.

Kinda makes you want to not give thanks, doesn't it?

The modern feast we all grew up with is in fact a savvy bit of dietary misdirection, one designed to give today's family table a more palatable protein choice while lining the pockets of the folks at Butterball and providing the nation with its only reason to watch those former college stars whose sad fate it was to be drafted by the Detroit Lions.

And Thanksgiving isn't the only holiday that's been corrupted by food marketers. The children nestled all snug in their beds in "The Night Before Christmas" weren't dreaming of giant chocolate Santas and gummies made of high-fructose corn syrup in the shape of Dora the Explorer. What danced in their heads were sugar-plums—a mixture of dried fruits, nuts, and spices with a light coating of sugar or coconut, and a lot healthier than what will be in your stocking this year. And Halloween? The original treats were roasted nuts, apples, pumpkin seeds, and potatoes.

So this year, don't think you're honoring your ancestors by downing every piece of candy corn, every leftover turkey sandwich, and every red- and green-foil-wrapped Hershey's Kiss. Yes, there are a lot of great holiday options.

But gorging yourself isn't one of them.

Thanksgiving

Protein

Ham
(4-oz bone-in rump)

148 calories
4 g fat (0 g saturated)
948 mg sodium

Ham is one of the leanest hoilday meats, but also one of the saltiest.

White turkey
(4 oz)

176 calories
4 g fat (0 g saturated)
372 mg sodium

A mean, lean, metabolism-boosting protein.

Dark turkey
(4 oz)

208 calories
8 g fat (4 g saturated)
388 mg sodium

The darker the meat, the more fat it harbors.

Fried turkey
(4 oz, white meat)

224 calories
14 g fat (6.8 g saturated)
532 mg sodium

Stick an otherwise healthy bird in a fryer and more than triple your fat intake.

Starchy Sides

Mashed potatoes
(½ cup made with whole milk)

87 calories
0.5 g fat
(0.5 g saturated)
317 mg sodium

To cut calories, prepare these with skim milk.

Roll with butter

130 calories
5 g fat (2 g saturated)
210 mg sodium

The pat of butter lowers this roll's glycemic index, helping to prevent dramatic spikes in blood sugar.

Candied sweet potatoes
(½ cup)

160 calories
4 g fat (0 g saturated)
80 mg sodium

These spuds cede the nutritional high ground when they're covered in sugar.

Stuffing
(½ cup)

175 calories
9 g fat (2 g saturated)
543 mg sodium

An appropriate name for a mash of refined carbohydrates basted with melted butter and turkey fat.

Corn bread
(2" x 2") with butter

190 calories
9 g fat (4 g saturated)
450 mg sodium

More calories, fat, and sodium than a regular roll.

Vegetable Sides

Roasted brussels sprouts
(½ cup)

28 calories
0 g fat
16 mg sodium

Low in calories, high in fiber. Enough said.

Roasted butternut squash
(½ cup, cubes)

40 calories
0 g fat
4 mg sodium

This squash's antioxidant carotenoid may help reduce the risk of lung cancer.

Green bean casserole
(½ cup)

100 calories
6 g fat (1 g saturated)
300 mg sodium

Replace the fried onions with caramelized ones and use fresh green beans.

Creamed spinach
(½ cup)

220 calories
14 g fat (7 g saturated)
440 mg sodium

Better off sautéing this nutritional powerhouse in olive oil and chopped garlic.

Condiments

Turkey gravy
(2 Tbsp)

16 calories
0 g fat
85 mg sodium

Oh so good for so few calories.

Fresh cranberry sauce
(2 Tbsp)

50 calories
0 g fat
11 g sugars

Fresh whole cranberries are some of the richest anticancer fighters.

Canned cranberry sauce
(½-inch slice)

85 calories
0 g fat
20 g sugars

Ban from your plate anything that shimmies like Jell-O.

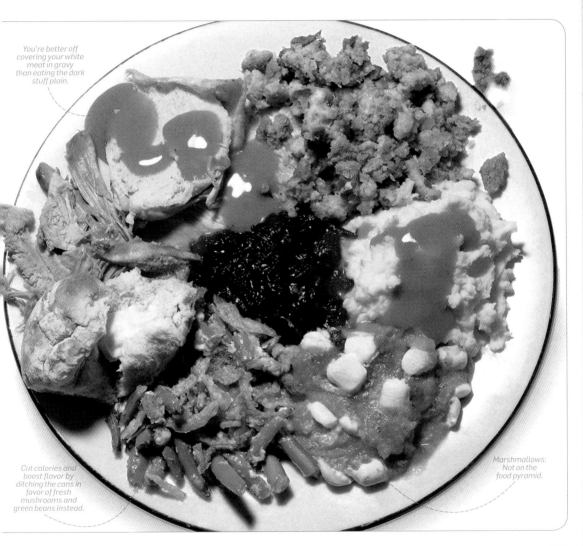

You're better off covering your white meat in gravy than eating the dark stuff plain.

Cut calories and boost flavor by ditching the cans in favor of fresh mushrooms and green beans instead.

Marshmallows: Not on the food pyramid.

christmas dinner

Protein

Beef tenderloin
(6 oz)

300 calories
15 g fat (6 g saturated)
400 mg sodium

Rubbed with olive oil, garlic, and rosemary, this is a protein powerhouse.

Leg of lamb
(6 oz)

408 calories
24 g fat (12 g saturated)
520 mg sodium

Switch to chops or loin if you want a leaner cut of lamb.

Duck breast
(6 oz)

480 calories
26 g fat (12 g saturated)
620 mg sodium

Peel off the skin and duck's protein-to-fat ratio is surprisingly impressive.

Prime rib
(6 oz)

600 calories
25 g fat (12 g saturated)
870 mg sodium

This cut is spiderwebbed with loads of intramuscular fat.

Vegetable Sides

Steamed green beans
(½ cup)

22 calories
0 g fat
0 mg sodium

These fiber-rich veggies will fend off the food coma.

Roasted red potatoes
(½ cup)

100 calories
5 g fat (1 g saturated)
170 mg sodium

Rule: Roasted over loaded. True always, especially with potatoes.

Salad Greens with croutons
(1 oz) and 2 Tbsp Italian dressing

240 calories
12 g fat (4 g saturated)
390 mg sodium

We applaud salad consumption as long as it's sans croutons and light on dressing.

Baked potato
with butter and sour cream (1 Tbsp each)

400 calories
14 g fat (6 g saturated)
500 mg sodium

This tater's only half stuffed and already bloated with calories.

Dessert

Chocolate-covered strawberries
(4)

164 calories
8.5 g fat
(4.5 g saturated)
24 g carbohydrates

Swap milk chocolate for dark to maximize antioxidant intake.

Coconut macaroons
(2)

195 calories
6 g fat (6 g saturated)
34 g sugars

The holiday perennial isn't the worst, but munch within reason.

Chocolate cake
(⅙ cake)

415 calories
13 g fat (5 g saturated)
45 g sugars

Better off eating a few squares of chocolate and calling it a night.

Cheesecake
(⅙ cake)

470 calories
26 g fat (13 g saturated)
39 g sugars

What do you expect from a dessert made almost entirely of cream cheese?

Wine

Sauvignon blanc
(5 fl oz)

119 calories
3 g carbohydrates
Resveratrol level: Very low

The driest white wine is still one of the best.

Chardonnay
(5 fl oz)

120 calories
4 g carbohydrates
Resveratrol level: Very low

Though white wines contain heart-strengthening resveratrol, they can't compete with reds on the antioxidant front.

Pinot noir
(5 fl oz)

121 calories
3 g carbohydrates
Resveratrol level: High

This big-bodied vino packs the most resveratrol.

Red zinfandel
(5 fl oz)

129 calories
4 g carbohydrates
Resveratrol level: Medium-high

Not as popular as merlot or cabernet, but it should be.

Dessert wine
(3.5 fl oz)

165 calories
14 g carbohydrates
Resveratrol level: Low

High in sugar, dessert wines always pack more calories than normal table wines.

BEST

WORST

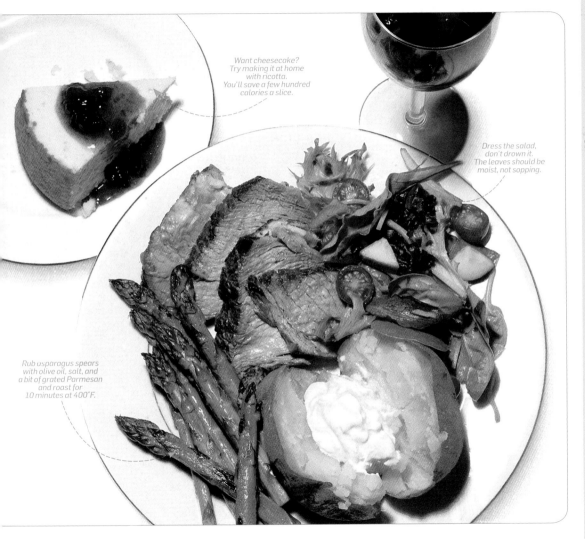

Want cheesecake? Try making it at home with ricotta. You'll save a few hundred calories a slice.

Dress the salad, don't drown it. The leaves should be moist, not sopping.

Rub asparagus spears with olive oil, salt, and a bit of grated Parmesan and roast for 10 minutes at 400°F.

New Year's Eve

Hors d'Oeuvres

Jumbo shrimp cocktail
(6) with 2 Tbsp cocktail sauce

60 calories
<1 g fat
470 mg sodium

*Indulge in the high-protein, virtually fat-free shrimp.
Limit the sodium-rich sauce.*

Cheddar cheese
(four ½-inch cubes)

140 calories
12 g fat (8 g saturated)
212 mg sodium

*High in fat, but also effective at squashing appetites.
If you want cheese, make it the first thing you eat.*

Tomato bruschetta
(2 pieces)

200 calories
4 g fat (1 g saturated)
230 mg sodium

Tomatoes, garlic, basil, and olive oil make this a potent party pick.

Crab cake with rémoulade

240 calories
18 g fat (4 g saturated)
600 mg sodium

*Bound with mayo and topped with a mayo-based sauce,
crab cakes don't offer the biggest bang for your caloric buck.*

Pigs in a blanket
(3)

400 calories
25 g fat (9 g saturated)
850 mg sodium

The real danger here is the calorie-dense pastry wrap.

Dips

Salsa
(½ cup and 8 chips)

156 calories
7 g fat (1 g saturated)
300 mg sodium

*You can't beat a dip made
entirely of produce.*

Guacamole
(¼ cup and 8 chips)

260 calories
15 g fat (3 g saturated)
325 mg sodium

*High in calories, but filled
with fiber and heart-healthy
monounsaturated fats.*

French onion
(¼ cup and 8 chips)

260 calories
17 g fat (7 g saturated)
440 mg sodium

*Nothing but spiked
sour cream. Better to spend
the calories on guac.*

Spinach artichoke
(¼ cup and 8 chips)

325 calories
19 g fat (9 g saturated)
625 mg sodium

*Woefully misnamed.
This is a cheese and
mayonnaise dip with a
sprinkling of vegetables.*

Booze

Champagne
(5 fl oz)

127 calories
8 g carbohydrates

*The standard New Year's drink
is also one of the lightest.*

Mojito
(8 fl oz)

180 calories
15 g carbohydrates

*Based almost entirely on
healthy ingredients:
lime juice, fresh mint, and
sugar-free club soda.*

Gin and tonic
(8 fl oz)

240 calories
16 g carbohydrates

*Adding tonic to anything
is like adding a
soda's worth of calories.*

Cosmopolitan
(8 fl oz)

300 calories
22 g carbohydrates

*Composed of high-sugar
additives that will slow
you down long before
the clock strikes midnight.*

Margarita
(8 fl oz)

450 calories
65 g carbohydrates

*The worst of all cocktails
for one reason: sugar.
Margarita mix is
nothing but dyed
high-fructose corn syrup.*

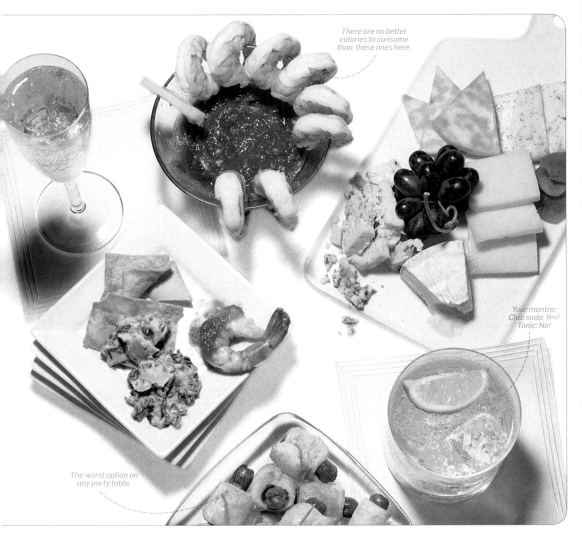

There are no better calories to consume than these ones here.

Your mantra: Club soda: Yes! Tonic: No!

The worst option on any party table.

Fourth of July

BEST

Off the Grill

Beef kabob
220 calories
9 g fat (4.5 g saturated)
120 mg sodium

Lean protein and fiber-rich veggies mean less need for unhealthy sides.

Hot dog
with relish, ketchup, and mustard
320 calories
18 g fat (8 g saturated)
960 mg sodium

While not the lowest-calorie choice, the frank is a relative winner on the grill.

Hamburger
(4 oz) with ketchup and mustard
462 calories
21.5 g fat (8 g saturated)
700 mg sodium

Cut 150 calories by using ground sirloin and a whole-wheat bun.

Baby back ribs
(½ rack)
490 calories
33 g fat (16 g saturated)
1,650 mg sodium

Universally the worst grill option, regardless of how little sauce has been slathered on top.

WORST

Sides

Canned baked beans
(½ cup)
120 calories
1 g fat (0 g saturated)
871 mg sodium

One serving is filled with 5 grams of fiber.

Coleslaw
(½ cup)
150 calories
8 g fat (1 g saturated)
350 mg sodium

Based on a formula similar to that for potato salad, but cabbage is healthier for you than potatoes. This number can climb, though, depending on the mayo application.

Corn on the cob
with butter
170 calories
11 g fat (7 g saturated)
190 mg sodium

Not the healthiest vegetable because most of its calories come from natural sugars, but not a terrible option on a hot summer day.

Homemade potato salad
(½ cup)
190 calories
12 g fat (3 g saturated)
560 mg sodium

Even the words "potato" and "salad" can be ruined by mayonnaise.

Dessert

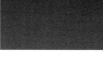

Grapes
(1 cup)
62 calories
0 g fat
15 g sugar

The phytonutrients in the skin of this fruit protect you against free-radical damage.

Cherry ice pop
50 calories
0 g fat
8 g sugars

A pretty harmless way to end a summer meal.

Ice cream sandwich
160 calories
5 g fat (3 g saturated)
13 g sugars

No matter the brand, this item's size dictates a restrained calorie load.

Chocolate ice cream bar
280 calories
20 g fat (13 g saturated)
20 g sugars

Bars from so-called premium brands like Häagen-Dazs and Dove pack a serious wallop.

Beer

Amstel Light
(12 fl oz)
95 calories
5 g carbohydrates

For when you desire the suds but don't want the heft.

Rolling Rock Premium
(12 fl oz)
132 calories
10 g carbohydrates

One of the lighter regular brews.

Budweiser
(12 fl oz)
145 calories
11 g carbohydrates

The king of beers is not a benevolent ruler.

Corona Extra
(12 fl oz)
148 calories
14 g carbohydrates

Light in flavor, not in calories.

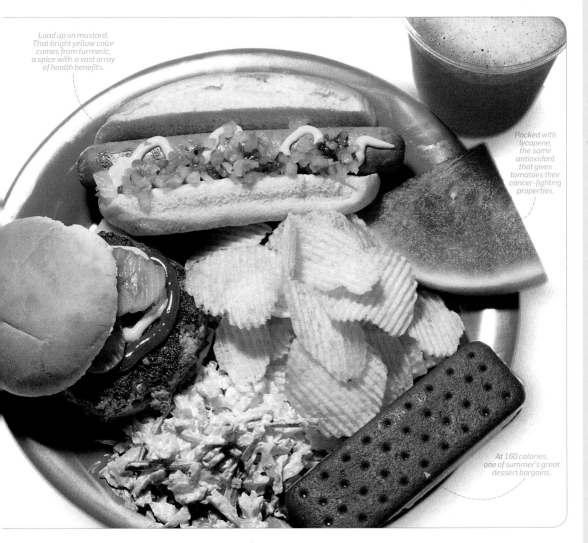

Load up on mustard. That bright yellow color comes from turmeric, a spice with a vast array of health benefits.

Packed with lycopene, the same antioxidant that gives tomatoes their cancer-fighting properties.

At 160 calories, one of summer's great dessert bargains.

H llow en

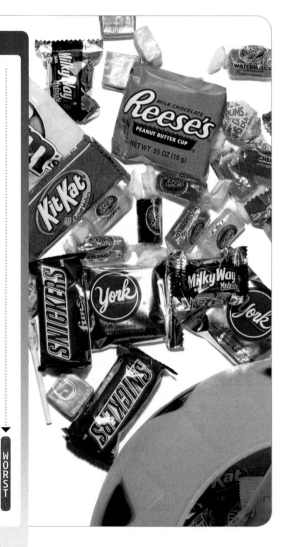

Candy

BEST

Sather's SweeTarts
(14 g, 10 pieces)

50 calories
0 g fat
12 g sugars

For tablets of refined sugar, these aren't that bad.

Smarties (14 g, 2 rolls)

50 calories
0 g fat
12 g sugars

Smarties are the intelligent candy choice.

Now and Later
(17 g, 4 pieces)

62 calories
0.5 g fat (0 g saturated)
11.5 g sugars

Opt for these now. Feel good about it later.

3 Musketeers
(15 g, "fun" size bar)

63 calories
2 g fat (1.5 g saturated)
10 g sugars

Compared to its "fun" size brethren, this bar is tame.

Brach's Candy Corn
(20 g, 11 pieces)

70 calories
0 g fat
14 g sugars

The only corn here is of the syrup variety.

Tootsie Roll
(20 g, 3 pieces)

70 calories
1.5 g fat (0.5 g saturated)
9.5 g sugars

Unroll too many of these and you'll add a roll to your midsection.

Snickers
(17 g, "fun" size bar)

80 calories
4 g fat (1.5 g saturated)
8.5 g sugars

Note: Does not actually satisfy.

Starburst (20 g, 4 pieces)

80 calories
2 g fat (1.5 g saturated)
11.5 g sugars

The fat comes from a weird combination of oils.

Skittles
(20 g, "fun" size pack)

80 calories
1 g fat (1 g saturated)
15 g sugars

Sugar, oil, and artificial coloring.

Butterfinger
(21 g, "fun" size bar)

100 calories
4 g fat (2 g saturated)
10 g sugars

Lives up to its name by being one of the fattiest bars out there.

Reese's Peanut Butter Cups
(1 cup)

105 calories
6.5 g fat (2.5 g saturated)
10.5 g sugars

More sugar than peanuts.

M&Ms Milk Chocolate
("fun" size bag)

106 calories
4.5 g fat (2.5 g saturated)
13.5 g sugars

Better off with peanut M&Ms.

WORST

Movie Theater

BEST ▲

WORST ▼

Salty Snacks

Homemade trail mix (¼ cup)
150 calories
7 g fat (3 g saturated)
325 mg sodium

Sometimes you need to bend the rules to eat well.

Soft pretzel
with mustard
290 calories
0 g fat
850 mg sodium

Skip the sludgy cheese dip to guarantee decent film fare.

Popcorn
(medium, 10–12 cups)
600 calories
39 g fat (12 g saturated)
1,120 mg sodium

Though movie theaters have begun to phase out trans fats in their "butter topping," it still packs a wallop.

Nachos
(40 chips and 4 oz cheese)
1,101 calories
59 g fat (18.5 g saturated)
1,580 mg sodium

As much sodium as 53 Saltine crackers.

Sweets

Good & Plenty
(33 pieces)
140 calories
0 g fat
25 g sugars

Licorice acts as an anti-inflammatory.

Junior Mints
(½ large box)
170 calories
3 g fat (2.5 g saturated)
32 g sugars

You can bet on mint candies to be the best chocolate choices.

Milk Duds
(½ large box)
230 calories
8 g fat (5 g saturated)
27 g sugars

They're called Duds for a reason.

Twizzlers
(½ 6-oz package)
320 calories
1 g fat
38 g sugars

Sure, they're "low fat,"—that's because they're pure sugar.

Drinks

Unsweetened iced tea
(from home or from theater; 16 fl oz)
Pack this in your purse for light, antioxidant-rich refreshment.
0 calories
0 g fat
0 g sugars

Cola (20 fl oz)
Nutritionally bankrupt soda is nothing but high-fructose corn syrup.
180 calories
0 g fat
46 g carbohydrates

Slushie (24 fl oz)
More sugar than 13 Double Stuf Oreos.
335 calories
0 g fat
88 g sugars

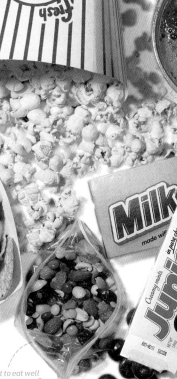

Pick the wrong popcorn and you could end up with 10 grams or more of trans fat.

Want to eat well and save money? Load up a sandwich bag with trail mix.

At the Mall

BEST

Main dish

Panda Express Potato Chicken
and Mixed Veggies

290 calories
11.5 g fat (2 g saturated)
1,340 mg sodium

You won't find a bowl of such lean proteins and nutrient-packed vegetables anywhere else in malls. Just be sure to skip the rice.

Subway Roast Beef
(6")

320 calories
5 g fat (1.5 g saturated)
700 mg sodium

Subway offers 14 sandwiches with 330 or fewer calories.

Sbarro Pepperoni Pizza
(1 slice)

591 calories
27 g fat (13 g saturated)
1,426 mg sodium

This one piece slices through 25 percent of your day's calories.

Quiznos Tuna Melt
(small)

690 calories
47 g fat (11 g saturated, 0.5 g trans)
840 mg sodium

From such a healthy fish is born a beastly sub.

Snacks

Chick-fil-A Fruit Cup
(medium)

70 calories
0 g fat
0 mg sodium

With this high fiber-to-calorie ratio, you're sure to get full without expanding your waistline.

Taco Bell Fresco Crunchy Taco

150 calories
7 g fat (2.5 g saturated)
350 mg sodium

The reasonable Fresco line includes four items with fewer than 200 calories.

Dairy Queen French Fries
(regular)

310 calories
13 g fat (2 g saturated)
640 mg sodium

You could have two tacos for the dietary cost of these fries.

Dessert

McDonald's Vanilla Reduced Fat Ice Cream Cone

150 calories
3.5 g fat (2 g saturated)
18 g sugars

In an era of colossal cone concoctions, McDonald's gets props for a sensible serving size.

Mrs. Fields Semi-Sweet Chocolate Chip Cookie

210 calories
10 g fat (5 g saturated)
19 g sugars

A step up from the food court's other dessert disasters.

Auntie Anne's Cinnamon Sugar Pretzel
without butter

380 calories
1 g fat (0 g saturated)
29 g sugars

Request your pretzel sans butter and save 90 calories of fat.

Cinnabon Classic Cinnamon Roll

880 calories
36 g fat (17 g saturated)
59 g sugars

A coronary catastrophe with as much fat as three McDonald's cheeseburgers.

Drinks

Orange Julius Raspberry Crush Premium Smoothie
(12 fl oz)

160 calories
0 g fat
32 g sugars

Jamba Juice Orange Dream Machine
(24 fl oz)

470 calories
1.5 g fat (1 g saturated)
97 g sugars

Smoothie King Cranberry Supreme Smoothie
(20 fl oz)

554 calories
1 g fat (0 g saturated)
96 g sugars

Its placement in the "Stay Healthy" section of the menu surely must be a mistake.

WORST

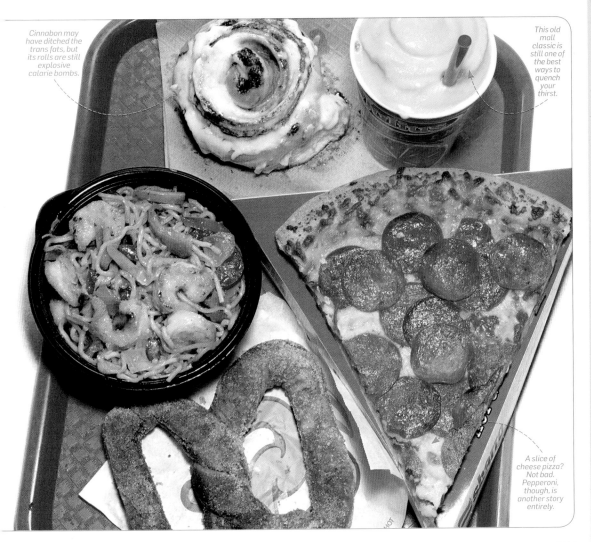

Cinnabon may have ditched the trans fats, but its rolls are still explosive calorie bombs.

This old mall classic is still one of the best ways to quench your thirst.

A slice of cheese pizza? Not bad. Pepperoni, though, is another story entirely.

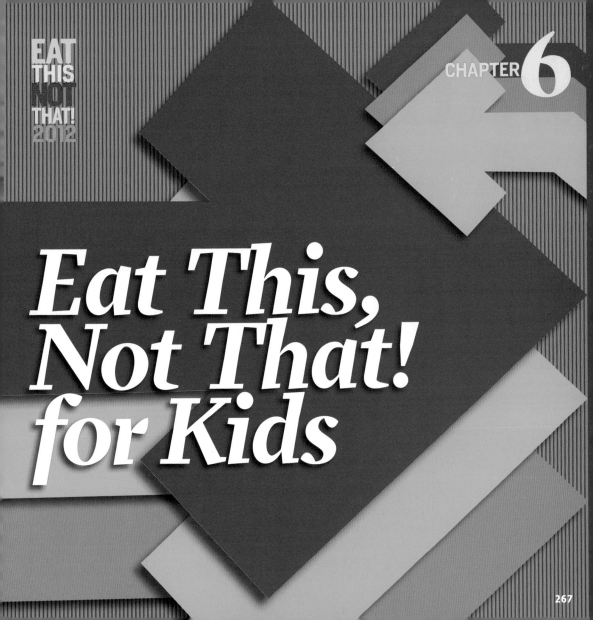

EAT
THIS
NOT
THAT!
2012

CHAPTER **6**

Eat This, Not That! for Kids

Raise an Advent Little Eater

LET'S SAY a new toy store opened in town, and it had a marvelous array of fascinating gadgets and gizmos that dazzled your eye and that of your towheaded toddler at prices that fit comfortably within your family budget. Sounds great, right?

Now, what if it turned out that more than 1 in every 3 toys you bought there was completely, irrevocably broken? The Rock 'Em Sock 'Em Robots couldn't rock or sock, the Mr. Potato Heads were total lemons, and the Barbies all came with Kirstie Alley's wardrobe. Oh, and there's a no-return policy on everything you buy.

You'd probably never shop at that store again, right?

Well, your local supermarket and fast-food joint have track records that are just as awful. Nearly a third of the foods our kids are consuming are utterly broken and useless. But we keep coming back and spending our money, week after week.

A 2010 study published by the American Dietetic Association found that nearly

urous

40 percent of the calories consumed by kids are empty calories. Forty percent of their food is worthless! For a 9-year-old boy consuming 1,400 calories a day, that's equivalent to chewing through 19 Starburst candies every single day of the week.

Now, food isn't exactly the same as toys. Getting kids to eat anything remotely nutritious is often a tug of war to the death. One of you emerges victorious. The other lands facedown in a pile of peas. But what if you just dropped the rope?

See, the food fight is not one you can win through will and force alone. Indeed, the best thing to do is not to fight at all. Do what the smartest parents do: Cheat. Dupe, deceive, dissemble, falsify, beguile, fabricate, prevaricate, exaggerate, and if that doesn't work, then just lie. Trix may be for kids, but tricks are for parents. Use these tactics to fool your kids into eating right, and you'll set them up for a lifetime of health and happiness. Bad daddy! Bad mommy! Lucky kid.

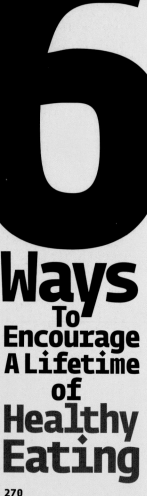

6

Ways To Encourage A Lifetime of Healthy Eating

Rule #1

PLAY PSYCHOLOGIST WITH YOUR KID

Nowadays, kids avoid vegetables like they're out-of-style sneakers; only one in five of them actually eats enough plant matter. If you want to reverse that trend, a little scheming can go a long way. Research out of England found that giving children a taste of a new vegetable daily for 2 weeks increased their enjoyment and consumption of that food.

Not all strategies sound as sinister as the exposure therapy. Giving kids ownership over what they eat is also a powerful play. Consider planting a garden. Studies show that kids' acceptance of fruits and vegetables increases after participating in growing them. No time to till? Simply letting your children choose their vegetables can lead to an 80 percent increase in their consumption.

Rule #2

NEVER SKIP BREAKFAST. EVER.

"Don't skip breakfast" is the persistent platitude heard 'round the world. Which may explain why so few pay attention—especially children. A 2005 study showed that kids skipped breakfast more than any other meal despite its reign as the king of meals. The effects of this epidemic are by now well known. Test after test shows that breakfast-eating students score higher on short-term memory and verbal fluency, among many other academic benefits.

Maybe breakfast's most important contribution, however, is found not in its own nutritional value, but in its impact on the rest of the day's eating habits. Research says children eating a meal in the

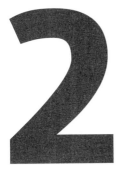

morning will themselves choose less soda and fewer fries while opting for more vegetables and milk throughout the rest of the day.

We know time can be an issue in the chaos of the early morning hours. But a nutritious bowl of cereal, cup of yogurt, or even microwaveable break-fast is never more than a few minutes away. Check out dozens of excellent options in Chapter 4.

Rule #3
FORGET ABOUT FORCE-FEEDING

Whether it's a Clean Plate Club membership drive or castigations about starving Africans, efforts by parents to get their children to eat healthy foods can backfire. In a 2009 study of 63 children, Cornell researchers found that those whose parents insisted on clean plates ate 35 percent more of a sweetened cereal later in the day. If kids ate 35 percent more than 1 serving of Froot Loops every day for a year, they'd gain 4 pounds.

There is a corollary. A Pennsylvania study indicated that the restric-tion of specific yummy foods from children's plates actually increased the kids' long-term prefer-ence for and consumption of those foods. It's also been found that kids who are barred from having certain indulgences tend to eat more when they're not hungry.

The lesson here is twofold: First, there is a fine line between encouraging your kids to try new foods and forcing them to eat against their will. The negative tone and tenor of all those warnings about not finishing our lima beans when we were kids is probably one of the reasons why most American adults still don't eat enough vegetables.

Set a house rule that your children need to try a new food three times before deciding whether they like it. If they still don't dig it after the third attempt, then Mom and Dad need to let it go. On the flip side, banning foods from your household can backfire, so rather than forbidding certain foods, set up specific parameters for when treats can be enjoyed.

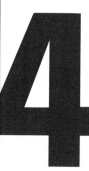

Rule #4
SHRINK YOUR SILVERWARE

According to another study from Cornell, portion size is the most powerful predictor of how much preschool-age children eat. And with the typical manufacturers' snack package being 2.5 times bigger than the appropriate amount for young kids, health-conscious parents fight an uphill battle.

Control what you can. Keep in mind that restaurant portions—even for kids—are egregiously oversized, so don't force them to wolf down every last tater tot. Splitting a dish with a sibling is never a bad idea (as long as you ask for two toys). At home, use smaller bowls, plates, and utensils. Jedi mind trick or not, there's plenty of evidence that kids will consume fewer calories when you downsize the dishes.

Rule #5
SET AN EXAMPLE (ESPECIALLY YOU, DAD)

The portion of America's food dollars spent on meals out increased from 34 percent to 48 percent between 1974 and 2008. Parents' increasing penchant for restaurant food can translate to nutritionally unsound decisions by kids. One recent study laid the heaviest blame on fathers. Researchers at Texas A&M University say dads carry the most influence largely because when they take their kids to the Mickey D's, it's often as a treat or some sort of celebration. This enforces the idea that unhealthy eating is positive. Mothers, on the other hand, often choose fast food due to time constraints, so the food doesn't hold as much psychological sway.

Rule #6
TURN OFF THE TUBE

Since 1970, the number of television ads aimed at children has doubled to 40,000 per year, and several studies suggest that the amount of time kids watch television is a strong predictor of how often they request specific foods. This spells big trouble for one reason: Half of all TV ads directed at children promote junk food.

The solution is simple: Shove your kids outside. Surprise them with a bike, a soccer dog, a Chihuahua dog—anything to get them moving. More time spent outdoors means less time being exposed to television marketing. Of course, the larger benefit is that they get more exercise, which decreases the risk of a lot of bad stuff: obesity, diabetes, heart disease, even boredom.

Eat This Plate, Not That One!

SIMPLICITY IS ELEGANT.
It's the case in nutrition as it is in design, and the USDA seems to have recognized these truths when it replaced the confusing, data-deluged food pyramid in June 2011. In its place, the government now dishes up a plate-shaped logo cut into smaller and bigger wedges connoting the food groups. Its spare design is meant to illustrate the ideal relative proportions for each category without overloading us with unnecessary details.

The growing need for clear parental guidance is starkly evident: Kids now consume more than a quarter of their daily calories in the form of empty snack calories, the vast majority of which are artery-clogging, blood-pressure-spiking, energy-jolting junk foods. And only one in four of our little ones consumes his or her daily recommended doses of fruits and vegetables. So we applaud the USDA's move. Yet, not all foods within a category are created equal, and plenty of room for error still exists with this stripped-down design. So in the name of true simplicity, we've broken down the best and worst options for each group.

Eat This

Meat, Poultry, Fish, Eggs, and Beans

- Grilled chicken breast
- Sirloin steak
- Grilled salmon or tilapia
- Deli turkey, ham, or roast beef
- Scrambled, poached, or boiled eggs
- Stewed black beans
- Hummus
- Natural, unsweetened peanut butter*

Dietary protein is the body's mechanic, repairing everything from cell walls to cuts to broken bones. It also drives metabolism, meaning that increasing your child's lean protein consumption will make his or her body more efficient at burning calories. For meats, the most important factors are that the cuts and the cooking methods are naturally lean. That means grilling or roasting chicken, pork loin, and less-marbled cuts of beef like sirloin, flank, and fillets.

Perfect for fruit and veggie dipping. Check the ingredients list and opt for a natural peanut butter without sugar and partially hydrogenated oils.

Fruits

- Sliced apples or pears
- Berries (straight, or on yogurt or cereal)
- Bananas
- Grapes
- 100 percent fruit smoothies

So much of the fruit consumed by children is heavily processed—either crushed to make juice or smashed into fruit snacks and bars. What you want is whole, unadulterated fruits in their most natural forms—even if that means buying them frozen. Actually, studies show that frozen fruit can be more nutrient packed because it's packaged during peak season.

Taken together, fruits and vegetables should compose at least half of your child's daily dietary plate.

Dairy

- **2% milk**
- **String cheese**
- **Cottage cheese**
- **Plain Greek yogurt with fresh fruit**

Dairy products are great sources of protein and bone-building calcium, but high fat content means they can pack plenty of calories. On the flip side, going fat free means your kid can lose out on some of the nutrients in dairy that your body needs a bit of fat to properly absorb. That's why we like low-fat dairy products like 2% milk and reduced-fat cheese: They have enough fat to make them tasty and nutritious, but not so much that dairy will pack on the pounds.

Grains

- **Brown rice**
- **Whole-grain bread**
- **Quinoa**
- **Whole-grain pasta**
- **Oatmeal**

11

Percentage of grain servings eaten by the average American that come from whole grains

Sure, this list's superiority is partially due to its lower glycemic index (meaning that the carbohydrates have less of an impact on the blood sugar level) and the occasional boost in protein provided by some of the foods. But it's the fiber that matters most. Many cram in double or triple what their non-whole-grain counterparts contain. For children, starting this habit now not only helps fend off diabetes, but also helps reduce the risk of cancer and heart disease later in life.

Vegetables

- **Steamed broccoli**
- **Mixed salad greens**
- **Sautéed mushrooms**
- **Roasted squash**
- **Grilled sweet peppers and onions**
- **Baby carrots**
- **Sweet potatoes**

Stick with raw vegetables or minimally cooked ones to retain the potent nutrients. And shop the rainbow. By choosing deep green, red, orange, and white vegetables, you're guaranteed to consume a balance of vitamins and minerals. One easy-to-make switch is from white potatoes to the sweet version, which lowers the impact on blood sugar levels and makes you feel fuller for longer.

Meat, Poultry, Fish, Eggs, and Beans

- Chicken nuggets
- Crispy chicken sandwich
- Fish sticks
- Deli salami, pepperoni, or bologna
- Burgers
- Fatty cuts of steak
- Peanut butter with added sugars and partially hydrogenated fats

An abnormally large percentage of kids' protein consumption is in the form of chicken nuggets. It doesn't take a genius to know that caked-on crumbs submerged in molten oil are a sure-fire way to jack up a meal's calories. So is opting for fatty cuts of beef like ground chuck (used to make burgers) and rib eyes (steaks loaded with intramuscular fat).

Fruits

- More than 8 ounces of juice a day
- More than a few tablespoons of dried fruits a day
- Smoothies made with sherbet, frozen yogurt, or added sugar
- Fruit-flavored yogurt

These choices might be better than a bag of Skittles, but not by much. Drinking your fruits in the form of juices or non-whole-fruit smoothies makes you miss out on one of fruits' biggest benefits—fiber. And fruit-flavored packaged foods are just that: industrially processed items heavy with sugar and light in actual fruit. On the entire plate, whole foods are better than processed ones.

5.5
Pounds gained over a year by eating one Chips Ahoy!'s worth of calories more than you expend every day

40
Percentage of 2- to 5-year-old kids' fruit intake that's in the form of juice

17
Teaspoons of added sugar most 5-year-olds eat every single day

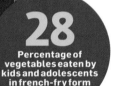

Dairy

- **Chocolate milk**
- **Ice cream**
- **Queso dip**
- **Yogurt processed with fruit**

Most people think about reducing the fat content of dairy products, and that can be helpful, since many of the listed foods are chock-full of it. But equally as significant nowadays are the spoonfuls of sugar added to so many milk products. One cup of Nesquik Chocolate Lowfat Milk has 28 grams of sugar—almost as much as a Snickers bar.

28

Percentage of vegetables eaten by kids and adolescents in french-fry form

Grains

- **White rice**
- **White bread**
- **Muffins**
- **Pasta**
- **Heavily sweetened cereals**

Quick-burning carbohydrates, the kind found in these refined grains, take a child's blood sugar on a bumpy ride. And that has short-term and long-term consequences. Increased sugar consumption has been linked not just to weight gain and obesity, but also to hyperactivity, ADHD, anxiety, and reduced school performance.

Vegetables

- **French fries**
- **Chips**
- **Onion rings**
- **White potatoes**

Don't negate the benefits of vegetables by frying them. The deep-fryer treatment not only zaps vegetables of most of their nutrients, but also subjects them mostly to oils loaded with excess calories and fat.

The 20 WORST Kids' Foods in America

The food industry has declared war on our kids' waistlines. It's time for parents to fight back.

WORST BREAKFAST CEREAL

20 Post
Fruity Pebbles (1 cup)
160 calories
1 g fat (1 g saturated)
15 g sugars
0 g fiber

This is Post's rosy appraisal of its flagship kids' cereal: "Fruity Pebbles is a wholesome, sweetened rice cereal. It is low in fat, cholesterol free, and provides 10 essential vitamins and minerals." Here's what it really meant to say: "Fruity Pebbles is a heavily manipulated, egregiously sweetened rice cereal. It is low in nutrients, fiber free, and the second and third ingredients in the cereal are sugar and hydrogenated vegetable oil, respectively." If you plan to feed your kids this stuff when they wake up, you may as well let them keep sleeping.

Eat This Instead!
Kellogg's
Froot Loops (1 cup)
110 calories
1 g fat (0.5 g saturated)
12 g sugars
3 g fiber

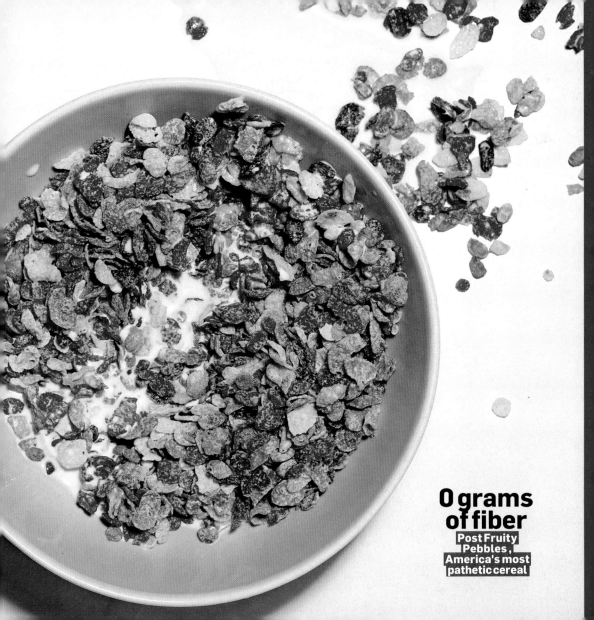

0 grams of fiber
Post Fruity Pebbles, America's most pathetic cereal

19 Denny's
Kids' Finish Line Fries

430 calories
23 g fat (5 g saturated)
50 g carbohydrates

As important as it is for your kids to choose healthy entrées, a bad side can bring down even the leanest dinner centerpiece. These fries (disturbingly, the exact same portion as the adult version) alone pack as many calories and grams of fat as a child should consume in an entire meal.

Eat This Instead!
Kids' Apple Dunkers

130 calories
0 g fat
30 g carbohydrates

18 Kid Cuisine
All American
Fried Chicken (286 g, 1 meal)

540 calories
24 g fat (6 g saturated, 1 g trans)
750 mg sodium

Busy parents understandably need to turn to the freezer section to look for quick dinner solutions when time is tight. Just know that danger lurks in the land of the deep freeze. Despite its cutesy packaging, this Kid Cuisine entrée sports not just excessive amounts of calories and fat, but also a dose of trans fats derived from partially hydrogenated oil—the last thing a growing body needs.

550 calories
Atlanta Bread Company pushes PB&J to the extreme

While icy blocks of meat and vegetables can never stack up to a fresh, home-cooked meal, there are plenty of solid options out there. Just by switching from Kid Cuisine to Banquet, you'll cut calories and fat nearly in half.

Eat This Instead!
Banquet Chicken Nuggets and Fries (142 g, 1 meal)

290 calories
13 g fat (2.5 g saturated)
520 mg sodium

17 Atlanta Bread
Company Kids' Peanut
Butter & Jelly

550 calories
15 g fat (3.5 g saturated)
89 g carbohydrates

It's hard to lose with the sturdy alliance of peanut butter and jelly—that is, unless you let your kid order it at Atlanta Bread Company. It would be easy to blame it on an excess of peanut butter, but sugary jelly is equally to blame here. Listed first on the sandwich's ingredients list, it accounts for a significant portion of the 89 grams of carbohydrates and helps to make this sandwich more caloric than the chain's grilled cheese.

Eat This Instead!
Kids' Grilled Cheese
390 calories
15 g fat (9 g saturated)
46 g carbohydrates

16 PF Chang's Kid's Chicken Fried Rice

580 calories
18 g fat (4 g saturated)
1,510 mg sodium

Chang's tries to shroud its nutrition numbers by breaking meals into multiple servings. Don't be fooled. The restaurant continues its usual sodium assault on its new kids' menu. There you find a dish whose potential (chicken and rice, what could possibly go wrong?) is outweighed only by the surplus of salt saturating every last greasy grain of rice.

Eat This Instead!
Kid's Stir-Fried Baby Buddha's Feast

180 calories
8 g fat (2 g saturated)
1,520 mg sodium

WORST FISH MEAL

15 Long John Silver's Popcorn Shrimp Kid's Meal with Pepsi

710 calories
28.5 g fat
(7 g saturated, 8.5 g trans)
1,155 mg sodium

There's plenty to dislike about this meal, but it's the explosive level of trans fats that caught our eye first. In fact, Silver's doesn't offer a single kids' meal with fewer than 5.5 grams of the dangerous fats—that's nearly three times the daily limit for a healthy adult. By simply switching fry oil, like so many other chains

have done, LJS can fix that problem. In the meantime, skip the kids' menu entirely and suggest the scampi—one of the few kid-friendly meals not spoiled with heart-threatening fats.

Eat This Instead!
Garlic Shrimp Scampi with Ice Water

200 calories
13.5 g fat (2.5 g saturated)
685 mg sodium

WORST BURGER

14 Applebee's Kids Mini Cheeseburgers (2)

740 calories
46 g fat
(16 g saturated, 2 g trans)
1,100 mg sodium

Just another sad example of Restaurant Law 172A, the Mini-Burger Paradox (MBP). The MBP states that the more diminutive the burger, the more potential it possesses for nutritional mayhem (see: Ruby Tuesday, Chili's, et al.). If restaurants stopped with one mini, you'd be fine, but these baby burgers normally come in groups of two or more—so you end up with two buns, two slices of cheese, two sets of condiments. The end result is a total package with more calories, fat, and sodium than you'd find in one normal-size burger.

Eat This Instead!
Kids Corn Dog

260 calories
14 g fat (4 g saturated)
440 mg sodium

WORST PIZZA

13 California Pizza Kitchen Kids Honey Chicken Pizza with Tomato Sauce

760 calories
N/A g fat (11 g saturated)
1,579 mg sodium
97 g carbohydrates

The sad truth is that we could have picked any of the kids' pizzas for this list. Even the cheese pizza has more than 600 calories, and the other four options go up from there. Thank the thick dough and heavy-handed cheese application. The little ones could eat two slices of Original BBQ Chicken pizza from a six-slice adult pie and save more than 300 calories.

Eat This Instead!
Kids Crispy Chicken with Broccoli

345 calories
N/A g fat (3 g saturated)
1,254 mg sodium
32 g carbohydrates

WORST BREAKFAST

12 Bob Evans Kids Plenty-o-Pancakes with Chocolate Chips

766 calories
22 g fat (13 g saturated fat)
1,281 mg sodium
137 g carbohydrates

As if five saucer-size pancakes studded with chocolate weren't bad enough, scoops of whip cream top each piece. The result is a load of refined carbohydrates that will have your kid bouncing in the booth (and crashing on the way home). And Bob's nutrition information doesn't even include the sugar dump found in the syrup or the additional fat and calories in the bacon or sausage that comes on the side.

Eat This Instead!
Kids Fruit Dippers
222 calories
1 g fat (0 g saturated)
62 mg sodium
51 g carbohydrates

WORST NACHOS
11 On the Border Kid's Bean & Cheese Nachos
770 calories
45 g fat (25 g saturated)
1,440 mg sodium

On the Border has scaled back this dish since *Eat This, Not That!* last attacked it, but the changes don't even come close to reining in this time bomb.

766 calories
Don't derail your kid's day with this trainwreck of a breakfast from Bob Evans.

The only thing worse than the 25 grams of saturated fat—nearly twice as much as an 8-year-old kid should consume in an entire day—is the fact that these nachos come with a complimentary sundae, pushing the meal total north of 1,100 calories.

Eat This Instead!
Kid's Grilled Chicken with Black Beans
270 calories
4 g fat (1 g saturated)
1,190 mg sodium

WORST DRINK
10 Applebee's Kids Oreo Cookie Shake
780 calories
41 g fat (26 g saturated)
97 g carbohydrates

Though Applebee's doesn't list it in its nutrition guide, we have a sneaking suspicion that nearly all of those 97 grams of carbohydrates are pure sugar. That's an insulin spike that

would make diabetes specialists cringe. (Not to mention dentists.) Your child would have to eat 15 Oreos to match this shake's caloric heft. Better off going with chocolate milk—or better yet, a single scoop of vanilla ice cream.

Eat This Instead!
Kids Chocolate Milk
270 calories
6 g fat (3 g saturated)
45 g carbohydrates

WORST FAST-FOOD CHICKEN MEAL
9 KFC Kids Meal with Popcorn Chicken, Potato Wedges, and Pepsi
800 calories
37.5 g fat (8 g saturated)
1,755 mg sodium

Fried chicken is almost always trouble, but the Potato Wedges constitute this meal's biggest calorie portion. And its most dangerous. Despite the Colonel's high-profile PR campaign touting its trans fat-free menu, these wedges are loaded with partially hydrogenated vegetable oils, the precursors to the perilous fats.

Eat This Instead!
Kids Meal with Grilled Chicken Drumstick, Mashed Potatoes (no gravy), and Capri Sun Roarin' Waters Tropical Fruit Juice Drink
250 calories
9.5 g fat (3 g saturated)
725 mg sodium

WORST GRILLED CHEESE

8 The Cheesecake Factory Kids Grilled Cheese Sandwich

810 calories
N/A g fat (21 g saturated)
1,656 mg sodium

Bread and cheese toasted into a warm, comforting meal. What's simpler than that? Well, the Factory shows it can ruin a simple kid favorite by oversizing every aspect of the sandwich. Its version is built with two thick slices of heavily buttered bread that bookend an even thicker layer of gooey cheese. This is just one of the many reasons the chain has for years resisted releasing comprehensive nutrition guides. The Grilled Chicken is the best alternative, but even that is far from danger free.

Eat This Instead!
Kids Grilled Chicken

510 calories
N/A g fat (16 g saturated)
1,204 mg sodium

WORST CHICKEN MEAL

7 The Cheesecake Factory Kids Southern Fried Chicken Sliders

820 calories
N/A g fat (10 g saturated)
2,049 mg sodium

When the Factory unveiled its kids' menu in 2009, its chief marketing officer said it was an effort to offer meals that fit kids' unique

"portion size requirement." On the surface, these sliders fit that bill. But if their size is humble, their nutritional numbers are not. These deep-fried slabs of chicken carry more than 2 days' worth of a child's sodium and more calories than a kid would get from eating 17 Chicken McNuggets.

Eat This Instead!
Kids Grilled Chicken

510 calories
N/A g fat (16 g saturated)
1,204 mg sodium

WORST FAST-FOOD BURGER MEAL

6 McDonald's Mighty Kids Meal with Double Cheeseburger, Fries (small), and 1% Chocolate Milk Jug

840 calories
37 g fat
(14 g saturated, 1.5 g trans)
1,460 mg sodium

The Golden Arches should be commended for increasing the number of healthy options in recent years. In particular, its Apple Dippers have inspired other large chains to offer alternatives to fried potatoes. Unfortunately, it's still easier to construct a lousy meal at McDonald's as it is a good one. This burger, fries, and milk combo chews through more than a half day's worth of calories, fat, and sodium. You might get a toy in the box, but you also get a lot

840 calories
A not-so-happy meal for parents who want to raise healthy kids

283

of empty calories, and that does not make a body happy.

Eat This Instead!
Happy Meal with Hamburger, Apple Dippers with Low-Fat Caramel Dip, and Apple Juice Box
450 calories
9.5 g fat
(3.5 g saturated, 0.5 g trans)
570 mg sodium

WORST SALAD
5 Friendly's Dippin' Chicken Salad
950 calories
50 g fat (12 g saturated)
1,880 mg sodium

It's an incredible thing to get a child excited about eating a salad. Just not this one. First off, this isn't so much a salad as a fried chicken dish with a few token veggies packed into a cone. Friendly's just doesn't know when to stop. On the side of the deep fried meat are bowls filled with croutons, cheese, and a honey mustard dipping sauce, which itself has 15 grams of fat. You end up with a "salad" that has more fat than three Snickers bars.

Eat This Instead!
Grilled Cheese Sandwich with Mandarin Oranges
370 calories
17 g fat (9 g saturated)
900 mg sodium

WORST MACARONI AND CHEESE
4 California Pizza Kitchen Kids Curly Mac n' Cheese with Edamame
1,088 calories
N/A g fat (33 g saturated)
750 mg sodium

Whereas most kid favorites—chicken fingers, cheeseburgers, even hot dogs—offer some redeeming nutritional value, macaroni and cheese brings nothing but cheese, cream, and refined carbohydrates to the table. CPK appears willing to solve that problem with the inclusion of protein- and fiber-rich edamame in its mac, but instead it stuffs its kiddy bowls to the brim with one of the most calorie-dense pastas we've ever seen. Another good opportunity squandered by the restaurant industry's penchant for excess.

Eat This Instead!
Kids Fusilli with Tomato Sauce
561 calories
N/A g fat (1 g saturated)
1,021 mg sodium

WORST DESSERT
3 Outback Steakhouse Joey Spotted Dog Sundae
1,216 calories
94 g fat (58.5 g saturated)
89 g carbohydrates

Nothing's more fun than seeing a small face transformed into a Jackson Pollack painting of ice cream and chocolate. So don't douse that joy with the bucket of guilt that comes with feeding your child more calories than two McDonald's Quarter Pounders with Cheese. This sundae has nearly 4 days' worth of saturated fat, which is fitting because the only way you should order it is with four spoons for sharing. Until Outback offers a decent dessert on its menu, either skip the sweet stuff or ask for a scoop of ice cream.

Eat This Instead!
Vanilla or chocolate ice cream (1 scoop)
Outback doesn't offer calorie counts for this, but you should have no trouble ordering it at any location.

WORST MEXICAN MEAL
2 On the Border Kid's Cheese Quesadilla with Mexican Rice
1,220 calories
75 g fat (31 g saturated)
1,930 mg sodium

On the Border's kids' menu mostly offers reasonable Mexican fare, but this cheese quesadilla, along with the nachos, stands out as a disturbing outlier. How the chain veers so far off course with this item, we don't know. Is it overloaded with cheese, or is the chicken poached in butter? Whatever the case, this quesadilla and rice provide more calories than should be in two kids' meals and enough sodium to cure a whole hog.

Eat This Instead!

Kid's Mexican Plate with Crispy Chicken Taco

260 calories
12 g fat (4 g saturated)
530 mg sodium

WORST KIDS' MEAL IN AMERICA

1 The Cheesecake Factory Kids Pasta with Alfredo Sauce

1,810 calories
N/A g fat (89 g saturated)
652 mg sodium

It's no surprise that America's worst restaurant for adult food also offers the Worst Kids' Meal in America. Heck, nine of its children's meals contain more than 800 calories. The Factory's blatant disregard for restraint is evidenced by the fact that this dish contains nearly a full day's calories for a grown adult —and that's not this meal's worst crime. The saturated fat content can only be fully understood by making grotesque comparisons: Taking in the 89 grams of saturated fat clinging to these noodles would require your child to consume nearly 2 pounds of Jimmy Dean Pork Sausage.

Eat This Instead!

Kids Pasta with Marinara Sauce

510 calories
N/A g fat (2 g saturated)
651 mg sodium

1,810 calories

With this Alfredo nightmare, Cheesecake Factory proves once again why it's America's Worst Restaurant.

The Eat This, Not That! No-Diet Cheat Sheets

Find the best and worst versions of all your kid's favorite foods

BURGERS

		CALORIES	FAT (g)	SATURATED (g)	SODIUM (mg)
1.	**Wendy's Kids' Meal Cheeseburger**	260	11	5	570
2.	**Red Robin Kids Rad Robin Burger**	286	12	N/A	380
3.	**Carl's Jr. Kid's Cheeseburger**	290	15	7	790
4.	**McDonald's Happy Meal Cheeseburger** (sandwich only)	300	12	6	750
5.	**Burger King Kids Cheeseburger**	300	14	6	710
6.	**Chili's Pepper Pals Little Mouth Cheeseburger**	400	24	10	950
7.	**Applebee's Kids Mini Cheeseburger**	430	30	9	610
8.	**Outback Steakhouse Joey Boomerang Cheese Burger**	488	21	11	949
9.	**IHOP Just for Kids Cheeseburger**	500	28	13	780
10.	**On the Border Kid's Cheeseburger**	530	42	15	300
11.	**Uno Chicago Grill Kid's Cheeseburger**	700	41	12	1,620
12.	**Ruby Tuesday Kid's Beef Minis**	776	41	N/A	1,559

FRIES

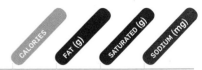

		CALORIES	FAT (g)	SATURATED (g)	SODIUM (mg)
1.	**Chili's Pepper Pals Side Homestyle Fries**	190	7	2	600
2.	**Red Robin Kids Steak Fries**	217	9	N/A	222
3.	**Burger King French Fries** (Value size)	220	11	2.5	340
4.	**McDonald's French Fries** (small)	230	11	1.5	160
5.	**Carl's Jr. Kids Natural-Cut Fries**	240	12	2	490
6.	**Bob Evans Kids' French Fries**	319	13	3	92
7.	**Romano's Macaroni Grill Kids Side Fries**	320	14	4	820
8.	**Friendly's My Meals Waffle Fries**	390	22	3	950
9.	**Applebee's Side Fries**	390	18	3.5	720
10.	**Olive Garden Children's Selections Fries**	400	21	2	880
11.	**Ruby Tuesday French Fries**	426	18	N/A	1,769
12.	**Denny's Kids' Finish Line Fries**	430	23	5	95

CHICKEN FINGER FOODS

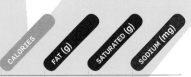

	CALORIES	FAT (g)	SATURATED (g)	SODIUM (mg)
1. **Wendy's Kids' Nuggets** (4)	180	11	2.5	370
2. **Burger King Chicken Tenders** (4)	190	11	2	310
3. **McDonald's Chicken McNuggets** (4, Happy Meal)	190	12	2	360
4. **Carl's Jr. Kid's Hand-Breaded Chicken Tenders** (2)	220	12	2.5	770
5. **Chick-fil-A Chicken Tenders** (2)	240	11	2	820
6. **Applebee's Kids Chicken Tenders**	240	14	3	600
7. **KFC Kids Popcorn Chicken**	260	17	3.5	690
8. **Olive Garden Children's Selections Chicken Fingers**	330	16	1.5	930
9. **Chili's Pepper Pals Crispy Chicken Crispers**	380	22	4	630
10. **Red Lobster Kids' Cove Chicken Fingers**	410	24	2	1,320
11. **Outback Steakhouse Joey Kookaburra Chicken Fingers**	676	41	12	1,942
12. **The Cheesecake Factory Kids Fried Chicken Strips**	810	N/A	8	1,306

PASTA

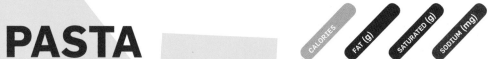

	CALORIES	FAT (g)	SATURATED (g)	SODIUM (mg)
1. **Olive Garden** Children's Selections Spaghetti	250	3	0.5	370
2. **Red Lobster Kids' Cove** Macaroni & Cheese	280	7	2	590
3. **Applebee's Kids' Kraft Macaroni & Cheese**	300	9	2.5	570
4. **Uno Chicago Grill** Kid's Macaroni & Cheese	440	14	4	820
5. **Ruby Tuesday Kid's Pasta Marinara**	469	7	N/A	978
6. **Chili's Pepper Pals** Kraft Macaroni & Cheese	500	18	6	930
7. **Olive Garden Children's Selections** Fettuccine Alfredo	510	32	19	450
8. **The Cheesecake Factory** Kids Pasta with Meat Sauce	580	N/A	5	612
9. **Outback Steakhouse** Joey Mac-A-Roo 'N Cheese	681	32	19	1,257
10. **Romano's Macaroni Grill** Kids Romano's Mac & Cheese	690	35	21	1,500
11. **The Cheesecake Factory** Kids Macaroni and Cheese	920	N/A	30	890
12. **California Pizza Kitchen Kids** Curly Mac N' Cheese	1,041	N/A	33	735

HEALTHY ENTRÉES

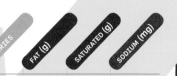

		CALORIES	FAT (g)	SATURATED (g)	SODIUM (mg)
1.	Red Lobster Kids' Cove Garlic Grilled Shrimp Skewer	60	1	0	580
2.	Subway Kids Black Forest Ham Sub	180	2.5	0.5	470
3.	Red Lobster Kids' Cove Grilled Chicken	210	4	1	710
4.	Bob Evans Kids Fruit Dippers	222	1	0	62
5.	Chili's Pepper Pals Grilled Chicken Sandwich	230	5	1	230
6.	Outback Steakhouse Joey Grilled Chicken on the Barbie	263	14	7	189
7.	Au Bon Pain Kid's Roasted Turkey Sandwich on Farmhouse Roll	270	7	2	780
8.	On the Border Grilled Chicken and Black Beans	270	4	1	1,190
9.	Panera Bread Kids Smoked Turkey Deli Sandwich	290	8	5	1,100
10.	Ruby Tuesday Kid's Chicken Breast	294	12	N/A	824
11.	Olive Garden Children's Selections Grilled Chicken with Pasta	310	5	1	680
12.	Uno Chicago Grill Kid's Chicken Caesar Salad	320	20	4	840

PIZZAS

	CALORIES	FAT (g)	SATURATED (g)	SODIUM (mg)
1. **Romano's Macaroni Grill** **Kids Pepperoni Pizza**	440	18	10	1,190
2. **Olive Garden** **Children's Selections** **Italian Cheese Pizza** (no toppings)	470	14	6	1,170
3. **Applebee's** **Kids' Cheese Pizza**	550	31	13	1,280
4. **Chili's Pepper Pals** **Cheese Pizza**	570	24	9	1,120
5. **Red Robin Red's** **Cheese Pizza**	605	27	N/A	1,465
6. **California Pizza Kitchen** **Kids Traditional** **Cheese Pizza**	637	N/A	8	1,337
7. **Uno Chicago Grill** **Kid's Deep Dish** **Cheese Pizza**	820	56	16	1,160
8. **The Cheesecake Factory** **Kids Cheese Pizza**	840	N/A	14	1,504

DESSERTS

		CALORIES	FAT (g)	SATURATED (g)	CARBS (g)
1.	**Red Lobster Kids' Cove Surf's Up Sundae**	170	9	6	20
2.	**Olive Garden Children's Selections Sundae**	180	9	6	21
3.	**Applebee's Kids' Vanilla Sundae with Hershey's Syrup**	330	14	9	49
4.	**On the Border Kiddie Sundae with Chocolate Syrup**	370	18	13	51
5.	**Uno Chicago Grill Kid's Sundae**	430	19	10	58
6.	**Chili's Pepper Pals Choc-A-Lot Shake**	460	22	14	61
7.	**California Pizza Kitchen Kids M&Ms Sundae**	509	N/A	21	43
8.	**Ruby Tuesday Kid Sundae**	574	29	N/A	71
9.	**TGI Friday's Kid's Sundae**	640	N/A	N/A	N/A
10.	**Denny's Kids' Oreo Blender Blaster**	690	33	17	88
11.	**Outback Steakhouse Joey Spotted Dog Sundae**	1,216	94	59	89

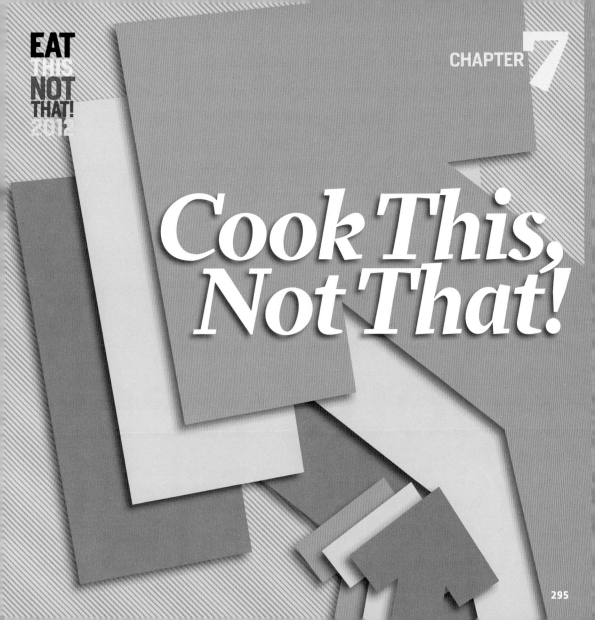

CHAPTER 7

EAT
THIS
NOT
THAT!
2012

Cook This,
Not That!

We know a long day. A long week. We understand that you're tired.

it's been

BUT SINCE WHEN is going out to eat any easier than cooking at home? By the time you've loaded up the family or coordinated with friends, you've already lost 30 minutes. You wait a few minutes or more for a table, another 10 to order, 20 minutes or more for your food. When all is said and done, you've invested 2 hours and about $25 dollars per person in a meal you could have bettered at home for a fraction of the cost, time, and effort. To wit: The average meal in this chapter takes approximately 17 minutes to prepare and costs $2.82 per serving.

On the flip side, the restaurant meals we replace average $10.75 (and that's without tax, tip, dessert, or drinks) and pack an astounding 1,087 calories per plate. That's three times more calories than you'll find in the average home-cooked meal in the pages to come. Fire up the stovetop just one more time a week and you and everyone at the table will drop nearly 11 pounds this year. Not bad.

But if shedding pounds and saving time and pocketing hard-earned cash aren't really your thing, we offer one last piece of motivation for experimenting with a few of these recipes: Every last morsel is down-right delicious. Good luck finding that at your neighborhood Applebee's.

297

Green Eggs & Ham

Anthony Bourdain famously wrote in his restaurant tell-all *Kitchen Confidential* that the hollandaise used to top that traditional breakfast favorite, eggs Benedict, is a breeding ground for bacteria. "Nobody I know has ever made hollandaise to order," he said. "And how long has that Canadian bacon been festering in the walk-in?" We take the basic conceit of a Benedict and clean things up a bit, replacing the Canadian bacon with prosciutto, adding roasted red peppers for a punch of sweetness, and, most crucially, ditching the hollandaise in favor of a simple pesto-yogurt sauce to drizzle over the top.

You'll Need:

- 8 eggs
- 1 Tbsp white vinegar
- 2 Tbsp prepared pesto
- 2 Tbsp plain Greek yogurt
- 4 English muffins, split and toasted
- 8 slices prosciutto, cooked ham, or cooked Canadian bacon
- ¼ cup bottled roasted red peppers, sliced
- Salt and cracked black pepper to taste

How to Make It:

- Bring 3 inches of water to a boil in a large sauté pan or saucepan. Turn down the heat to maintain a bare simmer and add the white vinegar. One at a time, crack each egg into a shallow cup and gently slide it into the water. Cook the eggs until the whites are just firm and the yolks are still runny, about 3 minutes, then use a slotted spoon to move the eggs to a plate.
- Mix together the pesto and yogurt. Top each English muffin half with a slice of meat, a few red pepper slices, and a poached egg. Season with a bit of salt and cracked black pepper. Divide the pesto-yogurt sauce among the eggs.

Makes 4 servings /
Cost per serving: $2.09

390 calories
18 g fat
(6 g saturated)
960 mg sodium

$$(\dashv + \vdash)^2$$

MEAL MULTIPLIER

The creamy texture of Greek yogurt serves as the perfect base for savory sauces, and the sharp lactic tang proves more flavorful than traditional sauce bases like mayo, cheese, and oil. Try mixing a cup of plain Greek yogurt with any of the following ingredients for a killer on-the-spot sauce.

- Minced garlic, chopped parsley, olive oil, lemon juice (great with grilled chicken; see page 316)
- Sun-dried tomatoes, olives, fresh basil, olive oil (doubles as a sauce and a dip for pitas)
- Blue cheese, chives, lemon juice (a low-cal replacement for blue cheese dressing)

Not That!
IHOP
Eggs Benedict
Price: $7.99

Save!
630 calories
and $5.90!

1,020 calories
57 g fat
(22 g saturated)
3,140 mg sodium

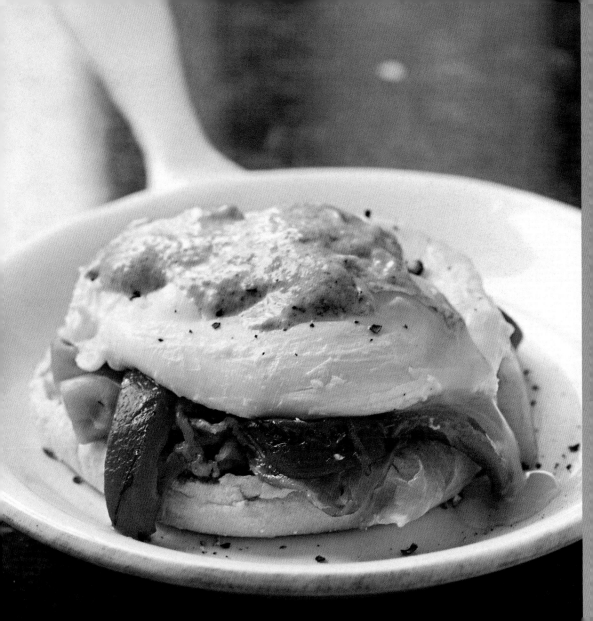

Baked Feta Cheese with Pita

Appetizer menus the country over are dens of decadence wherein lurk the biggest dietary dangers in the food chain. They hit diners when they're at their weakest: deliriously hungry, craving greasy, fatty sustenance to the point that anything fried or covered in cheese becomes a must-have. This bubbling cheese starter has all the flavors you crave when you're hungry—salt from the olives, sweetness from the red peppers and tomatoes, fat from the cheese—but delivers them for a fraction of the calories. Serve this at your next dinner party, and when they inevitably ask for the recipe, tell them it's an old family secret.

You'll Need:

- ½ lb feta cheese (in a single block, not crumbled)
- ¼ cup kalamata olives, pitted and chopped
- ¼ cup chopped sun-dried tomatoes
- ⅓ cup bottled roasted red peppers, cut into strips
- Ground black pepper to taste
- 1 Tbsp olive oil
- Juice of half a lemon
- 4 whole-wheat pitas

How to Make It:

- Preheat the oven to 375°F. Place the cheese in a baking dish or crock. Top with the olives, tomatoes, red peppers, and a sprinkle of black pepper. Bake until the cheese is hot and beginning to melt, about 12 to 15 minutes. Remove and drizzle with the olive oil, and squeeze the lemon over the top. While the oven is still hot, warm the pitas for a few minutes. Cut into quarters and serve with the cheese.

Makes 4 servings / Cost per serving: $2.23

290 calories
18 g fat
(9 g saturated)
1,020 mg sodium

1,710 calories
101 g fat
(37 g saturated)
3,490 mg sodium

Save!
1,420 calories and $3.06!

Not That!
Chili's Skillet Queso with Chips
Price: $5.29

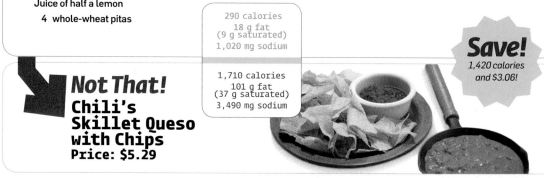

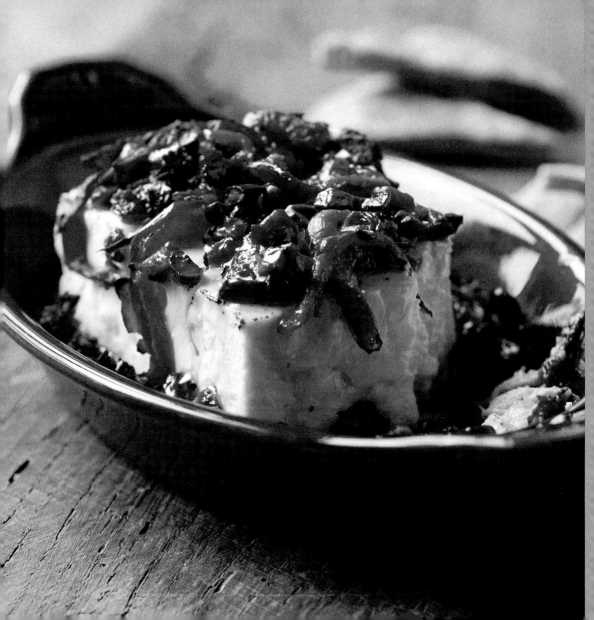

Asian Beef Salad with Sriracha-Honey Dressing

Restaurant salads suffer from a double dose of shamefulness: They are not only boring and sloppily executed, they also come with more calories and fat than your average bacon cheeseburger. Case in point: You'd be better off eating three full orders of Applebee's Asiago Peppercorn Steak than tussling with the tame-sounding Oriental Grilled Chicken Salad. Disgraceful. Here, we harbor the big flavors of the East—sweet, spicy, tart, cool—but leave all the excessive calories out of the equation. A generous portion of lean flank steak and creamy cubes of avocado make sure this salad truly satisfies.

You'll Need:

1 lb flank steak

Salt and ground black pepper to taste

1 tsp sriracha or other hot sauce

2 tsp honey

½ Tbsp low-sodium soy sauce

Juice of 1 lime

¼ cup canola oil

1 bag watercress (if your market doesn't stock watercress, a head of Bibb lettuce will work fine)

1 pint cherry tomatoes, sliced in half

1 small red onion, thinly sliced

½ English cucumber, thinly sliced

1 avocado, peeled, pitted, and chopped

Handful of fresh cilantro leaves

How to Make It:

● Preheat a grill, grill pan, or cast-iron skillet over medium-high heat. Season the flank steak all over with salt and pepper and cook until medium rare, about 3 to 4 minutes per side. Allow the steak to rest for at least 5 minutes before slicing thinly across the natural grain of the meat.

● While the meat rests, combine the sriracha, honey, soy sauce, and lime juice with a pinch of pepper in a mixing bowl. Slowly drizzle in the oil, whisking to combine.

● In a large salad bowl, combine the watercress, tomatoes, onion, cucumber, avocado, cilantro, and sliced steak and slowly drizzle in the dressing, tossing the ingredients gently with each addition, until everything is lightly coated.

Makes 4 servings / Cost per serving: $4.39

430 calories
31 g fat
(6 g saturated)
475 mg sodium

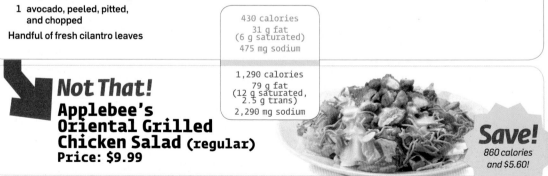

1,290 calories
79 g fat
(12 g saturated,
2.5 g trans)
2,290 mg sodium

Not That!
Applebee's Oriental Grilled Chicken Salad (regular)
Price: $9.99

Save!
860 calories
and $5.60!

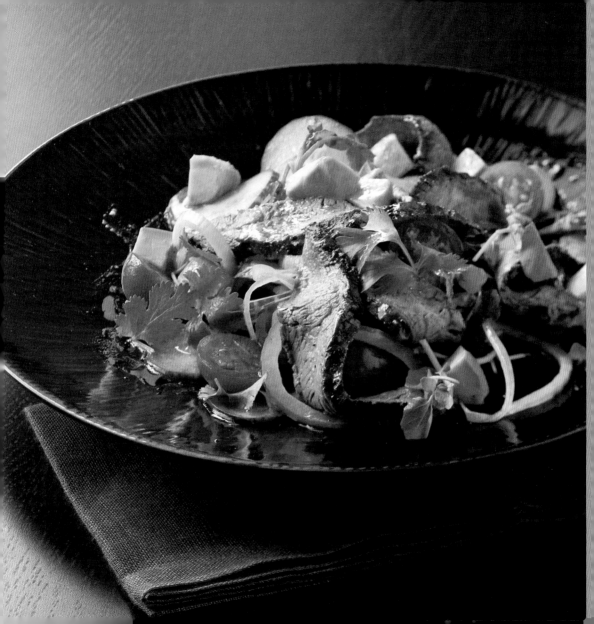

It lian Meatb ll Soup

Order a plate of spaghetti and meatballs in Italy and you'll likely leave your waiter dumbfounded, scratching his head for an answer. That's because one of America's favorite Italian dishes is a purely American invention, one that generally hinges on our typical tenets of excess. In Italy, *polpettine* are more likely to be enjoyed in a lighter fashion, either by themselves or in a soup like the one below. The pasta is still there (albeit a much smaller portion of it), but the broth houses a handful of stellar vegetables and serves to keep the meatballs moist and luscious. Though it's light in calories, this is still a potent bowl of goodness—served with a lightly dressed salad, it makes for an incredible weekday dinner.

You'll Need:

- 1 lb ground beef
- 2 medium eggs or 1 extra-large egg
- ¼ cup bread crumbs
- ½ cup finely grated Parmesan cheese

Salt and ground black pepper to taste

- ½ Tbsp olive oil
- 1 onion, chopped
- 2 carrots, peeled and chopped
- 2 ribs celery, chopped
- 8 cups low-sodium chicken stock
- 1 head escarole, chopped into bite-size pieces
- ¾ cup small pasta, like orzo, pastina, or spaghetti broken into ½-inch pieces

How to Make It:

- Combine the beef with the eggs, bread crumbs, cheese, and good-size pinches of salt and pepper in a mixing bowl. Being careful not to overwork the mixture, lightly form it into meatballs roughly ¾-inch in diameter, a bit smaller than a golf ball.

- Heat the olive oil in a large pot over medium-high heat. Add the onion, carrots, and celery and sauté until the vegetables have softened, about 5 minutes. Add the stock and the escarole and bring the soup to a simmer. Turn the heat down to low and add the meatballs and pasta. Simmer for another 8 to 10 minutes, until the meatballs are cooked through and the pasta is al dente. Taste and adjust the seasoning with salt and pepper.

- Serve the soup with extra cheese on top.

Makes 6 servings /
Cost per serving: $2.63

333 calories
14 g fat
(5 g saturated)
690 mg sodium

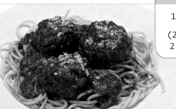

Not That!
Olive Garden
Spaghetti &
Meatballs
Price: $12.75

1,110 calories
50 g fat
(20 g saturated)
2,180 mg sodium

Save!
777 calories
and $10.12!

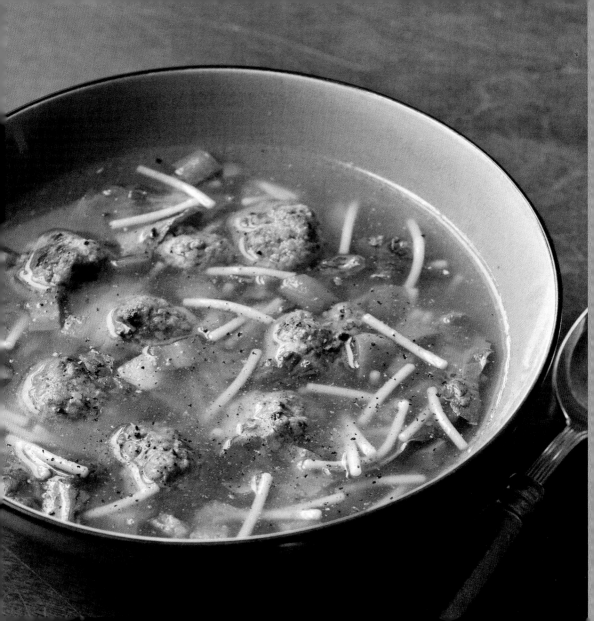

Turkey & Brie with Apple

It's a pretty simple concept: The more tricked-out a sandwich, the more calories it will contain. This holds true time and time again in the restaurant world, where subs rife with potential, like Panera's Sierra Turkey, go down in a burst of flames once bedecked with bells and whistles. It doesn't have to be that way. We've used add-ons to the greater good of this handheld wonder: Slices of apple add coolness and crunch; a quick honey-mustard mix provides sweetness and spice; and a few slices of brie bring that intense creaminess we all crave. All told, the condiment treatment here tacks onto the sandwich about 100 calories—not bad for a trio that also bolsters fiber, antioxidants, and, above all, flavor.

You'll Need:

- 2 Tbsp plain mustard
- 2 Tbsp honey
- 4 seeded whole-wheat rolls, split and lightly toasted
- 1 Fuji or Gala apple, thinly sliced
- 4 cups baby spinach or arugula or other lettuce
- 4 thin slices red onion
- 1 lb sliced smoked turkey
- 2 oz brie cheese, thinly sliced

How to Make It:

- Combine the mustard and honey in a small bowl and spread on the bottom half of each roll. Divide the apple among the rolls, then top with the divided spinach, red onion, turkey, and cheese.

*Makes 4 sandwiches /
Cost per serving: $3.40*

410 calories
10 g fat
(4 g saturated)
910 mg sodium

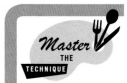

Master THE TECHNIQUE

Sweet and Savory Sandwiches

Nothing wrong with standard turkey, ham, or roast beef, but we like to push the culinary boundaries in the sandwich genre. A favorite technique is to pair savory meats with sweet fruits to create a yin-yang balance that will keep your taste buds at full attention. A few of our favorites:

- Prosciutto or other good ham with sliced figs and crumbled goat cheese

- Grilled chicken, grilled pineapple, and melted pepper jack cheese

- Peanut butter, banana, and crispy bacon (Elvis has never steered us wrong!)

920 calories
49 g fat
(12 g saturated,
1 g trans)
1,900 mg sodium

Not That!
Panera Sierra Turkey on Asiago Cheese Focaccia
Price: $6.59

Save!
*510 calories
and $3.19!*

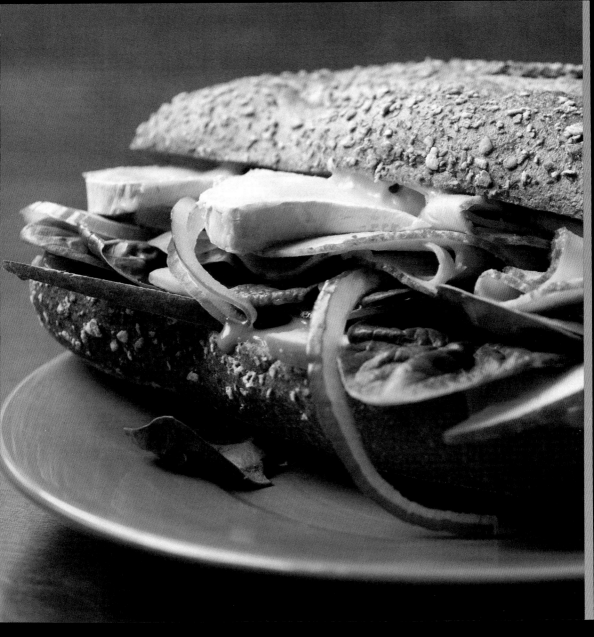

Eat This!

o st d H libut Wrapped in Prosciutto

We've seen a preponderance of "crusted" and "wrapped" fish dishes come to market in recent years, and despite the diversity of purveyors laying claim to this hot new restaurant trend, the results are universally abysmal. The ingredients doing the crusting are normally cheese or bread crumbs and the technique used for cooking is some form of frying, hence the 810-calorie price tag on Red Lobster's tilapia (and that's before sides). We skip the crusting and frying and instead opt for a simpler, healthier, and (we think) more delicious alternative: wrapping. It looks fancy and tastes like a sophisticated fine-dining dish, but the truth is that this is the simplest recipe in this chapter.

You'll Need:

4 pieces (4–6 oz) halibut, cod, sea bass, or other flaky white fish

Salt and ground black pepper to taste

4 thin slices prosciutto

1 lemon, quartered

2 Tbsp prepared pesto

How to Make It:

- Preheat the oven to 375°F. Season the fish all over with salt and pepper. Lay the slices of prosciutto on a cutting board and wrap each piece of fish tightly with one of the slices. Place the fish on a baking sheet and position it on the middle rack of the oven. Roast until the prosciutto begins to crisp up and the fish flakes with gentle pressure from your finger, about 10 to 12 minutes. Serve each with a wedge of lemon and the pesto drizzled over the top.

Makes 4 servings / Cost per serving: $4.89

230 calories
8 g fat
(2 g saturated)
580 mg sodium

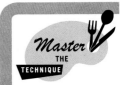

Master THE TECHNIQUE

Wrapping Fish and Meat

Rather than smothering meat or fish with viscous, calorie-dense sauces or, worse yet, deep-frying it, encasing it in a thin sheet of prosciutto or Spanish-style jamón is an excellent way to keep the flesh moist and tender without adding more than 50 calories to the final dish. Place a chicken breast, pork loin, or meaty fish fillet in the center of a strip of prosciutto, season with salt and pepper, and wrap tightly. Roast on a baking sheet in the oven at 400°F until cooked all the way through.

810 calories
41 g fat
(17 g saturated)
2,590 mg sodium

Not That!
Red Lobster Parmesan-Crusted Tilapia
Price: $17.99

Save!
580 calories
and $13.10!

308

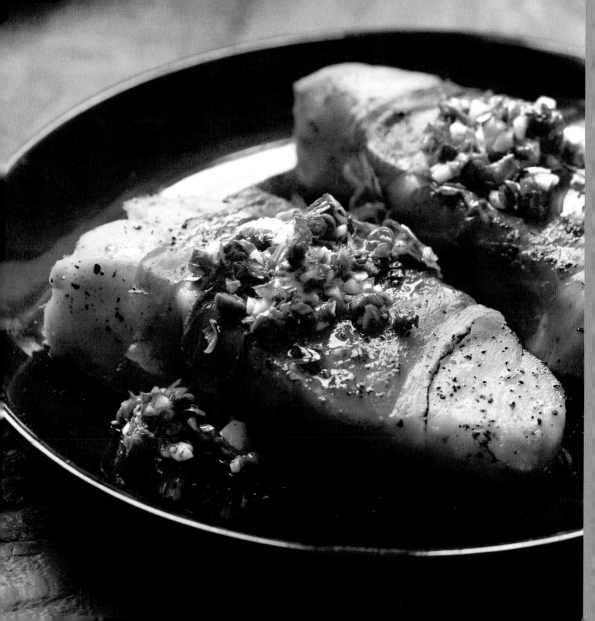

Eat This!
Poor Man's Steak with Garlicy Gravy

This country has fallen on lean times in recent years, but unfortunately the figurative belt-tightening doesn't seem to be accompanied by a literal one. That's because the most potent sources of calories and seasoning (oil, butter, sugar, salt) are still cheap and more common in restaurant cooking than ever. A few of these are showcased prominently in Outback's mushroom-smothered filet, which, with sides, packs more than a day's worth of sodium and saturated fat and requires a small loan to afford. Here, we mimic its taste and tenderness with inexpensive lean ground sirloin and cover it with a soy-spiked sauce good enough to make your doormat taste delicious. Serve this hot, decadent mess over a velvety bed of mashed potatoes, or for a healthier, easier sidekick, try spinach sautéed in olive oil and chopped garlic.

You'll Need:

- 1 lb ground sirloin or chuck, shaped into 4 equal patties
- 1 Tbsp canola oil
- Salt and ground black pepper to taste
- 2 cloves garlic, minced
- 1 yellow onion, sliced
- 4 oz white or cremini mushrooms, stems removed, sliced
- ½ Tbsp flour
- ½ cup beef or chicken stock
- 1 Tbsp ketchup
- 1 Tbsp low-sodium soy sauce
- 1 tsp Worcestershire sauce

How to Make It:

- Preheat the oven to 200°F.
- Heat a large cast-iron skillet or sauté pan over medium-high heat. Season the patties all over with salt and pepper. Add the oil to the pan and cook until a nicely browned crust forms on the patties, about 3 to 4 minutes, then flip and continue cooking for another 3 to 4 minutes for medium-rare. Move the patties to a baking sheet and place in the oven to keep warm.
- Add the remaining oil and the garlic, onions, and mushrooms to the same pan, and cook until the vegetables begin to brown nicely, about 5 to 7 minutes. Sprinkle the flour over the vegetables, stir so that it coats them evenly, then add the stock, using a whisk to keep lumps from forming. Stir in the ketchup, soy sauce, and Worcestershire sauce and continue cooking until the gravy thickens, another 2 to 3 minutes. Serve the patties on a bed of mashed potatoes or sautéed spinach (or both) with the gravy drizzled over the top.

Makes 4 servings /
Cost per serving: $1.81

220 calories
9 fat
(3 g saturated)
470 mg sodium

922 calories
52 g fat
(26 g saturated)
3,045 mg sodium

Not That!
Outback Steakhouse Filet with Wild Mushroom Sauce
Price: $15.99

Save!
702 calories
and $14.18!

310

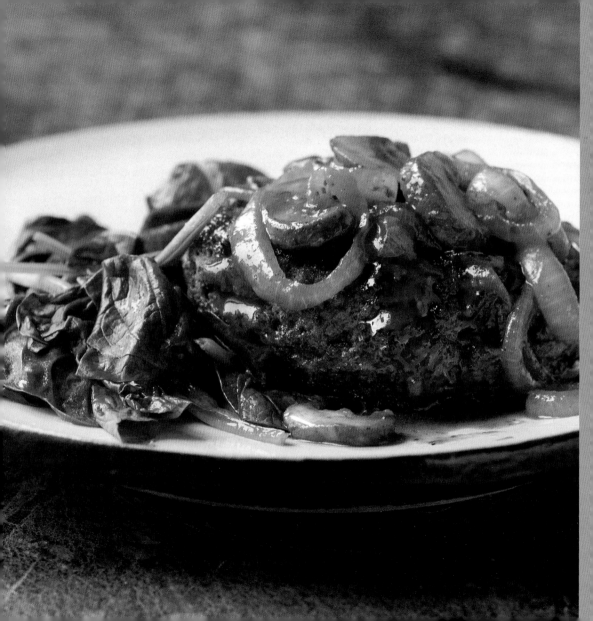

Garbanzos with Chorizo and Spinach

The Spanish have one of the longest life spans on the planet, and when you look at their eating habits, it's not hard to see why. Meat plays a secondary role to fish and vegetables, often being used as a supporting actor rather than the star of the dish. That's the philosophy behind this classic stew, which uses a few chunks of chorizo to infuse an entire pot of fiber-rich garbanzos and wilted spinach with smoky, meaty flavor.

You'll Need:

- ½ Tbsp olive oil
- 2 links chorizo or chicken chorizo, chopped
- 1 large onion, chopped
- 2 cloves garlic, minced
- ¼ tsp dried red pepper flakes
- 1 tsp paprika (preferably the smoked Spanish kind, also called pimentón)
- 2 bay leaves
- 2 Tbsp tomato paste
- 1 lb Yukon gold potatoes, cut into ½-inch chunks
- 1½ cups low-sodium chicken stock
- Salt and ground black pepper to taste
- 2 cans (14 oz) garbanzo beans, drained and rinsed
- 8 cups baby spinach

How to Make It:

- Heat the oil in a large pot or saucepan over medium heat. Add the chorizo and sauté until the meat is lightly browned. Move to a plate and reserve.
- Add the onion, garlic, red pepper flakes, paprika, and bay leaves to the pan and cook until the onion begins to brown, about 5 minutes. Stir in the tomato paste and cook for another few minutes, until it evenly coats the onions and garlic. Add the potatoes and stock, and simmer the vegetables until the potatoes are just tender, about 10 minutes. Add the garbanzos and cook for another 5 minutes. Season with salt and black pepper to taste.
- Just before you're ready to serve, stir in the reserved chorizo and the spinach and cook until the spinach wilts.

Makes 6 servings /
Cost per serving: $2.04

360 calories
11 g fat
(3.5 g saturated)
825 mg sodium

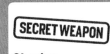

SECRET WEAPON

Chorizo

There are two types out there: Mexican-style chorizo, which is a spicy, uncooked sausage lashed with ground chili; and Spanish chorizo, which is cured, but derives most of its flavor (and color) from smoked paprika. While Mexican chorizo is excellent and will work in this dish, the latter is really what you're looking for here. A few hunks sautéed with onions and garlic form a brilliant base for a pot of black beans, lentils, chili, or even scrambled eggs. If you can't find chorizo in your local market, order it online at www.latienda.com.

Not That!
Red Robin Red's Homemade Chili Chili (bowl)
Price: $4.99

Save!
191 calories
and $2.95!

551 calories
32 g fat
1,329 mg sodium

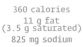

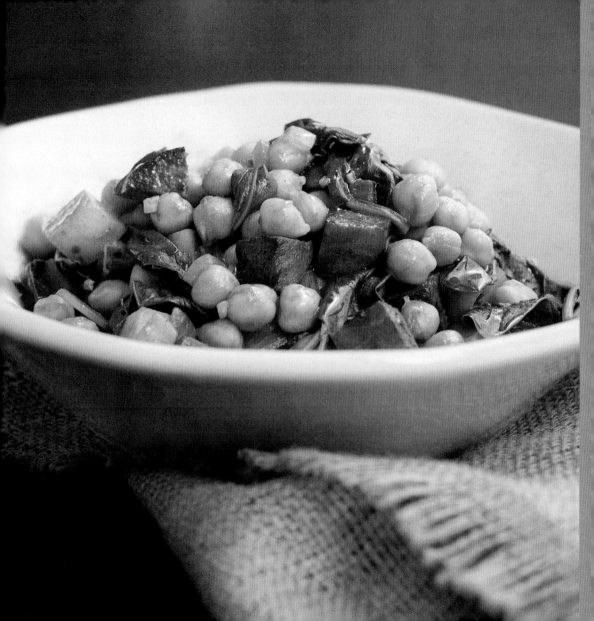

Sausage Penne
with Zucchini and Goat Cheese

The average dinner plate of pasta at Olive Garden, the largest Italian restaurant chain in America, contains 976 calories. Other restaurants, from huge chains to your neighborhood red sauce joint, fare even worse. All of this is to say that it's tough to leave your house for a bowl of noodles without doing damage to your waistline. Our suggestion? Stop leaving the house. With low-calorie, big-flavor dishes like this, there's just no need to.

You'll Need:

- **12 oz penne** (we like Ronzoni Smart Taste)
- **1 Tbsp olive oil**
- **8 oz uncooked chicken or turkey sausage,** casing removed
- **1 medium yellow onion,** chopped
- **2 cloves garlic, thinly sliced**
- **1 medium zucchini,** sliced into half-moons
- **Salt and ground black pepper** to taste
- **¼ cup sun-dried tomatoes,** reconstituted in hot water if not oil-packed
- **½ cup chicken stock**
- **½ cup goat cheese**

How to Make It:

- Bring a large pot of generously salted water to a boil and cook the pasta until just al dente. As always, rely on your taste buds—not the package instructions—to make this determination.
- While the water heats and the pasta cooks, heat the oil in a large sauté pan over medium-high heat. Add the sausage and sauté until cooked all the way through, about 5 minutes. Remove and reserve. Add the onion and garlic and cook for a few minutes, until the onion is translucent, then add the zucchini and cook until lightly caramelized, about 5 more minutes. Season with salt and pepper.
  Add the sun-dried tomatoes, the stock, and the reserved sausage and keep warm until the pasta is ready.
- Drain the pasta and add it directly to the pan with the sausage and vegetables. Cook together for 30 seconds, cut the heat, and sprinkle on the cheese just before serving.

Makes 4 servings / Cost per serving: $2.41

480 calories
11 g fat
(4 g saturated)
600 mg sodium

1,270 calories
67 g fat
(24 g saturated)
3,090 mg sodium

Not That!
Olive Garden Spaghetti & Italian Sausage
Price: $12.75

Save!
790 calories and $10.34!

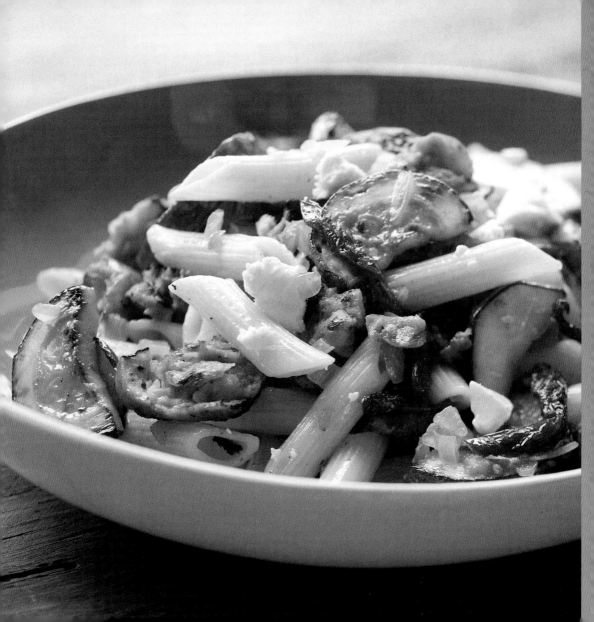

Greek·nik with Lemon-Yogurt Sauce

Grilled chicken is one of those great dishes that needs very little help. Fire up the grill (charcoal, preferably, but gas will do), add some salt and pepper, and cook until the skin is lightly charred and smoky and the meat is moist and tender. It's a backyard miracle, re-created year after year. We don't want to tweak the formula too much, but with a simple marinade and a 1-minute sauce, you can turn a dish that's consistently good into something truly magical.

You'll Need:

- 1 cup 2% Greek yogurt
- 6 cloves garlic, minced and divided
- Juice of two lemons, divided
- 3 Tbsp olive oil, divided
- 2 lb bone-in, skin-on chicken thighs and drumsticks
- 1 tsp dried oregano
- ¾ tsp salt
- ½ tsp ground black pepper

How to Make It:

- Combine the yogurt, one-third of the garlic, the juice of half a lemon, and 1 tablespoon of the olive oil. Mix thoroughly and reserve in the refrigerator.

- Combine the chicken with the oregano, salt, pepper, and the remaining garlic, lemon juice, and olive oil. Cover and marinate in the refrigerator for at least 30 minutes and up to 4 hours.

- Preheat a grill or grill pan. Remove the chicken from the marinade and grill over a medium flame until the skin is nicely caramelized and the meat is cooked all the way through, about 15 to 20 minutes. Serve with the yogurt on the side or drizzled over the top.

Makes 4 servings / Cost per serving: $2.31

395 calories
30 g fat
(7 g saturated)
510 mg sodium

1,160 calories
67 g fat
(16 g saturated,
1 g trans)
3,190 mg sodium

SECRET WEAPON

Chicken Skin

Popular belief has it that chicken skin is flat-out bad for you. Indeed, many prominent nutritionists and organizations (including the American Heart Association) continue to regurgitate the antiquated mantra that all animal fat is bad for you, despite reams of evidence suggesting otherwise. Despite its reputation, chicken skin contains a heavy dose of mono-unsaturated oleic acid, the very same heart-healthy kind you find in olive oil. Still, calories come with fat, and if cutting calories is your first priority, grill the chicken with the skin on (it will keep the meat moist and tender), then remove it before eating.

Not That!
Applebee's Fiesta Lime Chicken
Price: $11.99

Save!
765 calories
and $9.68!

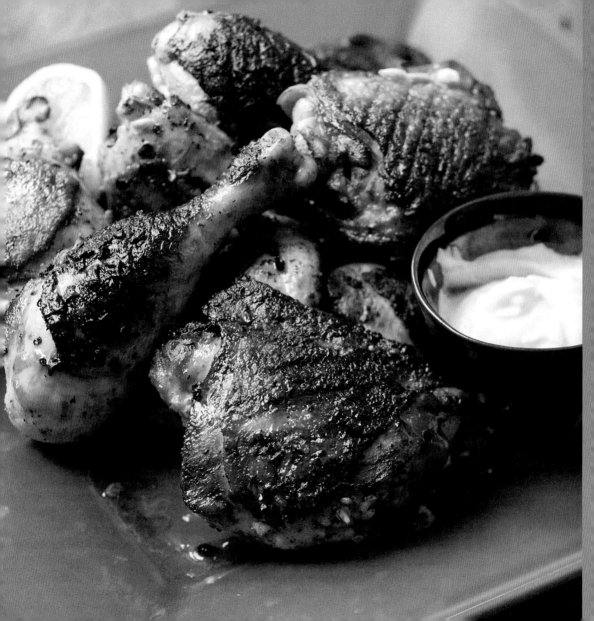

Spicy Turkey Burger with Sharp Cheddar

Restaurant turkey burgers are never the health havens they pretend to be (with the exception of the line of turkey burgers we helped create for Carl's Jr. and Hardee's, but that's another story). Unfortunately, home-cooked turkey burgers suffer from the opposite problem: They're nearly always dry and boring. We think this creation solves both problems. A touch of cumin adds smokiness, chipotle brings heat, and sharp Cheddar brings the whole package together.

You'll Need:

- 2 Tbsp ketchup
- 2 Tbsp olive oil mayonnaise
- ½ Tbsp chipotle pepper puree
- 1 lb ground turkey
- ¼ tsp ground cumin
- Salt and ground black pepper to taste
- 4 slices (¼ inch thick) red onion
- 4 slices sharp Cheddar cheese
- 4 potato or sesame seed hamburger buns
- Bibb lettuce or arugula
- 4 thick tomato slices (optional)

How to Make It:

- Preheat a grill, grill pan, or cast-iron skillet over medium-high heat.

- Combine the ketchup, mayonnaise, and chipotle in a mixing bowl, stir, and set aside. In a separate bowl, gently combine the ground turkey with the cumin and a few generous pinches of salt and pepper. Being careful not to overwork the meat, form four patties of equal size.

- Place the burgers and the onions on the grill. Cook the burgers for 4 minutes on the first side, flip, and immediately crown each with a slice of cheese. Cook for another 4 to 5 minutes, until firm but gently yielding to the touch. Grill the onions until lightly charred and soft. If you like, toast the buns.

- Dress the bottom part of each bun with lettuce and tomato (if using). Top with a burger, grilled onions, and a generous spoonful of the spicy ketchup.

Makes 4 servings /
Cost per serving: $2.88

445 calories
19 g fat
(6 g saturated)
690 mg sodium

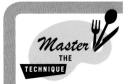

Master
THE
TECHNIQUE

Perfect Patties

Proper patty formation is key to the texture and taste of a good burger. Start with very cold meat, season, and very gently form patties; if you overwork the meat, you'll end up with a dense, chewy burger. Once the patty is formed, use your thumb to make a small indentation in the center. As it cooks, ground meat swells in the center, creating a rounded, oblong burger. The cavity will ensure a flat, evenly cooked burger.

1,200 calories
27 g saturated fat
1,544 mg sodium

Not That!

The Cheesecake Factory Grilled Turkey Burger
Price: $11.95

Save!
755 calories
and $9.07!

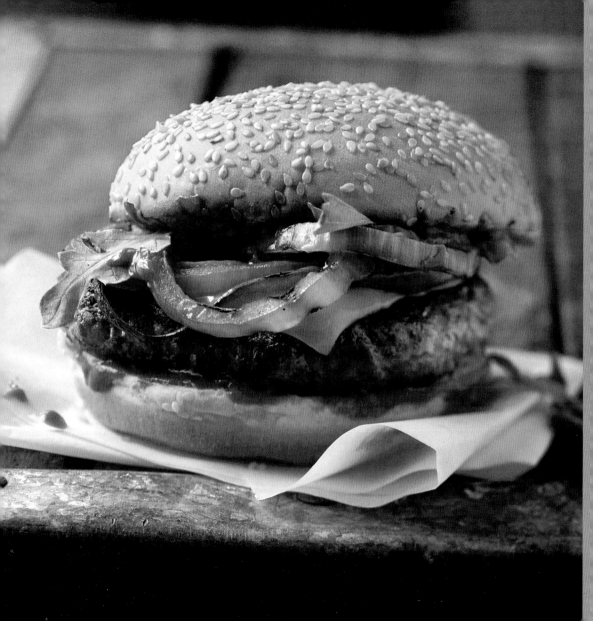

Molten Chocolate Cake

The idea of baking and frosting a multitiered chocolate cake is daunting for most, but these little self-contained parcels of joy are the lazy man's cake, the type of dessert that makes a non-baker feel like a pastry king when they emerge from the oven, pregnant with a tide of melted chocolate. Crack the middle and watch the flood of lava flow freely onto your plate—and eventually into your eagerly awaiting mouth. Did we mention these have only 360 calories?

You'll Need:

5 oz bittersweet chocolate (at least 60 percent cacao), plus 4 chunks for the cake centers

2 Tbsp butter

2 eggs

2 egg yolks

¼ cup sugar

Pinch of salt

2 Tbsp flour

1 tsp vanilla extract

½ Tbsp instant coffee or espresso (optional)

How to Make It:

- Preheat the oven to 425°F. Lightly butter four 6-ounce ramekins or custard cups.

- Bring a few cups of water to a boil in a medium saucepan over low heat. Place a glass mixing bowl over the pan (but not touching the water) and add the chocolate and butter. Cook, stirring occasionally, until both the chocolate and butter have fully melted. Keep warm.

- Use an electric mixer to beat the eggs, egg yolks, sugar, and salt until pale yellow and thick, about 5 minutes. Stir in the melted chocolate mixture, the flour, vanilla, and instant coffee if using.

- Pour the mixture into the prepared ramekins. Stick one good chunk of chocolate in the center of each ramekin. Bake the cakes on the center rack for 8 to 10 minutes, until the exterior is just set (the center should still be mostly liquid). The cakes can be eaten straight from the ramekins, but it's more dramatic to slide them on to plates (after letting them rest for a minute or two), where the molten chocolate can flow freely.

Makes 4 servings / Cost per serving: $1.20

360 calories
26 g fat
(13 g saturated)
34 mg sodium

1,070 calories
51 g fat
(28 g saturated)
143 g carbohydrates

Not That!
Chili's Molten Chocolate Cake
Price: $5.99

Save!
710 calories
and $4.79!

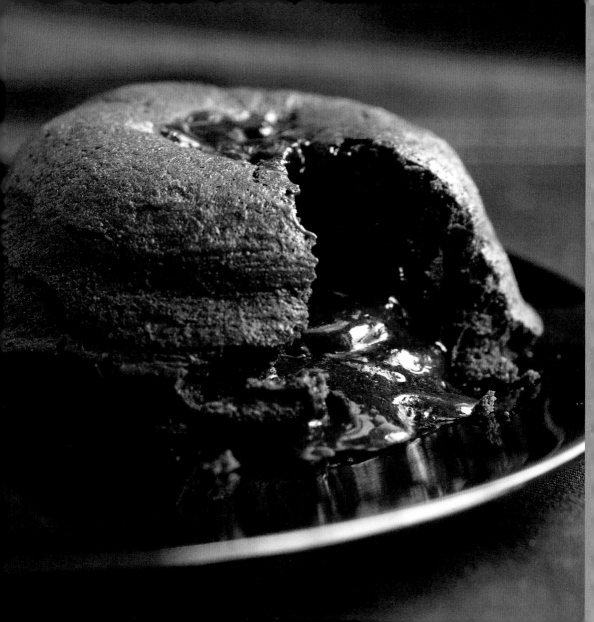

Index

Boldface page references indicate photographs.
Underscored references indicate boxed text.